Handbook for Stoelting's Anesthesia and Co-Existing Disease

Handbook for Stoelting's Anesthesia and Co-Existing Disease

Third Edition

Roberta L. Hines, MD
Nicholas M. Greene Professor and Chair
Department of Anesthesiology
Yale University School of Medicine
New Haven, Connecticut

Katherine E. Marschall, MD
Assistant Professor
Department of Anesthesiology
Yale University School of Medicine
New Haven, Connecticut

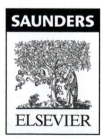

SAUNDERS

ELSEVIER

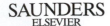

SAUNDERS
ELSEVIER

1600 John F. Kennedy Blvd.
Ste 1800
Philadelphia, PA 19103-2899

HANDBOOK FOR STOELTING'S ANESTHESIA
AND CO-EXISITING DISEASE, THIRD EDITION   ISBN: 978-1-4160-3997-6
Copyright © 2009, 2002, 1993 by Saunders, an imprint of Elsevier Inc.

Notice

Knowledge and best practice in this field are constantly changing. As new research and experience broaden our knowledge, changes in practice, treatment, and drug therapy may become necessary or appropriate. Readers are advised to check the most current information provided (i) on procedures featured or (ii) by the manufacturer of each product to be administered, to verify the recommended dose or formula, the method and duration of administration, and contraindications. It is the responsibility of the practitioner, relying on their own experience and knowledge of the patient, to make diagnoses, to determine dosages and the best treatment for each individual patient, and to take all appropriate safety precautions. To the fullest extent of the law, neither the Publisher nor the Editors assume any liability for any injury and/or damage to persons or property arising out of or related to any use of the material contained in this book.

The Publisher

Library of Congress Cataloging-in-Publication Data

Handbook for Stoelting's anesthesia and co-existing disease / [edited by] Roberta L. Hines, Katherine E. Marschall. -- 3rd ed.
    p. ; cm.
    Includes index.
    Rev. ed. of : Handbook for anesthesia and co-existing disease / [edited by] Robert K. Stoelting, Stephen F. Dierdorf. 2nd ed. c2002.
    ISBN 978-1-4160-3997-6
    1. Anesthesia--Complications--Handbooks, manuals, etc. 2. Therapeutics, Surgical--Handbooks, manuals, etc. I. Stoelting, Robert K. II. Hines, Roberta L. III. Marschall, Katherine E. IV. Handbook for anesthesia and co-existing disease. V. Stoelting's anesthesia and co-existing disease.
    [DNLM: 1. Anesthesia--adverse effects--Handbooks. 2. Anesthesia--adverse effects--Outlines. 3. Anesthetics--Handbooks. 4. Anesthetics--Outlines. WO 245 H236 2009]
    RD87.A53 2009 Suppl.
    617.9'6041--dc22

                                    2008047123

Executive Publisher: Natasha Andjelkovic
Developmental Editor: Liliana Kim
Design Direction: Steven Stave

Printed in the United States of America

Last digit is the print number: 9 8 7 6 5 4 3 2

Working together to grow
libraries in developing countries
www.elsevier.com | www.bookaid.org | www.sabre.org

ELSEVIER   BOOK AID International   Sabre Foundation

Contributors

Shamsuddin Akhtar, MD
Associate Professor
Department of Anesthesiology
Yale University School of Medicine
New Haven, Connecticut

Michael S. Avidan, MB BCh
Assistant Professor
Department of Anesthesiology
Washington University School of Medicine
Barnes Jewish Hospital
St. Louis, Missouri

Bruno Bissonnette, BSc, MD, FRCP(C)
Professor
Department of Anesthesiology
University of Toronto Faculty of Medicine
Director, Neurosurgical Anesthesia
Hospital for Sick Children
Toronto, Ontario
Canada

Ferne R. Braveman, MD
Professor and Chief of Obstetric Anesthesia
Department of Anesthesiology
Yale University School of Medicine
New Haven, Connecticut

Susan Garwood, MB ChB
Associate Professor
Department of Anesthesiology
Yale University School of Medicine
New Haven, Connecticut

Marbelia Gonzalez, MD
Assistant Professor
Department of Anesthesiology
Yale University School of Medicine
New Haven, Connecticut

Alá Sami Haddadin, MD
Assistant Professor
Department of Anesthesiology
Yale University School of Medicine
New Haven, Connecticut

Adriana Herrera, MD
Assistant Professor
Department of Anesthesiology
Yale University School of Medicine
New Haven, Connecticut

Zoltan G. Hevesi, MD
Associate Professor
Departments of Anesthesiology and
Surgery
University of Wisconsin Medical School
Madison, Wisconsin

Roberta L. Hines, MD
Nicholas M. Greene Professor and Chair
Department of Anesthesiology
Yale University School of Medicine
New Haven, Connecticut

Viji Kurup, MD
Assistant Professor
Department of Anesthesiology
Yale University School of Medicine
New Haven, Connecticut

William L. Lanier, Jr., MD
Professor
Department of Anesthesiology
Mayo Clinic College of Medicine
Rochester, Minnesota

Charles Lee, MD
Assistant Professor
Department of Anesthesiology
Loma Linda University
Director of Acute and Perioperative
Pain Service
Loma Linda University Medical Center
Loma Linda, California

Igor Luginbuehl, MD
Assistant Professor
Department of Anesthesiology
University of Toronto Faculty of Medicine
Staff Anesthesiologist
Hospital for Sick Children
Toronto, Ontario
Canada

Inna Maranets, MD
Assistant Professor
Department of Anesthesiology
Yale University School of Medicine
New Haven, Connecticut

Katherine E. Marschall, MD
Assistant Professor
Department of Anesthesiology
Yale University School of Medicine
New Haven, Connecticut

Linda J. Mason, MD
Professor of Anesthesiology and Pediatrics
Loma Linda University
Director of Pediatric Anesthesia
Loma Linda University Medical Center
Loma Linda, California

Raj K. Modak, MD
Assistant Professor
Department of Anesthesiology
Yale University School of Medicine
New Haven, Connecticut

Jeffrey J. Pasternak, MD
Assistant Professor
Department of Anesthesiology
Mayo Clinic College of Medicine
Rochester, Minnesota

Wanda M. Popescu, MD
Assistant Professor
Department of Anesthesiology
Yale University School of Medicine
Department of Anesthesiology
New Haven, Connecticut

Christine S. Rinder, MD
Associate Professor
Department of Anesthesiology
Yale University School of Medicine
New Haven, Connecticut

Jeffrey J. Schwartz, MD
Associate Professor
Department of Anesthesiology
Yale University School of Medicine
New Haven, Connecticut

Hossam E. Tantawy, MD
Assistant Professor
Department of Anesthesiology
Yale University School of Medicine
New Haven, Connecticut

Nalini Vadivelu, MD
Assistant Professor
Department of Anesthesiology
Yale University School of Medicine
New Haven, Connecticut

Gail A. Van Norman, MD
Professor
Director, Pre-Anesthesia Clinic
Department of Anesthesiology
University of Washington
Seattle, Washington

Russell T. Wall III, MD
Professor
Department of Anesthesiology
Georgetown University
Washington, DC

Matthew C. Wallace, MD
Major, Medical Corps, USAF
Staff Anesthesiologist
Wilford Hall Medical Center
Lackland Air Force Base, Texas

Kelley Teed Watson, MD
Assistant Clinical Professor
Yale University School of Medicine
New Haven, Connecticut;
Cardiac Anesthesiologist
Carolina Cardiac Surgery at
Self Regional Healthcare
Greenwood, South Carolina

This third edition of the *Handbook for Anesthesia and Co-Existing Disease* is intended to provide a ready source of information about the impact of the pathophysiology of disease states on the management of patients in the perioperative period. The Handbook utilizes an outline format that follows the chapters and headings of the fifth edition of *Anesthesia and Co-Existing Disease*, thus allowing students and clinicians to refer to corresponding areas in the textbook for more detailed information. As such, the intent of the Handbook is to serve as a portable counterpart to *Anesthesia and Co-Existing Disease*. There is an emphasis on the presentation of information in tables, illustrations, and algorithms. This format provides for rapid accessibility of pertinent aspects of a particular medical condition that can be reviewed on site in the operating room or at other anesthetizing locations that are remote from one's personal library.

We wish to thank Dr. Gail A. Van Norman for her invaluable help in redacting the text.

Roberta L. Hines
Katherine E. Marschall

Contents

Handbook for Stoelting's Anesthesia and Co-Existing Disease

Ischemic Heart Disease

Ischemic heart disease affects approximately 30% of patients undergoing surgery in the United States. Angina pectoris, acute myocardial infarction, and sudden death are often the first manifestations of this disease. Cardiac dysrhythmias are the major cause of sudden death. The two most important risk factors for the development of coronary artery atherosclerosis are male gender and increasing age (**Table 1-1**). Patients with ischemic heart disease can present with chronic stable angina or with an acute coronary syndrome (ACS). ACS can present as ST-elevation myocardial infarction (STEMI) or unstable angina/non-ST-segment elevation myocardial infarction (UA/NSTEMI) (**Fig. 1-1**).

I. ANGINA PECTORIS

Angina pectoris occurs when there is a mismatch of oxygen delivered to the myocardium (supply) and myocardial oxygen consumption (demand). Stable angina typically develops in the setting of partial occlusion or chronic narrowing of a segment of coronary artery. When the imbalance between myocardial oxygen supply and demand becomes critical, congestive heart failure, electrical instability with dysrhythmias, and myocardial infarction (MI) can result. Atherosclerosis is the most common cause of impaired coronary blood flow resulting in angina pectoris.

    A. Diagnosis. The pain of angina pectoris is generally described as retrosternal chest discomfort, pain, pressure, or heaviness that often radiates to the neck, left shoulder, left arm, or jaw and occasionally to the back or down both arms. Angina may also present as epigastric discomfort resembling indigestion, chest tightness, or shortness of breath. Discomfort usually lasts several minutes and follows a crescendo/decrescendo pattern; a sharp pain lasting only a few seconds or a dull ache lasting for hours is rarely angina. *Stable* angina is unchanged in frequency or severity over 2 months or longer. *Unstable angina* (UA) is angina at rest, of new onset, or of increased severity or frequency compared with previously stable angina. Chest wall tenderness suggests a musculoskeletal origin. Sharp retrosternal

TABLE 1-1	Risk Factors for Development of Ischemic Heart Disease
Male gender	
Increasing age	
Hypercholesterolemia	
Hypertension	
Cigarette smoking	
Diabetes mellitus	
Obesity	
Sedentary lifestyle	
Genetic factors/family history	

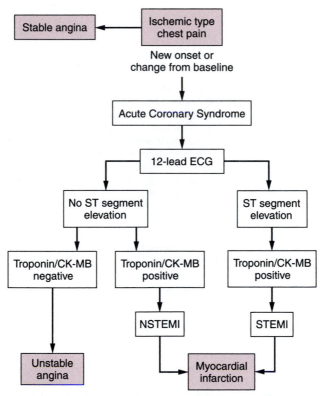

Figure 1-1 • Terminology of acute coronary syndrome. CK-MB, creatine kinase, myocardial bound isoenzyme; ECG, electrocardiogram. NSTEMI, non–ST elevation myocardial infarction; STEMI, ST elevation myocardial infarction. (Adapted from Alpert JS, Thygesen K, Antman E, Bassand JP: Myocardial infarction redefined—a consensus document of The Joint European Society of Cardiology/American College of Cardiology Committee for the redefinition of myocardial infarction. *J Am Coll Cardiol* 2000;36:959–969.)

pain exacerbated by deep breathing, coughing, or change in body position suggests pericarditis. Esophageal spasm can produce discomfort similar to angina pectoris and may be similarly relieved by administration of nitroglycerin.

1. Electrocardiography

a. Standard Electrocardiography (ECG). Subendocardial ischemia is associated with ST-segment depression during anginal pain. Variant angina (angina that results from coronary vasospasm) is characterized by ST elevation during anginal pain.

b. Exercise ECG. Exercise ECG can detect signs of myocardial ischemia in relationship to chest pain. A new murmur of mitral regurgitation or decrease in blood pressure during exercise increases the diagnostic value of this test. Exercise testing may be contraindicated in some conditions (e.g., severe aortic stenosis) and may not be possible in patients who cannot exercise or if other conditions interfere with interpretation of the exercise ECG (e.g., paced rhythm, left ventricular hypertrophy, digitalis administration, or pre-excitation syndrome). A minimum criterion for an abnormal ST-segment response is 1 mm or more of horizontal or down-sloping ST-segment depression during or within 4 minutes after exercise.

2. Noninvasive Imaging Tests.
Noninvasive imaging tests are recommended when exercise electrocardiography is not possible or interpretation of ST-segment changes would be difficult. Cardiac stress can be induced by administration of atropine or dobutamine, by cardiac pacing to increase heart rate, or by administration of a coronary vasodilator such as adenosine or dipyridamole.

a. Echocardiography. Wall motion analysis is performed immediately after stressing the heart. Ventricular wall motion abnormalities induced by stress correspond to the site of myocardial ischemia.

b. Nuclear Stress Imaging. Nuclear tracers (thallium, technetium) are injected into the bloodstream and detected over the myocardium by single-photon emission computed tomography techniques. Areas of reduced tracer activity during cardiac stress that are not present at rest indicate regions of reversible ischemia.

c. Electron Beam Computed Tomography. Coronary artery calcifications can be detected by electron beam computed tomography. Sensitivity is high but specificity is low, and routine use is not recommended.

3. Invasive Methods

a. Coronary Angiography. Coronary angiography provides the most information about the condition of the coronary arteries. It is indicated in patients who continue to have angina pectoris despite maximal medical therapy, in those who are being considered for coronary revascularization, and for the definitive diagnosis of coronary disease in individuals whose occupations could place others at risk (e.g., airline pilots).

    1.) The most important prognostic determinants are the extent of atheromatous coronary artery disease, the stability of coronary plaque, and left ventricular function (ejection fraction).

    2.) Left main coronary artery disease is the most dangerous anatomic lesion.

    3.) Plaques most likely to rupture and initiate ACS have a thin fibrous cap and large lipid core.

4.) Left ventricular ejection fraction of less than 40% is associated with poorer prognosis.

B. Treatment

1. Lifestyle Modification. Progression of atherosclerosis may be slowed by cessation of smoking; maintenance of an ideal body weight through a low-fat, low-cholesterol diet; regular aerobic exercise; and treatment of hypertension (HTN). Lowering the low-density lipoprotein level to less than 100 mg/dL by diet and/or drugs such as statins reduces risk of cardiac death. Lowering blood pressure from hypertensive levels to normal levels decreases the risk of MI, congestive heart failure (CHF), and cerebrovascular accident.

2. Medical Treatment of Myocardial Ischemia (Table 1-2)

3. Revascularization. Revascularization by coronary artery bypass grafting (CABG) or percutaneous coronary intervention (PCI) with or without placement of intracoronary stents is indicated when optimal medical therapy fails to control angina pectoris. Revascularization is also indicated for specific anatomic lesions (left main stenosis of >70%, combinations of two-vessel or three-vessel disease that include a proximal left anterior descending artery stenosis of >70%) and decreased left ventricular ejection fraction (EF).

II. ACUTE CORONARY SYNDROME

Acute coronary syndrome is a hypercoagulable state caused by to focal disruption of an atheromatous plaque, generation of thrombin, and partial or complete occlusion of the coronary artery. Patients presenting with ischemic chest pain are categorized by ECG characteristics and the presence of cardiac-specific biomarkers. Patients presenting with ST-segment elevation have ST-segment-elevation myocardial infarction. Those with ST-segment depression or nonspecific ECG changes and ischemic pain are classified as having non-ST-segment elevation MI when cardiac biomarkers are positive and as having unstable angina if biomarkers are negative.

A. ST-Elevation Myocardial Infarction (STEMI). One in 25 patients who survive hospitalization with acute MI will die within 1 year, with most deaths occurring within 3 months. Long-term prognosis is determined principally by left ventricular EF (determined 2 to 3 months after MI), the degree of residual ischemia, and the potential for malignant ventricular dysrhythmias.

1. Pathophysiology. Inflammation plays an important role in events leading to rupture of atherosclerotic plaque. Serum markers of inflammation are increased in those at greatest risk of development of coronary artery disease. STEMI occurs when coronary blood flow decreases abruptly because of acute thrombus formation after a plaque fissures, ruptures, or ulcerates.

a. Plaques with rich lipid cores and thin fibrous caps are most prone to rupture; such plaques are rarely large enough to cause coronary obstruction by themselves.

b. Flow-restrictive plaques that cause angina pectoris and stimulate development of collateral circulation are less likely to rupture.

c. Rarely, STEMI is the result of acute coronary spasm or coronary artery embolization.

2. Diagnosis. Diagnosis of acute MI requires the presence of at <u>least</u> two of these three criteria: (1) chest pain, (2) serial ECG changes indicative of MI, and (3) increase and decrease of serum cardiac enzymes. Two thirds of

TABLE 1-2	Medical Treatment of Myocardial Ischemia	
Classification	**Drugs**	**Comments**
Antiplatelet drugs	• Low-dose aspirin • Adenosine diphosphate receptor blockers: clopidogrel (Plavix), ticlopidine (Ticlid) • Platelet glycoprotein IIb/IIIa receptor antagonists (abciximab, eptifibatide, tirofiban)	Decrease risk of cardiac events in patients with stable or unstable angina. Particularly useful after intracoronary stent placement.
β-blockers	• β_1-blockers (atenolol, metoprolol, acebutolol, bisoprolol) • β_2-blockers (propranolol, nadolol)	Principal drug treatment for angina. Long-term use decreases risks of death and repeat MI. Used even in patients with congestive heart failure and pulmonary disease.
Calcium channel blockers (CCBs)	• Long-acting: amlodipine, nicardipine, isradipine, felodipine, long-acting nifedipine • Short-acting: nifedipine, verapamil, diltiazem	Long-acting CCBs are effective at relieving anginal pain; short-acting CCBs are not. Not as effective as β-blockers in reducing risk of MI. Contraindicated in CHF; use with caution in patients already on β-blockers.
Nitrates	• Sublingual nitroglycerine, isosorbide dinitrate	Decrease frequency, duration, and severity of angina. Contraindicated in obstructive cardiomyopathy and severe aortic stenosis. Must not be used within 24 hours of sildenafil (Viagra), tadalafil, (Cialis) or vardenafil (Levitra) due to potential hypotension.
Angiotensin-converting enzyme inhibitors	• Captopril, enalapril	Recommended for all patients with coronary artery disease, especially those with HTN, diabetes, or left ventricular dysfunction. Contraindicated in patients with renal failure and bilateral renal artery stenosis.

patients describe new-onset angina or change in anginal pattern during the 30 days preceding acute MI (**Table 1-3**).

a. Laboratory Studies. Cardiac troponins (troponin T or I) increase within 4 hours after myocardial injury and remain elevated for 7 to 10 days. They are more specific than CK-MB for determining myocardial injury.

b. Imaging Studies. Echocardiography to look for regional wall motion abnormalities is useful in patients with left bundle branch block or an abnormal ECG (but without ST-segment elevation) in whom the diagnosis of acute MI is uncertain.

3. Acute Treatment (Table 1-4)

TABLE 1-3 Signs and Symptoms of Acute MI
Anginal pain that does not resolve with rest
Anxiety
Pallor
Diaphoresis
Sinus tachycardia
Hypotension
Pulmonary rales
New cardiac murmur
Dysrhythmia
Abnormal ECG
Increased cardiac biomarkers (CPK, troponins)

CPK, creatine phosphokinase.

TABLE 1-4 Acute Treatment of Myocardial Infarction	
Immediate	• Evaluate hemodynamic stability • Obtain 12-lead ECG • Supplemental oxygen • Pain relief: nitroglycerin, morphine • Aspirin (clopidogrel if aspirin intolerant)
Within 30–60 minutes of arrival	• Thrombolytic therapy (streptokinase, tissue plasminogen activator, reteplase, tenecteplase) • Note: NOT recommended in patients with UA or NSTEMI
Within 90 minutes of arrival and 12 hours of symptom onset	• Coronary angioplasty • Coronary stenting with glycoprotein IIb/IIIa inhibitor
If coronary anatomy precludes a percutaneous intervention or angioplasty fails	• CABG (also indicated with acute mitral regurgitation or infarction-related ventricular septal defect)

4. Adjunctive Medical Therapy for Acute MI (Table 1-5)
B. Unstable angina/non-ST-segment elevation myocardial infarction (NSTEMI). UA/NSTEMI results from a reduction in myocardial oxygen supply caused by rupture or erosion of an atherosclerotic coronary plaque with thrombosis, inflammation, and vasoconstriction. Most affected arteries have less than 50% stenosis.

   1. Diagnosis. UA/NSTEMI has three principal presentations: (1) angina at rest, (2) chronic angina pectoris that becomes more frequent and more easily provoked, and (3) new-onset angina that is severe, prolonged, or disabling. UA/NSTEMI can also present with hemodynamic instability or CHF. ECG findings can include ST-segment depression and T-wave inversions. Elevation of cardiac biomarkers, troponins, and/or CK-MB distinguishes NSTEMI from UA.
   2. Treatment of UA/NSTEMI (Table 1-6)

III. COMPLICATIONS OF ACUTE MYOCARDIAL INFARCTION (Table 1-7)

IV. PERIOPERATIVE MYOCARDIAL INFARCTION

Approximately 500,000 to 900,000 perioperative MIs occur annually worldwide. The incidence of perioperative MI in patients who undergo elective high-risk vascular surgery is 5% to 15%.

TABLE 1-5	Adjunctive Medical Therapy in Acute Myocardial Infarction
Drug	**Indication/timing**
Heparin (unfractionated or low molecular weight)	• For 24–48 hours after thrombolytic therapy to reduce thrombin regeneration
Bivalirudin, hirudin	• For 24–48 hours in patients with heparin-induced thrombocytopenia
β-blockers	• For ALL patients without specific contraindications, starting as early as possible and continued indefinitely
ACEIs	• Large anterior MI • Clinical evidence of left ventricular failure • EF <40% • Diabetes
Angiotensin II receptor blockers	• Patients with indications who are intolerant of ACEIs
Calcium channel blockers	• Only in patients with persistent ischemia despite aspirin, β-blockers, nitrates, and IV heparin
Hypoglycemic agents	• Glycemic control in patients with diabetes
Magnesium	• Only in torsades de pointes ventricular tachycardia
Statins	• Should be started as soon as possible after acute MI

TABLE 1-6	Treatment of UA/NSTEMI
Decrease oxygen demand and increase oxygen supply	• Bed rest • Supplemental oxygen • Analgesia • β-blockers • Sublingual or IV nitroglycerin • Treat severe anemia
Reduce further thrombus formation	• Aspirin or clopidogrel • IV unfractionated heparin or subcutaneous low-molecular-weight heparin for 48 hours
For high-risk patients:	• Coronary angiography • Revascularization by PCI or CABG
For lower-risk patients:	• Medical therapy • Later stress testing

A. Pathophysiology. Most perioperative MIs occur within 24 to 48 hours after surgery. Two mechanisms appear to play a role in perioperative MI: (1) increased myocardial oxygen demand relative to supply and (2) thrombosis associated with vulnerable plaque rupture. These processes are not mutually exclusive. However, one process or the other can predominate in a particular patient (**Fig. 1-2**).

B. Diagnosis of Perioperative MI. The diagnosis of acute MI traditionally requires the presence of at least two of the following three elements: (1) ischemic chest pain, (2) evolutionary changes on the ECG, and (3) increase and decrease in cardiac biomarker levels. In the perioperative period, ischemic episodes are often not associated with chest pain, and many postoperative ECGs are nondiagnostic. An acute increase in troponin levels should be considered an MI in the perioperative setting, requiring careful attention and referral to a cardiologist for further evaluation and management.

V. PREOPERATIVE ASSESSMENT OF PATIENTS WITH KNOWN OR SUSPECTED ISCHEMIC HEART DISEASE

A. History (Table 1-8)

1. Silent Myocardial Ischemia. A history of ischemic heart disease or an abnormal ECG suggestive of a previous MI is associated with an increased incidence of silent myocardial ischemia. Treatment of silent myocardial ischemia is the same as that for classic angina pectoris.

2. Previous Myocardial Infarction. Acute (1–7 days) and recent MI (8–30 days) and UA incur the highest risk of perioperative myocardial ischemia, MI, and cardiac death.

    a. Elective surgery should be delayed at least 6 weeks after acute MI.

    b. Elective noncardiac surgery should be delayed for 4 to 6 weeks after coronary angioplasty.

    c. Elective noncardiac surgery should be delayed for 6 weeks after PCI with bare metal stent placement and as long as 12 months after

TABLE 1-7 Complications of Acute Myocardial Infarction

Complication	Treatment
Dysrhythmia	Ventricular fibrillation: rapid defibrillation, amiodarone, β-blockers, treatment of hypokalemia Ventricular tachycardia: cardioversion if sustained, amiodarone and/or lidocaine Atrial fibrillation: cardioversion if hemodynamically unstable, β-blocker or calcium channel blocker to control rate Sinus bradycardia: atropine, temporary cardiac pacing Second- or third-degree heart block: temporary cardiac pacing
Pericarditis—acute and delayed (Dressler's syndrome)	Aspirin or indomethacin, corticosteroids only for refractory symptoms
Severe mitral regurgitation	IV nitroprusside or other therapies to decrease left ventricular afterload Intra-aortic balloon pump Prompt surgical repair
Ventricular septal rupture	Intra-aortic balloon pump Prompt surgical repair
Congestive heart failure and cardiogenic shock	Treat reversible causes Support blood pressure Decrease left ventricular overload Treat pulmonary edema Restore coronary blood flow via thrombolytic therapy, PCI, or CABG Consider circulatory assist device, IAPB
Myocardial rupture	Emergency surgery
Right ventricular infarction	Intravascular volume replacement Inotropic support devices
Cerebrovascular accident	Echocardiography and immediate initiation of anticoagulation for left ventricular thrombus if present, followed by 6 months of warfarin therapy

drug-eluting stent placement to allow complete endothelialization of the stent and completion of antiplatelet therapy with gIIb/IIIa inhibitors such as clopidogrel.

3. Coexisting Noncardiac Diseases. The history should elicit symptoms of relevant coexisting noncardiac diseases (peripheral vascular disease, syncope, cough, dyspnea, orthopnea, paroxysmal nocturnal dyspnea, history of cigarette smoking, renal insufficiency, and diabetes mellitus).

4. Current Medications. The presence of effective β-blockade is suggested by a resting heart rate of 50 to 60 bpm. Many recommend withholding angiotensin-converting enzyme inhibitors (ACEIs) for 24 hours before surgical procedures involving significant fluid shifts

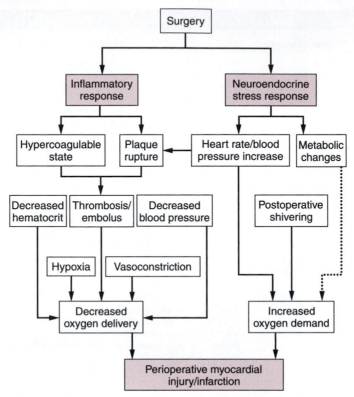

Figure 1-2 • Factors that can contribute to perioperative myocardial infarction.

or blood loss. A history of current use of clopidogrel and ticlopidine precludes neuraxial anesthesia. Both can also increase the risk of perioperative bleeding and necessitate platelet transfusion in urgent clinical situations.

B. Physical Examination. The physical examination of patients with ischemic heart disease is often normal (**Table 1-9**).

C. Specialized Preoperative Testing (Table 1-10)

VI. MANAGEMENT OF ANESTHESIA IN PATIENTS WITH KNOWN OR SUSPECTED ISCHEMIC HEART DISEASE UNDERGOING NONCARDIAC SURGERY

The preoperative assessment of patients with ischemic heart disease or risk factors for ischemic heart disease is geared toward the following goals: (1) determining the extent of ischemic heart disease and any previous interventions (CABG, PCI),

TABLE 1-8 Clinical Predictors of Increased Perioperative Cardiovascular Risk

Major

Unstable coronary syndromes

Acute or recent MI with evidence of important ischemic risk by clinical symptoms or noninvasive study

Unstable or severe angina

Decompensated heart failure

Significant dysrhythmias

High-grade atrioventricular block

Symptomatic ventricular dysrhythmias in the presence of underlying heart disease

Supraventricular dysrhythmias with uncontrolled ventricular rate

Severe valvular heart disease

Intermediate

Mild angina pectoris

Previous MI by history or Q waves on ECG

Compensated or previous heart failure

Diabetes mellitus (particularly insulin dependent)

Renal insufficiency

Minor

Advanced age (older than 70 years)

Abnormal ECG (left ventricular hypertrophy, left bundle branch block, ST-T abnormalities)

Rhythm other than sinus

Low functional capacity

History of stroke

Uncontrolled systemic hypertension

Adapted from Fleisher LA, Beckman JA, Brown KA, et al: ACC/AHA 2006 guideline update on perioperative cardiovascular evaluation for noncardiac surgery: Focused update on perioperative beta-blocker therapy: A report of the American College of Cardiology/American Heart Association Task Force on Practice Guidelines. Circulation 2006;113:2662–2674, with permission.

TABLE 1-9 Possible Physical Exam Findings in Patients with Ischemic Heart Disease

Left ventricular failure (S_3 gallop, rales)

Right ventricular failure (jugular venous distension, peripheral edema)

Cerebrovascular disease (carotid bruit)

Orthostatic hypotension (due to antihypertensive medication)

TABLE 1-10	Specialized Preoperative Testing in Patients with Ischemic Heart Disease

Preoperative stress test—usually not indicated in patients with stable coronary disease and acceptable exercise tolerance.

Echocardiography—can assess left ventricular EF and valve function

Stress echocardiography—wall motion abnormalities during pharmacologic stress testing (atropine, dipyridamole, dobutamine) can indicate presence and extent of ischemic heart disease

Radionuclide ventriculography—can evaluate left ventricular EF

Thallium scintigraphy—"cold spots" show areas of possible ischemia or infarction

Computed tomography and magnetic resonance imaging—can visualize coronary artery calcifications

Positron emission tomography—demonstrates regional myocardial blood flow and metabolism

(2) determining the severity and stability of the disease, and (3) reviewing medical therapy and noting drugs that can increase the risk of surgical bleeding or contraindicate a particular anesthetic technique.

A. Risk Stratification. In stable patients undergoing elective major noncardiac surgery, six independent predictors of major cardiac complications have been described in the Lee Revised Cardiac Risk Index (**Table 1-11**). The presence of several risk factors increases the incidence of postoperative cardiac complications (**Fig. 1-3**). These risk factors have been incorporated into the American College of Cardiology/American Heart Association (ACC/AHA) guidelines for perioperative cardiovascular evaluation for noncardiac surgery. Preoperative intervention is rarely necessary just to lower the risk of surgery. Interventions are indicated or not indicated irrespective of the need for surgery. Preoperative testing should be performed only if it is likely to influence perioperative management. The need for perioperative cardiac evaluation is determined in several steps.

1. Assess the Urgency of Surgery. The need for emergency surgery takes precedence over the need for additional workup (**Fig. 1-4**).

2. Assess Whether the Patient Has Undergone Revascularization and whether and when the patient underwent invasive or noninvasive cardiac evaluation (**Fig. 1-5**).

3. If No Prior Revascularization Was Performed, stratify risk according to clinical risk factors (**Table 1-12**), surgery-specific risk factors (**Table 1-13**) and functional capacity ($>$ or $<$4 metabolic equivalent tasks [METs]). Patients able to meet a 4-MET demand during normal daily activities without chest pain or dyspnea have good functional capacity. Patients with two of the following three factors—high-risk surgery, low exercise tolerance, and moderate clinical risk factors—could be considered for further cardiac evaluation. Patients who have low functional capacity or in whom it is difficult to assess functional capacity are good candidates for further evaluation (**Fig. 1-6**).

TABLE 1-11	**Cardiac Risk Factors in Patients Undergoing Elective Major Noncardiac Surgery**

I. High-risk surgery

    Abdominal aortic aneurysm

    Peripheral vascular operation

    Thoracotomy

    Major abdominal operation

II. Ischemic heart disease

    History of myocardial infarction

    History of a positive exercise test

    Current complaints of angina pectoris

    Use of nitrate therapy

    Q waves on electrocardiogram

III. Congestive heart failure

    History of congestive heart failure

    History of pulmonary edema

    History of paroxysmal nocturnal dyspnea

    Physical examination showing rales or S3 gallop

    Chest radiograph showing pulmonary vascular redistribution

IV. Cerebrovascular disease

    History of stroke

    History of transient ischemic attack

V. Insulin-dependent diabetes mellitus

VI. Preoperative serum creatinine concentration >2 mg/dL

Adapted from Lee TH, Marcantonio ER, Mangione CM, et al: Derivation and prospective validation of a simple index for prediction of cardiac risk of major noncardiac surgery. Circulation 1999;100:1043–1049, with permission.

B. Management After Risk Stratification. Three therapeutic options are available before elective noncardiac surgery: (1) revascularization by surgery, (2) revascularization by PCI, and (3) optimal medical management.

    1. Coronary Artery Bypass Grafting. The indications for preoperative coronary revascularization are the same as those in the nonoperative setting. There is no value in preoperative coronary intervention in patients with stable ischemic heart disease.

    2. Percutaneous Coronary Intervention. Angioplasty is now often accompanied by stenting, which requires postprocedure antiplatelet therapy to prevent acute coronary thrombosis and maintain long-term vessel patency. Discontinuation of antiplatelet therapy predisposes to stent thrombosis with significant morbidity and mortality. The following precautions should be adopted: (1) determine the date of placement, kind of stent, and any

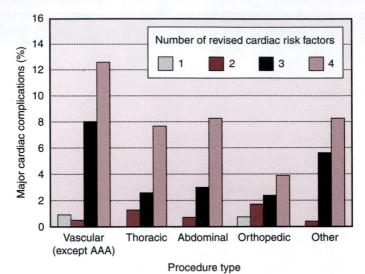

Figure 1-3 • Bars represent the rate of major cardiac complications in patients in Revised Cardiac Risk Index classes according to the type of surgery performed. Note that by definition, patients undergoing AAA (abdominal aortic aneurysm), thoracic, and abdominal procedures are excluded from class I because these operations are all considered high-risk surgery. In all subsets, there was a statistically significant trend toward greater risk with higher risk class. (Reproduced with permission from Lee TH, Marcantonio ER, Mangione CM, et al: Derivation and prospective validation of a simple index for prediction of cardiac risk of major noncardiac surgery. Circulation 1999;100:1043–1049.)

stent-related complications in patients with a history of PCI with coronary stenting; (2) consider patients with recent stent placement (<6 weeks for bare metal stents and <1 year for drug-eluting stents) as high risk and consult an interventional cardiologist for recommendations; (3) review the timing of the proposed surgery. Discontinuing or modifying antiplatelet therapy should involve a multidisciplinary team of cardiologist, surgeon, and anesthesiologist.

3. Pharmacologic Management

a. β-blockers reduce perioperative morbidity and mortality in selected patients (**Table 1-14**).

b. α_2-agonists have analgesic, sedative, and sympatholytic effects and may be useful in patients in whom β-blockers are contraindicated.

c. Perioperative hyperglycemia must be controlled.

d. Anxiety must be treated.

e. ACEIs, statins, and aspirin may also prove beneficial.

C. Intraoperative Management. Goals are (1) to prevent myocardial ischemia by optimizing myocardial oxygen supply and reducing myocardial oxygen demand and (2) to monitor for and treat ischemia. Factors influencing

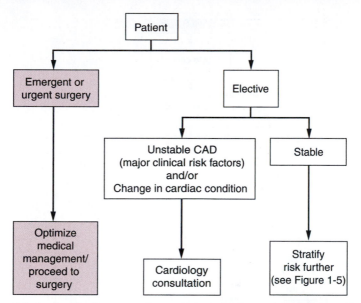

Figure 1-4 • An algorithm for preoperative assessment of patients with ischemic heart disease. Identify patients for urgent or emergent surgery and proceed to the operating room with medical management. In patients scheduled for elective surgery, the presence of major clinical risk factors or a change in medical condition may prompt further evaluation before surgery. CAD, coronary artery disease.

the balance of myocardial oxygen demand and supply are summarized in **Table 1-15**. Avoid persistent and excessive changes in heart rate and systemic blood pressure. A common recommendation is to keep the heart rate and blood pressure within 20% of the normal awake value. Increased heart rate increases myocardial oxygen requirements while decreasing supply because of decreased diastolic coronary artery perfusion time. Hypertension results in increased myocardial oxygen demand that is only partially offset by increased coronary perfusion pressure. Maintenance of the balance between myocardial oxygen supply and demand is more important than the specific anesthetic technique or drugs selected to produce anesthesia and muscle relaxation.

1. Induction of Anesthesia. Induction of anesthesia in patients with ischemic heart disease can be accomplished with many intravenous induction drugs. (Ketamine is an unlikely choice because resultant increases in heart rate and systemic blood pressure.) Myocardial ischemia may accompany the sympathetic nervous system stimulation that results from direct laryngoscopy and tracheal intubation. This can be mitigated by short-duration direct laryngoscopy (≤15 seconds) and/or administration of drugs to minimize the pressor response, such as laryngotracheal lidocaine, intravenous lidocaine, esmolol, and/or fentanyl.

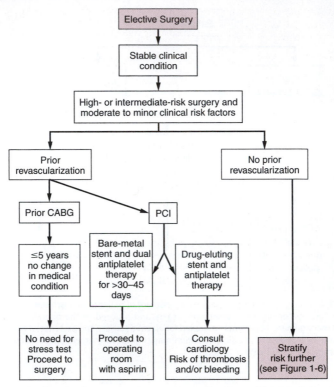

Figure 1-5 • An algorithm for preoperative assessment of patients with ischemic heart disease scheduled for elective intermediate- to high-risk surgery who are in stable clinical condition with moderate clinical risk factors. Determine previous coronary intervention and stability of cardiac condition. If no interval change in cardiac condition occurs, proceed with surgery with medical management. For patients with intracoronary stents, determine the date of insertion and location of the stent(s), the kind of stent(s), and the status of current antiplatelet therapy. Patients on antiplatelet therapy may require consultation with the cardiologist and the surgeon. CABG, coronary artery bypass grafting; PCI, percutaneous coronary intervention.

TABLE 1-12	Clinical Risk Factors for Perioperative Cardiac Risk	
Major Risk Factors: may require delay of elective surgery and cardiology evaluation	Unstable coronary syndrome, decompensated heart failure, significant dysrhythmias, severe valvular heart disease
Intermediate Risk Factors: well-validated markers of increased cardiac risk	Stable angina, previous MI, compensated or previous heart failure, insulin-dependent diabetes mellitus, renal insufficiency
Minor Risk Factors: markers of coronary disease not proven to increase perioperative risk	Hypertension, left bundle branch block, nonspecific ST-T wave changes, history of stroke

TABLE 1-13	Surgery-Specific Risk Factors for Perioperative Cardiac Complications	
High-Risk Surgery	Emergency major surgery, aortic or other major vascular surgery, peripheral vascular surgery, prolonged surgery involving large fluid shifts and/or blood loss
Intermediate-Risk Surgery	Carotid endarterectomy, head and neck surgery, intraperitoneal and intrathoracic surgery, orthopedic surgery, prostate surgery
Low-Risk Surgery	Endoscopic surgery, superficial surgery, cataract surgery, breast surgery

2. Maintenance of Anesthesia. Drug selection for maintenance of anesthesia is based in part on the patient's presumed left ventricular function.

   a. In patients with normal left ventricular function, controlled myocardial depression with a volatile anesthetic (with or without nitrous oxide) may minimize sympathetic nervous system activity during intense stimulation, such as laryngoscopy or surgical manipulation. However, volatile agents can be detrimental if drug-induced hypotension leads to decreases in coronary perfusion pressure. Equally acceptable is use of a nitrous oxide–opioid technique with the addition of a volatile anesthetic to treat undesirable increases in blood pressure at critical points.

   b. In patients with severely impaired left ventricular function, opioids may be selected for maintenance anesthesia. The addition of nitrous oxide, a benzodiazepine, or a low-dose volatile anesthetic should be considered because total amnesia cannot be ensured with an opioid alone, although the addition of nitrous oxide or a volatile anesthetic may be associated with myocardial depression.

   c. Regional anesthesia is acceptable in patients with ischemic heart disease, but decreases in blood pressure associated with epidural or spinal anesthesia must be controlled. Hypotension that exceeds 20% of the preblock blood pressure should be treated promptly. Despite presumed benefits of regional anesthesia, the postoperative cardiac morbidity and mortality does not appear to be significantly different between general and regional anesthesia.

3. Choice of Muscle Relaxant. Muscle relaxants with minimal or no effect on heart rate and systemic blood pressure (vecuronium, rocuronium, cisatracurium) are preferred. Histamine release and resulting decrease in blood pressure caused by atracurium are less desirable. Glycopyrrolate is preferred to atropine for the anticholinergic component in combination therapy to reverse neuromuscular blockade, because it is associated with less increase in heart rate.

4. Monitoring. Intraoperative monitoring should aim for early detection of myocardial ischemia. However, most myocardial ischemia occurs in the absence of hemodynamic alterations, so one should be cautious when endorsing routine use of expensive or complex monitors to detect myocardial ischemia (**Table 1-16**).

5. Intraoperative Management of Myocardial Ischemia. Treatment of myocardial ischemia should be instituted when there are 1-mm or greater

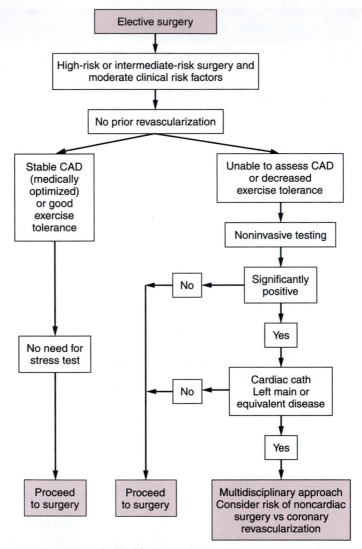

Figure 1-6 • For patients scheduled for intermediate- to high-risk surgery who have moderate clinical risk factors and poor exercise tolerance (or inability to determine exercise tolerance), consider noninvasive stress testing to determine whether significant myocardium is at risk. If significant myocardium is at risk, consider coronary angiogram. CAD, coronary artery disease.

TABLE 1-14   Recommendations for Perioperative β-Blocker Use

	Already Receiving β-Blockers	Clinical Risk Factors			
		Major Clinical Risk Factors or Positive Ischemia on Preoperative Stress Testing	Multiple Moderate Clinical Risk Factors	Single Moderate Clinical Risk Factor	Minor Clinical Risk Factors
Vascular surgery	++	++	+	±	*
High- or intermediate-risk surgery	++	+	+	±	*
Low-risk surgery	*	*	*	*	*

* , Insufficient data available; ++, class I recommendation, β-blockers should be used; +, class IIa recommendation, β-blockers should probably be used; ±, class IIb recommendation, β-blockers may be used.

Adapted from Fleisher LA, Beckman JA, Brown KA, et al: ACC/AHA 2006 guideline update on perioperative cardiovascular evaluation for noncardiac surgery: Focused update on perioperative beta-blocker therapy: A report of the American College of Cardiology/American Heart Association task force on practice guidelines: Circulation 2006;113:2662–2674, with permission.

TABLE 1-15	Intraoperative Events That Influence the Balance Between Myocardial Oxygen Delivery and Myocardial Oxygen Requirements
Decreased Oxygen Delivery	
Decreased coronary blood flow	
Tachycardia	
Diastolic hypotension	
Hypocapnia (coronary artery vasoconstriction)	
Coronary artery spasm	
Decreased oxygen content	
Anemia	
Arterial hypoxemia	
Shift of the oxyhemoglobin dissociation curve to the left	
Increased Oxygen Requirements	
Sympathetic nervous system stimulation	
Tachycardia	
Hypertension	
Increased myocardial contractility	
Increased afterload	
Increased preload	

ST-segment changes on the ECG. A persistent increase in heart rate can be treated by intravenous administration of a β-blocker (e.g., esmolol). Nitroglycerin is appropriate when myocardial ischemia is associated with a normal to modestly elevated blood pressure. Hypotension is treated with sympathomimetic drugs to restore coronary perfusion pressure. Fluid infusion can be useful to help restore blood pressure.

TABLE 1-16	Intraoperative Monitoring for Myocardial Ischemia
ECG	• Ischemia is characterized ST-segment elevation or depression of ≥1 mm • The degree of ST change parallels the severity of ischemia • Monitoring of three leads (either II, V_4, V_5 or V_3, V_4, and V_5) is recommended
Pulmonary artery catheter (PAC)	• Increase pulmonary capillary wedge pressure may indicate ischemia • V waves indicate mitral regurgitation and papillary muscle dysfunction • PAC can guide treatment of myocardial dysfunction
Transesophageal echocardiography	• Development of regional wall motion abnormalities precedes ECG changes

D. Postoperative Management
1. Prevent or treat events that increase myocardial oxygen demand, such as pain, shivering, hypercarbia, and sepsis.
2. Avoid or treat conditions that lead to decreased myocardial oxygen supply, such as anemia, hypoxemia, hypovolemia, and hypotension.
3. Continue treatments in the perioperative period that reduce the risks of adverse cardiac events, such as β-blockers.
4. Manage the timing of weaning and tracheal extubation to avoid detrimental alterations in blood pressure and heart rate.
5. Continuous ECG monitoring is useful for detecting postoperative myocardial ischemia, which is often silent.

VII. CARDIAC TRANSPLANTATION

Heart transplantation is most often used in patients with end-stage heart failure due to dilated cardiomyopathy or ischemic heart disease. Preoperatively, the ejection fraction is often less than 20%. Irreversible pulmonary hypertension is a contraindication to cardiac transplantation.

A. Management of Anesthesia
1. Etomidate is a preferred induction agent because it has little effect on hemodynamics. Opioids are often chosen for maintenance of anesthesia. Volatile anesthetics may produce undesirable degrees of myocardial depression and peripheral vasodilation. Nitrous oxide is rarely used because of its additive effects on myocardial depression, detrimental effects on pulmonary artery pressure, and potential to enlarge air emboli.
2. Following cardiopulmonary bypass, isoproterenol is commonly administered to support heart rate and lower pulmonary artery pressure. Additional treatments of pulmonary hypertension may include a prostaglandin, nitric oxide, or a phosphodiesterase inhibitor.
3. The denervated transplanted heart initially assumes an intrinsic heart rate of about 110 bpm, which is unresponsive to anticholinergic drugs. These patients tolerate hypovolemia poorly. The transplanted heart responds to direct-acting catecholamines, but drugs that act by indirect mechanisms such as ephedrine have less effect. Vasopressin may be needed to treat severe hypotension unresponsive to catecholamines.

B. Postoperative Complications
1. Early postoperative morbidity after heart transplantation surgery is usually related to sepsis and rejection. The most common early cause of death after cardiac transplantation is opportunistic infection as a result of immunosuppressive therapy. CHF and development of dysrhythmias can be late signs of rejection. Nephrotoxicity is a potential complication of cyclosporine therapy. Long-term corticosteroid use can result in skeletal demineralization and glucose intolerance.
2. Late complications of cardiac transplantation include development of coronary artery disease in the allograft and an increased incidence of cancer.

C. Anesthetic Considerations in Heart Transplant Recipients
1. Cardiac innervation
  a. The transplanted heart has no sympathetic, parasympathetic, or sensory innervation, and the loss of vagal tone results in a higher than

normal resting heart rate. Carotid sinus massage and the Valsalva maneuver have no effect on heart rate. There is no sympathetic response to direct laryngoscopy and tracheal intubation, and the denervated heart has a blunted heart rate response to light anesthesia or intense pain. The transplanted heart is unable to increase its heart rate immediately in response to hypovolemia or hypotension but responds instead with an increase in stroke volume (Frank-Starling mechanism).

b. Adrenergic receptors are intact on the transplanted heart, which will eventually respond to circulating catecholamines.

c. First-degree atrioventricular block is common after cardiac transplantation. Some patients may require a cardiac pacemaker for treatment of bradydysrhythmias.

2. Responses to Drugs

a. Responses to direct-acting sympathomimetic drugs are intact. Epinephrine, isoproterenol, and dobutamine have similar effects in normal and denervated hearts.

b. Indirect-acting sympathomimetics such as ephedrine have a blunted effect on denervated hearts.

c. Vagolytic drugs such as atropine do not increase the heart rate. Pancuronium does not increase the heart rate, and neostigmine and other anticholinesterases do not slow the heart rate of transplanted hearts.

3. Preoperative Evaluation

a. Heart transplant recipients may present with ongoing rejection manifesting as myocardial dysfunction, accelerated coronary atherosclerosis, or dysrhythmias.

b. All preoperative drug therapy must be continued, and proper functioning of a cardiac pacemaker, if in place, must be confirmed. Cyclosporine-induced hypertension may require treatment with calcium channel–blocking drugs or ACEIs. Cyclosporine-induced nephrotoxicity may present as an increased creatinine concentration, and anesthetic drugs excreted mainly by renal clearance mechanisms should then be avoided.

c. Proper hydration is important and should be confirmed preoperatively because heart transplant patients are preload dependent.

4. Management of Anesthesia

a. Maintain Intravascular Volume. These patients are preload dependent, and the denervated heart is unable to respond to sudden shifts in blood volume with an increase in heart rate.

b. General anesthesia is often preferable to spinal or epidural anesthesia because of potentially impaired response to hypotension associated with vasodilation. Avoid significant vasodilation and acute reductions in preload. Volatile agents are usually well tolerated in heart transplant patients who do not have significant heart failure.

c. Pay Careful Attention to Aseptic Technique and Antibiotic Prophylaxis. Patients are immunosuppressed and have increased susceptibility to infection.

2

Valvular Heart Disease

Management of the patient with valvular heart disease during the perioperative period requires an understanding of the hemodynamic alterations that accompany valvular dysfunction. The most commonly encountered cardiac valve lesions produce pressure overload (mitral stenosis, aortic stenosis) or volume overload (mitral regurgitation, aortic regurgitation) on the left atrium or left ventricle. Anesthetic management during the perioperative period is based on the likely effects of drug-induced changes in cardiac rhythm, heart rate, preload, afterload, myocardial contractility, systemic blood pressure, systemic vascular resistance, and pulmonary vascular resistance relative to the pathophysiology of the heart disease.

I. PREOPERATIVE EVALUATION

Preoperative evaluation of patients with valvular heart disease includes assessment of (1) the severity of the cardiac disease, (2) the degree of impaired myocardial contractility, and (3) the presence of associated major organ system disease. Recognition of compensatory mechanisms for maintaining cardiac output (increased sympathetic nervous system activity, cardiac hypertrophy) and knowledge of current drug therapy are important. The presence of prosthetic heart valves requires special considerations in the preoperative evaluation, especially if noncardiac surgery is planned.

  A. History and Physical Examination. Defining exercise tolerance is necessary to evaluate cardiac reserve in the presence of valvular heart disease and to provide a functional classification according to the criteria established by the New York Heart Association (**Table 2-1**). CHF is a common complication of chronic valvular heart disease. Elective surgery should be deferred until CHF can be treated and myocardial contractility optimized. The character, location, intensity, and direction of radiation of a heart murmur provide clues to the location and severity of the valvular lesion. Cardiac dysrhythmias, especially atrial fibrillation, are common. Valvular heart disease and ischemic heart disease often coexist.

TABLE 2-1	New York Heart Association Functional Classification of Patients with Heart Disease	
Class	**Description**	
I	Asymptomatic	
II	Symptoms with ordinary activity but comfortable at rest	
III	Symptoms with minimal activity but comfortable at rest	
IV	Symptoms at rest	

B. Drug Therapy. Modern drug therapy for valvular heart disease may include β-blockers, calcium channel blockers, and digitalis for heart rate control; angiotensin-converting enzyme inhibitors (ACEIs) and vasodilators to control blood pressure and afterload; and diuretics, inotropes, and vasodilators as needed to control heart failure. Antidysrhythmic therapy may also be necessary.

C. Laboratory Data

1. The Electrocardiogram (ECG) often exhibits broad and notched P waves (P mitrale), left and/or right axis deviation, and high voltage.

2. Chest Radiograph may show cardiomegaly (heart size exceeds 50% of the internal width of the thoracic cage on a posteroanterior chest radiograph).

3. Echocardiography with Doppler Color Flow Imaging is essential for noninvasive evaluation of valvular heart disease (**Table 2-2**).

4. Cardiac Catheterization can demonstrate the presence and severity of valvular stenosis and/or regurgitation, coronary artery disease, intracardiac shunting, transvalvular pressure gradients, the presence of pulmonary hypertension, and the presence of right-sided heart failure.

D. Presence of Prosthetic Heart Valves

1. Assessment of Prosthetic Heart Valve Function. Prosthetic heart valve dysfunction is suggested by the appearance of a new murmur or a change in an existing murmur. Transesophageal echocardiography is indicated for evaluation of the mitral valve. Cardiac catheterization permits measurement of transvalvular pressure gradients.

TABLE 2-2	Doppler Echocardiography in Evaluation of Valvular Heart Disease
Determine significance of cardiac murmurs.	
Identify hemodynamic abnormalities associated with physical findings.	
Determine transvalvular pressure gradient.	
Determine valve area.	
Determine ventricular ejection fraction.	
Diagnose valvular regurgitation.	
Evaluate prosthetic valve function.	

2. Complications Associated with Prosthetic Heart Valves (Table 2-3). Patients with mechanical prosthetic heart valves require long-term anticoagulant therapy. Antibiotic prophylaxis is necessary in certain situations to decrease the risk of endocarditis.

3. Management of Anticoagulation in Patients with Prosthetic Heart Valves

a. Anticoagulation can be continued for minor surgery in which blood loss is expected to be minimal.

b. Discontinue warfarin 2 to 3 days preoperatively.

c. Substitute intravenous unfractionated heparin or subcutaneous low-molecular-weight (LMW) heparin until the day before surgery (LMW heparin) or 2 to 4 hours prior to surgery on the day of (intravenous unfractionated heparin).

d. Warfarin is contraindicated during pregnancy; administer subcutaneous unfractionated or LMW heparin. Low-dose aspirin may also be used in conjunction with heparin therapy.

E. Prevention of Bacterial Endocarditis

1. New American Heart Association (AHA) guidelines focus endocarditis prophylaxis *only on patients with conditions listed in* **Table 2-4**.

2. The recommendations regarding which antibiotic to use for endocarditis prophylaxis are not dissimilar from previous recommendations and are listed in **Table 2-5**.

3. Antibiotic prophylaxis *is* recommended for the following procedures:

a. Dental procedures that involve manipulation of gingival tissues or the periapical regions of teeth or perforation of the oral mucosa.

b. Invasive procedures (i.e., those that involve incision or biopsy) on the respiratory tract or infected skin, skin structures, or musculoskeletal tissue.

4. Antibiotic prophylaxis *is not* recommended for genitourinary (GU) or gastrointestinal (GI) tract procedures.

II. MITRAL STENOSIS (MS)

A. Pathophysiology. MS causes progressive mechanical obstruction to left ventricular diastolic filling, with resulting increase in left atrial volume and pressure. Pulmonary venous pressure increases with the increase in left atrial pressure. Transudation of fluid into the pulmonary interstitial space results in decreased pulmonary compliance, increased work of breathing, and dyspnea on

TABLE 2-3 Complications Associated with Prosthetic Heart Valves
Valve thrombosis
Systemic embolization
Structural failure
Hemolysis
Paravalvular leak
Endocarditis

TABLE 2-4 Cardiac Conditions Associated with Higher Risk of Adverse Outcomes from Endocarditis; Prophylaxis for Dental Procedures Is Reasonable

1. Prosthetic cardiac valve or prosthetic material used for cardiac valve repair

2. Previous infective endocarditis

3. Congenital heart disease:

Unrepaired cyanotic congenital heart disease, including palliative shunts and conduits

Completely repaired congenital heart defect with prosthetic material or device, whether placed by surgery or by catheter intervention, during the first 6 months after the procedure[*]

Repaired congenital heart disease with residual defects at the site or adjacent to the site of a prosthetic patch or prosthetic device (which inhibit endothelialization)

4. Cardiac transplantation recipients who develop cardiac valve pathology

Except for the conditions listed above, antibiotic prophylaxis is no longer recommended for any other form of congenital heart disease.
[*] Prophylaxis is reasonable because endothelialization of prosthetic material occurs within 6 months after the procedure.
From Wilson W, Taubert KA, Gewitz M, et al: Prevention of infective endocariditis. Guidelines from the American Heart Association. Circulation 2007;116:1736–1754, with permission.

TABLE 2-5 Antibiotic Prophylaxis for Dental Procedures

Situation	Agent	Regimen: Single Dose 30 to 60 min Before Procedure	
		Adults	Children
Oral	Amoxicillin	2 g	50 mg/kg
Unable to take oral medication	Ampicillin OR Cefazolin or ceftriaxone	2 g IM or IV 1 g IM or IV	50 mg/kg IM or IV 50 mg/kg IM or IV
Allergic to penicillins or ampicillin—oral	Cephalexin[*,†] OR Clindamycin[*,†] OR Azithromycin or clarithromycin	2 g 600 mg 500 mg	50 mg/kg 20 mg/kg 15 mg/kg
Allergic to penicillins or ampicillin and unable to take oral medication	Cefazolin or ceftriaxone[†] OR Clindamycin	1 g IM or IV 600 mg IM or IV	50 mg/kg IM or IV 20 mg/kg IM or IV

IM, intramuscularly.
[*] Or other first- or second-generation oral cephalosporin in equivalent adult or pediatric dosage.
[†] Cephalosporins should not be used in an individual with a history of anaphylaxis, angioedema, or urticaria with penicillins or ampicillin.
From Wilson W, Taubert KA, Gewitz M, et al: Prevention of infective endocarditis. Guidelines from the American Heart Association. Circulation 2007;116:1736–1754, with permission.

exertion. Overt pulmonary edema occurs when the pulmonary venous pressure exceeds the oncotic pressure of plasma proteins.

B. Diagnosis. Echocardiography is used to assess the severity of MS and calculating valve area. Pulmonary hypertension is likely if the left atrial pressure is chronically above 25 mm Hg, which is common when the mitral valve area is less than 1 cm^2. Clinically, MS is recognized by the characteristic opening snap that occurs early in diastole and by a rumbling diastolic heart murmur best heard at the apex or in the axilla.

C. Treatment (Table 2-6)

D. Management of Anesthesia (Table 2-7)

    1. Preoperative Medication is used to decrease anxiety-induced tachycardia. Drugs used for heart rate control should be continued. Diuretic-induced hypokalemia should be treated preoperatively. Anticoagulation should be discontinued for major surgery with anticipated significant blood loss.

TABLE 2-6	Treatment of Mitral Stenosis
1.	Diuretics to reduce left atrial pressure
2.	Heart rate control (β-blockers, digoxin, calcium channel blockers)
3.	Anticoagulation therapy
4.	Surgical correction (commissurotomy, valvuloplasty, valve reconstruction, valve replacement) when symptoms increase or evidence of pulmonary hypertension appears

TABLE 2-7	Anesthetic Considerations for Patients with Mitral Stenosis	
Problem		**Management**
Sinus tachycardia or rapid ventricular response to atrial fibrillation decreases cardiac output and can cause pulmonary edema		Administer cardioversion or intravenous β-blocker, calcium channel blocker, or digoxin
Congestive heart failure due to central blood volume changes		Avoid excessive fluid administration, do not place patient in Trendelenberg's position
Sudden decrease in systemic vascular resistance with hypotension and increased heart rate decreases cardiac output		Administer sympathometic amines. Ephedrine may increase cardiac output but also increase heart rate; phenylephrine may be preferable because it avoids increases in heart rate.
Pulmonary hypertension and right-sided heart failure		Avoid hypercarbia, hypoxemia, lunge hyperinflation. Right-sided heart failure may require inotropic support and pulmonary vasodilating agents.

2. Induction of Anesthesia. Avoid drugs likely to increase heart rate (e.g., ketamine) or to precipitate hypotension from histamine release.

3. Maintenance of Anesthesia should be designed to minimize minimal sustained changes in heart rate, myocardial contractility, and systemic and pulmonary vascular resistance. A nitrous/narcotic anesthetic or a balanced anesthetic with low concentrations of a volatile anesthetic usually achieve this goal. Nitrous oxide may cause pulmonary vasoconstriction, particularly if pulmonary hypertension is present.

4. Monitoring. Use of invasive monitoring depends on the complexity of the procedure and the severity of MS. Asymptomatic patients without evidence of pulmonary congestion do not generally require special monitoring. In patients with symptomatic MS, transesophageal echocardiography and/or continuous monitoring of intra-arterial pressure, pulmonary artery pressure, and left atrial pressure should be considered.

5. Postoperative Management. In patients with MS, the risk of pulmonary edema and right-sided heart failure continues into the postoperative period. Pain and hypoventilation can cause increased heart rate and pulmonary vascular resistance. Patients may require continued mechanical ventilation, particularly after major thoracic or abdominal surgery.

III. MITRAL REGURGITATION (MR)

A. Pathophysiology. MR is characterized by decreases in forward left ventricular stroke volume and cardiac output associated with increased left atrial pressure. Volume and pressure overload of the left atrium are especially increased in patients with combined MS and MR.

B. Diagnosis. MR is recognized clinically by the presence of a holosystolic apical murmur with radiation to the axilla. ECG and chest radiograph may indicate left ventricular hypertrophy. Echocardiography documents the presence, severity, and sometimes the cause of MR (**Table 2-8**). The presence of a V wave in a pulmonary artery occlusion pressure waveform reflects regurgitant flow through the mitral valve.

C. Treatment. Surgical repair or replacement is indicated when the ejection fraction is less than 0.6 or before the left ventricle end-systolic dimension is 45 mm or greater. Symptomatic patients should undergo mitral valve surgery even if ejection fraction is normal. There is no apparent benefit to long-term use of vasodilator drugs in asymptomatic patients with chronic MR. ACEIs or β-blockers and biventricular pacing have been shown to decrease functional MR and improve symptoms and exercise tolerance in symptomatic patients.

TABLE 2-8	Grading of Mitral Regurgitation by Echocardiography		
	Mild	**Moderate**	**Severe**
Area of MR jet (cm^2)	<3	3.0-6.0	>6
MR jet area as percentage of left atrial area	20–30	30–40	>40
Regurgitant fraction (%)	20–30	30–50	>55

D. Management of Anesthesia (Table 2-9). Modest increases in heart rate and reduction in left ventricular afterload (e.g., with nitroprusside) with or without inotropic drugs improve left ventricular output. The decrease in systemic vascular resistance caused by regional anesthesia may be beneficial in some patients.

    1. Induction of Anesthesia. Avoid increases in systemic vascular resistance or decreases in heart rate. Pancuronium may be a useful muscle relaxant, due to a modest increase in heart rate.

    2. Maintenance of Anesthesia. The increase in heart rate and decrease in systemic vascular resistance plus the minimal negative inotropic effects of isoflurane, desflurane, and sevoflurane make them all acceptable choices for maintenance of anesthesia. When myocardial function is severely compromised, opioid-based anesthesia may be considered, although caution is advised because narcotics can produce significant bradycardia that is very deleterious in severe MR.

    3. Monitoring. Invasive monitoring is not needed for minor surgery in asymptomatic patients. In patients with severe MR, pulmonary artery occlusion pressure monitoring may be helpful.

IV. MITRAL VALVE PROLAPSE

Mitral valve prolapse (MVP) is defined as the prolapse of one or both mitral leaflets into the left atrium during systole with or without MR. It is usually a benign condition, affecting 1% to 2.5% of the population; however, MVP can have devastating complications, such as cerebral embolic events, infective endocarditis, severe mitral regurgitation requiring surgery, dysrhythmias, and sudden death.

  A. Diagnosis. The diagnosis of MVP is based on echocardiographic findings of valve prolapse of 2 mm or more above the mitral annulus. Cardiac dysrhythmias associated with MVP include both supraventricular and ventricular dysrhythmias and respond well to β-blocker therapy. Cardiac conduction abnormalities are not uncommon.

  B. Management of Anesthesia. Management of anesthesia in patients with MVP follows the same principles outlined earlier for patients with mitral regurgitation (**Table 2-9**). The degree of MVP is adversely affected by increased ventricular emptying, decreased left ventricular filling, and smaller ventricular dimensions, such as occur with increased myocardial contractility, decreased systemic vascular resistance, upright posture, and hypovolemia.

    1. Preoperative Evaluation. Preoperative evaluation should focus on distinguishing patients with purely functional disease (often women

TABLE 2-9	Anesthetic Considerations in Patients with Mitral Regurgitation
Prevent bradycardia.	
Prevent increases in systemic vascular resistance.	
Minimize drug-induced myocardial depression.	
Monitor the magnitude of regurgitant flow with a pulmonary artery catheter (size of the V wave) and/or echocardiography.	

younger than 45 years treated with β-blockers) from patients with significant MR (older men who present with symptoms of mild to moderate CHF). Patients taking β-blockers should have them continued perioperatively. Anxiolytic medications should be used to avoid tachycardia. Antithrombotic medications such as aspirin or warfarin may be continued in patients undergoing minor surgery when significant blood loss is not expected.

2. Selection of Anesthetic Technique. Most patients with MVP have normal left ventricular function; volatile agents are well tolerated. The decrease in systemic vascular resistance associated with regional anesthesia should be offset by fluid administration to avoid changes in left ventricular volume that could adversely affect MVP and MR.

3. Induction of Anesthesia. Avoid sudden decreases in systemic vascular resistance. Etomidate is an attractive choice for induction in patients with significant MVP, because it causes minimal myocardial depression or alterations in sympathetic nervous system activity. Ketamine stimulates the sympathetic nervous system and enhances MVP and MR.

4. Maintenance of Anesthesia. Minimize sympathetic nervous system activation due to surgical stimuli (volatile anesthetics with or without nitrous oxide and/or opioids). Unexpected ventricular dysrhythmias can occur, especially during operations performed in the head-up or sitting position, presumably due to increased left ventricular emptying and accentuation of MVP. Generous intravenous fluid therapy and prompt replacement of intraoperative blood loss is indicated. If vasopressors are needed, an α-agonist such as phenylephrine is more desirable than inotropes, which may enhance MVP and MR.

5. Monitoring. Routine monitoring is all that is necessary in the vast majority of patients with MVP. An intra-arterial catheter and pulmonary artery catheter are only needed in patients with significant MR and left ventricular dysfunction.

V. AORTIC STENOSIS (AS)

A. Pathophysiology. Obstruction to ejection of blood into the aorta due to decreases in the aortic valve area necessitates an increase in left ventricular pressure to maintain forward stroke volume. Angina pectoris may occur in patients with AS despite the absence of coronary disease. Critical AS is defined as transvalvular pressure gradients greater than 50 mmHg.

B. Diagnosis. The classic symptoms of critical AS are: angina pectoris, syncope, and dyspnea on exertion. Physical exam reveals a characteristic systolic murmur heard best in the aortic area, possibly radiating to the neck. Because many patients with AS are asymptomatic, it is important to listen for the systolic murmur of AS in older patients scheduled for surgery. The ECG may demonstrate left ventricular hypertrophy.

1. Echocardiography with Doppler examination of the aortic valve provides a more accurate assessment of the severity of aortic stenosis (**Table 2-10**) than does clinical evaluation.

2. Cardiac Catheterization and coronary angiography may be necessary when the severity of AS cannot be determined by echocardiography.

TABLE 2-10	Severity of Aortic Stenosis Measured by Echocardiography		
	Mild	Moderate	Severe
Mean transvalvular pressure gradient (mm Hg)	<20	20–50	>50
Peak transvalvular pressure gradient (mm Hg)	<36	>50	>80
Aortic valve area (cm²)	1.0–1.5	0.8–1.0	<0.8

3. Exercise Stress Testing may be useful in risk-stratifying asymptomatic patients with moderate to severe AS. Patients with exercise-induced symptoms might benefit from aortic valve replacement.

C. Treatment. In asymptomatic patients with AS, it appears to be safe to continue medical management and delay valve replacement surgery until symptoms develop. Surgical/procedural interventions include valve replacement and balloon valvotomy.

D. Management of Anesthesia. Management of anesthesia in patients with AS includes the prevention of hypotension and any hemodynamic change that will decrease cardiac output (**Table 2-11**). Cardiopulmonary resuscitation is unlikely to be effective in patients with AS because it is difficult, if not impossible, to create an adequate stroke volume across a stenotic aortic valve with cardiac compressions.

1. Induction of Anesthesia. General anesthesia is usually preferable to epidural or spinal anesthesia, which can decrease systemic vascular resistance and precipitate significant hypotension. Induction of anesthesia can be accomplished with an intravenous induction drug that does not decrease systemic vascular resistance.

2. Maintenance of Anesthesia can be accomplished with a combination of nitrous oxide and volatile anesthetic and opioids or by opioids alone. Decreases in systemic vascular resistance are undesirable. Intravascular fluid volume should be maintained at normal levels. The onset of junctional rhythm or bradycardia requires prompt treatment with glycopyrrolate, atropine, or ephedrine. Persistent tachycardia can be treated with β-antagonists such as esmolol. Supraventricular tachycardia should be promptly terminated with electrical cardioversion. Lidocaine and a

TABLE 2-11	Anesthetic Considerations in Patients with Aortic Stenosis
Maintain normal sinus rhythm.	
Avoid bradycardia or tachycardia.	
Avoid hypotension.	
Optimize intravascular fluid volume to maintain venous return and left ventricular filling.	

defibrillator should be kept available, as these patients have a propensity to develop ventricular dysrhythmias.

3. Monitoring. The use of invasive monitoring is determined by the complexity of the surgery and severity of AS and may include continuous arterial blood pressure monitoring, a pulmonary artery catheter, and/or transesophageal echocardiography.

VI. AORTIC REGURGITATION (AR)

A. Pathophysiology. Regurgitation of some of the ejected stroke volume from the aorta back into the left ventricle during diastole results in a combined pressure and volume overload on the left ventricle. The magnitude of the regurgitant volume depends on (1) the duration of diastole, which is determined by heart rate, and (2) the pressure gradient across the aortic valve, which is dependent on systemic vascular resistance. The magnitude of AR is decreased by tachycardia and peripheral vasodilation. Patients with acute AR experience severe left ventricular volume overload before compensation can occur and therefore may present with coronary ischemia, rapid deterioration in left ventricular function, and heart failure.

B. Diagnosis. AR is recognized clinically by a characteristic diastolic murmur heard best along the left sternal border, and peripheral signs of a hyperdynamic circulation (widened pulse pressure, decreased diastolic blood pressure, bounding pulses). Signs of left ventricular hypertrophy may be seen on the chest radiograph and ECG. Echocardiography with Doppler examination identifies the presence and severity of AR (**Table 2-12**).

C. Treatment. Surgical replacement of a diseased aortic valve is recommended before the onset of permanent left ventricular dysfunction, even in asymptomatic patients. Medical therapy of AR is directed at decreasing systolic hypertension and ventricular wall stress and improving left ventricular function.

D. Management of Anesthesia (Table 2-13). Management of anesthesia in patients with AR is directed toward maintaining forward left ventricular stroke volume. The heart rate should be kept at greater than 80 bpm because bradycardia increases the amount of backward blood flow; leading to left ventricular volume overload. Abrupt increases in systemic vascular resistance

TABLE 2-12	Severity of Aortic Regurgitation Measured by Echocardiography		
	Mild	**Moderate**	**Severe**
Regurgitant jet width as percentage of LVOT width	25–46	47–64	>65
Regurgitant jet area as percentage of LVOT area	4–24	25–59	>60
Aortic diastolic flow reversal	None		Holodiastolic retrograde flow in the descending aorta

LVOT, left ventricular outflow tract.

TABLE 2-13	Anesthetic Considerations in Patients with Aortic Regurgitation

Avoid bradycardia.
Avoid increases in systemic vascular resistance.
Minimize myocardial depression.

can precipitate left ventricular failure, requiring treatment with a vasodilator for afterload reduction and an inotrope to increase contractility. Overall, modest increases in heart rate and modest decreases in systemic vascular resistance are reasonable hemodynamic goals.

1. Induction of Anesthesia. Induction of anesthesia in the presence of AR can be achieved with any intravenous induction drugs with or without inhalation anesthesia that ideally do not decrease heart rate or increase systemic vascular resistance.

2. Maintenance of Anesthesia is often provided with nitrous oxide plus a volatile anesthetic and/or opioid. Intravascular fluid volume should be maintained at normal levels to provide for adequate cardiac preload. Bradycardia and junctional rhythm may require prompt treatment with intravenous atropine.

3. Monitoring. Minor surgery in patients with asymptomatic AR does not require invasive monitoring. For severe AR, monitoring with a pulmonary artery catheter or transesophageal echocardiography is helpful to monitor myocardial depression, facilitate intravascular volume replacement, and measure the response to vasodilating drugs.

VII. TRICUSPID REGURGITATION (TR)

A. Pathophysiology. Right atrial volume overload results in only a minimal increase in right atrial pressures even in the presence of a large regurgitant volume, due to high compliance of the right atrium and vena cavae. Clinical signs include jugular venous distension, hepatomegaly, ascites, and peripheral edema.

B. Management of Anesthesia. Intravascular fluid volume and central venous pressure should be maintained in the high normal range to facilitate adequate right ventricular preload and left ventricular filling. Events known to increase pulmonary artery pressure (e.g., hypoxemia, hypercarbia) should be avoided. Nitrous oxide can be a weak pulmonary artery vasoconstrictor and could increase the degree of TR. Right atrial pressure monitoring may help to guide intravenous fluid replacement and to detect changes in the amount of TR during anesthesia.

VIII. TRICUSPID STENOSIS (TS)

TS is rare in the adult population and may be associated with a history of rheumatic fever, carcinoid syndrome, and endomyocardial fibrosis. TS increases right atrial pressure and the pressure gradient between the right atrium and right ventricle.

IX. PULMONIC REGURGITATION (PR)

PR results from pulmonary hypertension and annular dilation of the pulmonic valve. Other causes include connective tissue diseases, carcinoid syndrome, infective endocarditis, and rheumatic heart disease. It is rarely symptomatic.

X. PULMONIC STENOSIS (PS)

PS is usually congenital and detected and corrected in childhood. An acquired form can be due to rheumatic fever, carcinoid syndrome, or infective endocarditis. Significant obstruction can cause syncope, angina, right ventricular hypertrophy, and right ventricular failure. Surgical valvotomy can be used to relieve the obstruction.

CHAPTER 3

Congenital Heart Disease

Congenital anomalies of the heart and cardiovascular system occur in 7 to 10 per 1000 live births (**Table 3-1**). Signs and symptoms of congenital heart disease in infants and children (**Table 3-2**) are apparent during the first week of life in approximately 50% of afflicted neonates and before 5 years of age in virtually all remaining patients. Echocardiography is the initial diagnostic step. Certain complications are likely to accompany the presence of congenital heart disease (**Table 3-3**). Cardiac dysrhythmias are not usually a prominent feature.

I. ACYANOTIC CONGENITAL HEART DISEASE

Acyanotic congenital heart disease is characterized by a left-to-right intracardiac shunt (**Table 3-4**). Such shunts, regardless of their locations, often result in increased pulmonary blood flow with pulmonary hypertension, right ventricular hypertrophy, and eventually congestive heart failure (CHF). The onset and severity of clinical symptoms vary with the site and magnitude of the vascular shunt.

A. Atrial Septal Defect (ASD) accounts for about one third of the congenital heart disease detected in adults and is two to three times more common in females than males. The physiologic consequences of ASDs reflect the shunting of blood from one atrium to the other; the direction and magnitude of the shunt are determined by the size of the defect and the relative compliance of the ventricles. When the diameter of the ASD approaches 2 cm, it is likely that left-to-right shunt has led to increased pulmonary blood flow. A systolic ejection murmur audible in the second left intercostal space may be mistaken for an innocent flow murmur. Transesophageal echocardiography and Doppler color flow echocardiography are both useful for detecting and determining the location and size of ASDs.

    1. Signs and Symptoms. ASDs initially produce no symptoms or signs and may remain undetected for years. Symptoms due to large ASDs include dyspnea on exertion, supraventricular dysrhythmias, right-sided heart failure,

TABLE 3-1 Classification and Incidence of Congenital Heart Disease	
Disease	**Incidence (%)**
Acyanotic Defects	
Ventricular septal defect	35
Atrial septal defect	9
Patent ductus arteriosus	8
Pulmonary stenosis	8
Aortic stenosis	6
Coarctation of the aorta	6
Atrioventricular septal defect	3
Cyanotic Defects	
Tetralogy of Fallot	5
Transposition of the great vessels	4

paradoxical embolism, and recurrent pulmonary infections. When pulmonary blood flow is 1.5 times the systemic blood flow, closure of the ASD is indicated to prevent right ventricular dysfunction and irreversible pulmonary hypertension. Prophylaxis against infective endocarditis is not indicated for ASD.

2. Management of Anesthesia (Table 3-5)

TABLE 3-2 Signs and Symptoms of Congenital Heart Disease
Infants
Tachypnea
Failure to gain weight
Heart rate >200 bpm
Heart murmur
Congestive heart failure
Cyanosis
Children
Dyspnea
Slow physical development
Decreased exercise tolerance
Heart murmur
Congestive heart failure
Cyanosis
Clubbing of digits
Squatting
Hypertension

TABLE 3-3	Common Problems Associated with Congenital Heart Disease

Infective endocarditis
Cardiac dysrhythmias
Complete heart block
Hypertension (systemic or pulmonary)
Erythrocytosis
Thromboembolism
Coagulopathy
Brain abscess
Increased plasma uric acid concentration
Sudden death

TABLE 3-4	Congenital Heart Defects Resulting in a Left-to-Right Intracardiac Shunt or Its Equivalent

Secundum atrial septal defect
Primum atrial septal defect (endocardial cushion defect)
Ventricular septal defect
Aorticopulmonary fenestration

TABLE 3-5	Anesthetic Considerations in Patients with Left-to-Right Intracardiac Shunts

- Pharmacology of inhaled anesthetics is not altered as long as systemic blood flow remains normal.
- Avoid increases in systemic vascular resistance; this increases left-to-right shunting.
- Avoid measures that decrease pulmonary vascular resistance (e.g., high FiO_2, pulmonary vasodilators); this increases left-to-right shunt.
- Decreased systemic vascular resistance and increased pulmonary vascular resistance decrease left-to-right shunt.
- Positive-pressure ventilation is well tolerated.
- Antibiotic prophylaxis is only indicated for ASD when a valvular abnormality is also present. Antibiotic prophylaxis *is* indicated for VSD and PDA.
- Avoid introducing air into the circulation, such as through IV solutions.
- Transient supraventricular dysrhythmias and atrioventricular conduction changes are common after closure of the ASD.

B. Ventricular Septal Defect (VSD) is the most common congenital cardiac abnormality in infants and children and many close spontaneously by 2 years of age. Echocardiography with Doppler flow ultrasonography confirms the presence and location of the VSD, and color-flow mapping provides information about the magnitude and direction of the intracardiac shunt.

1. Signs and Symptoms. The physiologic significance of a VSD depends on the size of the defect and the relative resistance in the systemic and pulmonary circulations. If the defect is large, over time the pulmonary vascular resistance increases; the direction of the shunt may reverse, resulting in cyanosis. Adults with small defects and normal pulmonary arterial pressures are generally asymptomatic, and pulmonary hypertension is unlikely. The murmur of a VSD is holosystolic and loudest at the lower left sternal border. Closure of the defect is recommended in patients with large VSDs, in whom the magnitude of the pulmonary hypertension is not prohibitive (pulmonary/systemic vascular resistance ratio < 0.7).

2. Management of Anesthesia for VSD is similar to management for ASD in most respects (**Table 3-5**). Right ventricular infundibular hypertrophy may be present in patients with VSDs and increased myocardial contractility, or hypovolemia may exaggerate right ventricular obstruction. Third-degree atrioventricular heart block may follow surgical closure if the cardiac conduction system is near the VSD.

C. Patent Ductus Arteriosus (PDA) is present when the ductus arteriosus (which arises just distal to the left subclavian artery and connects the descending aorta to the left pulmonary artery) fails to close spontaneously shortly after birth, resulting in continuous flow of blood from the aorta to the pulmonary artery. The PDA can usually be visualized on echocardiography, with Doppler studies confirming the continuous flow into the pulmonary circulation.

1. Signs and Symptoms. Most patients are asymptomatic, and most PDAs are recognized by the presence of a characteristic continuous systolic and diastolic murmur. If severe pulmonary hypertension develops, closure of the PDA is contraindicated.

2. Treatment. The PDA is treated by either medical (cyclooxygenase inhibitors such as indomethacin) or surgical closure.

3. Management of Anesthesia includes the same considerations for other patients with left-to-right cardiac shunts (**Table 3-5**). Ligation of the PDA is often associated with significant systemic hypertension during the postoperative period, which can be managed with vasodilator drugs such as nitroprusside. Long-acting antihypertensive drugs can be gradually substituted for nitroprusside if systemic hypertension persists.

D. Aorticopulmonary Fenestration is characterized by a communication between the ascending aorta and the main pulmonary artery. The physiologic consequences and anesthesia management are similar to those associated with a large PDA.

E. Aortic Stenosis (AS). Bicuspid aortic valves occur in 2% to 3% of the U.S. population, and about 20% of these patients have other cardiovascular abnormalities, such as PDA or coarctation of the aorta. Transthoracic echocardiography with Doppler flow studies permits assessment of the severity of the aortic stenosis and of left ventricular function.

1. Signs and Symptoms. AS is associated with a systolic murmur that is audible over the aortic area (second right intercostal space) and often radiates into the neck. Most patients are asymptomatic until adulthood. Infants with severe AS may present with CHF. The electrocardiogram (ECG) may show left ventricular hypertrophy. Angina in the absence of coronary artery disease reflects the inability of coronary blood flow to meet increased myocardial oxygen requirements of the hypertrophied left ventricle. Syncope can occur when the pressure gradient across the aortic valve exceeds 50 mm Hg. In patients with supravalvular AS, associated findings can include prominent facial bones, rounded forehead, pursed upper lip, strabismus, inguinal hernias, dental abnormalities, and developmental delay.

2. Treatment of symptomatic congenital AS is valve replacement.

F. Pulmonic Stenosis (PS) producing obstruction to right ventricular outflow is valvular in 90% of patients and supravalvular or subvalvular in the remainder. Supravalvular PS often coexists with other congenital cardiac abnormalities (e.g., ASD, VSD, PDA, tetralogy of Fallot). Valvular PS is typically an isolated abnormality, but it may occur in association with a VSD. Echocardiography and Doppler flow studies can determine the site of the obstruction and the severity of the stenosis. Treatment of pulmonic stenosis is with percutaneous balloon valvuloplasty.

1. Signs and Symptoms. In asymptomatic patients, the presence of pulmonic stenosis is identified by the presence of a loud systolic ejection murmur, best heard at the second left intercostal space. Dyspnea may occur on exertion, and eventually right ventricular failure with peripheral edema and ascites develops.

2. Treatment is percutaneous balloon valvuloplasty.

3. Management of Anesthesia. Management of anesthesia is designed to avoid increases in right ventricular oxygen requirements (tachycardia, increased myocardial contractility). Decreases in systemic blood pressure should be promptly treated with sympathomimetic drugs.

G. Coarctation of the Aorta is usually due to a discrete, diaphragm-like ridge extending into the aortic lumen just distal to the left subclavian artery (postductal coarctation).

1. Signs and Symptoms. Most adults are asymptomatic, and the diagnosis is made when systemic hypertension is detected in the arms in association with diminished or absent femoral arterial pulses. The ECG shows left ventricular hypertrophy. Clinical symptoms include headache, dizziness, epistaxis, and palpitations.

2. Treatment. Surgical resection of the coarctation of the aorta is indicated for patients with a transcoarctation pressure gradient of more than 30 mm Hg. Balloon dilation is a therapeutic alternative.

3. Management of Anesthesia (Table 3-6)

4. Postoperative Management. Immediate postoperative complications include paradoxical hypertension, aortic regurgitation, and paraplegia. Administration of intravenous (IV) nitroprusside with or without esmolol usually controls systemic blood pressure during the early postoperative period. Paraplegia may result from ischemic damage to the spinal cord during the aortic cross-clamping. Abdominal pain may occur, presumably due to sudden increases in blood flow to the gastrointestinal tract.

TABLE 3-6	Anesthetic Considerations for Patients with Coarctation of the Aorta

- Maintain adequate perfusion to the lower body during aortic cross-clamping (mean arterial pressure ≥40 mm Hg); consider partial circulatory bypass if pressure cannot be maintained.
- Continuously monitor systemic pressure above and below the coarctation (right radial and femoral artery catheterization).
- Upper body systemic hypertension during cross-clamping can cause increased work load to the heart and make surgical repair more difficult (consider nitroprusside).
- Consider somatosensory evoked potentials to monitor spinal cord function and adequacy of blood flow to the spinal cord during cross-clamping of the aorta.

II. CYANOTIC CONGENITAL HEART DISEASE

Cyanotic congenital heart disease is characterized by a right-to-left intracardiac shunt (**Table 3-7**) with associated decreases in pulmonary blood flow and the development of arterial hypoxemia.

A. **Tetralogy of Fallot (TOF),** the most common cyanotic congenital heart defect, is characterized by a large single VSD, an aorta that overrides the right and left ventricles, obstruction to right ventricular outflow, and right ventricular hypertrophy. The resistance to flow across the right ventricular outflow tract is relatively fixed; changes in systemic vascular resistance may affect the magnitude of the shunt. Decreases in systemic vascular resistance increase right-to-left shunt and arterial hypoxemia, whereas increases in systemic vascular resistance (e.g., by squatting) decrease left-to-right shunt and increase pulmonary blood flow.

   1. **Diagnosis.** Echocardiography is used to establish the diagnosis and assess the presence of associated abnormalities. Cardiac catheterization further confirms the diagnosis and permits confirmation of anatomic and hemodynamic data.

   2. **Signs and Symptoms (Table 3-8)**

   3. **Treatment** of TOF is complete surgical correction (closure of the VSD with a Dacron patch and relief of right ventricular outflow obstruction by placing a synthetic graft) when patients are extremely young.

   4. **Management of Anesthesia** for patients with TOF aims to avoid events that acutely increase the magnitude of the right-to-left shunt (**Table 3-9**).

TABLE 3-7	Congenital Heart Defects Resulting in a Right-to-Left Intracardiac Shunt

Tetralogy of Fallot

Eisenmenger's syndrome

Ebstein's anomaly (malformation of the tricuspid valve)

Tricuspid atresia

Foramen ovale

TABLE 3-8 Signs and Symptoms of Tetralogy of Fallot

- Cyanosis
- Systolic ejection murmur along the left sternal border
- Squatting (particularly in children; increases systemic vascular resistance)
- Right axis deviation and right ventricular hypertrophy on ECG
- Compensatory erythropoiesis
- Hypercyanotic attacks (sudden episode of arterial hypoxemia, tachypnea, syncope, seizures, often precipitated by crying or exercise; treatment is esmolol and/or phenylephrine)
- Cerebrovascular accident due to cerebrovascular thrombosis or arterial hypoxemia
- Cerebral abscess
- Infective endocarditis

a. Preoperative Preparation. Avoid dehydration by maintaining oral feedings in extremely young patients or by providing IV fluids before the patient's arrival in the operating room. Crying associated with intramuscular administration of drugs used for preoperative medication can lead to hypercyanotic attacks. Continue β-adrenergic antagonists in patients receiving these drugs for prophylaxis against hypercyanotic attacks.
b. Induction of Anesthesia is often with ketamine, which preserves systemic vascular resistance. Induction of anesthesia with a volatile anesthetic such as sevoflurane is acceptable but must be accomplished with caution and careful monitoring of systemic oxygenation.
c. Maintenance of Anesthesia is often achieved with nitrous oxide combined with ketamine. The principal disadvantage of using nitrous oxide is the associated decrease in the inspired oxygen concentration. Ventilation of the patient's lungs should be controlled, but excessive positive airway pressure may increase the resistance to blood flow through the lungs. Intravascular fluid volume must be maintained because acute hypovolemia increases right-to-left intracardiac shunt. Meticulous care must be taken to avoid infusion of air through IV tubing because of the risk of systemic

TABLE 3-9 Events That Increase Right-to-Left Intracardiac Shunting

Decreased systemic vascular resistance	• Volatile anesthetic agents • Histamine release • Ganglionic blockade • β-adrenergic blockade
Increased pulmonary vascular resistance	• Intermittent positive airway pressure • Positive end-expiratory pressure • Negative intrapleural pressure
Increased myocardial contractility (accentuates infundibular obstruction to right ventricular ejection)	• Surgical stimulation • Inotropic agents

air embolization. α-Adrenergic agonist drugs (phenylephrine) are used to treat decreases in systemic vascular resistance.

5. Patient Characteristics after Repair of TOF. Ventricular cardiac dysrhythmias and atrial fibrillation or flutter are common. Right bundle branch block is common, but third-degree atrioventricular heart block is uncommon.

B. Eisenmenger's Syndrome refers to patients in whom a left-to-right intracardiac shunt is reversed when pulmonary vascular resistance increases to a level that equals or exceeds the systemic vascular resistance. It occurs in approximately 50% of patients with an untreated VSD and approximately 10% of patients with an untreated ASD. The murmur associated with these cardiac defects disappears when Eisenmenger's syndrome develops.

1. Signs and Symptoms (Table 3-10)

2. Treatment. Epoprostenol may help decreased pulmonary vascular resistance. Hyperviscosity can be treated with phlebotomy and isovolemic replacement. Pregnancy is discouraged in women with Eisenmenger's syndrome. Lung transplantation with repair of the cardiac defect or combined heart-lung transplantation may be an option. Surgical correction of the underlying heart defect is contraindicated in the presence of irreversible pulmonary hypertension.

3. Management of Anesthesia. Management of anesthesia is based on maintenance of preoperative levels of systemic vascular resistance, recognizing that increases in right-to-left shunt are likely if sudden vasodilation occurs. Continuous IV infusions of norepinephrine may be useful, but β-adrenergic agonists that may decrease systemic vascular resistance should be avoided. Minimizing blood loss and hypovolemia and the prevention of iatrogenic paradoxical embolization are important considerations. If epidural anesthesia is selected, it seems prudent to avoid epinephrine in the local anesthetic solution due to its peripheral β-agonist effects.

C. Ebstein's Anomaly is an abnormality of the tricuspid valve in which the valve leaflets are malformed or displaced downward into the right ventricle.

1. Signs and Symptoms (Table 3-11). The severity of the hemodynamic derangements depends on the degree of displacement and the functional

TABLE 3-10 Signs and Symptoms of Eisenmenger's Syndrome
Arterial hypoxemia
• Cyanosis
• Erythrocytosis
• Increased blood viscosity
Decreased exercise tolerance
Atrial fibrillation
Hemoptysis (pulmonary infarction)
Thrombosis
Cerebrovascular accident
Brain abscess
Syncope
Sudden death

TABLE 3-11	Signs and Symptoms of Ebstein's Anomaly

Cyanosis

Congestive heart failure

Paradoxical embolization

Hepatomegaly (due to passive hepatic congestion secondary to increased right atrial pressure)

Massive enlargement of the right atrium

First-degree atrioventricular block

Paroxysmal arrhythmias, both supraventricular and ventricular

Brain abscess

Sudden death

status of the tricuspid valve leaflets and can vary from CHF in neonates to asymptomatic adults. Echocardiography is used to assess right atrial dilation, distortion of the tricuspid valve leaflets, and the severity of the tricuspid regurgitation or stenosis.

2. Treatment of Ebstein's anomaly is based on preventing associated complications. It includes antibiotic prophylaxis against infective endocarditis, diuretics and digoxin to manage congestive heart failure, pharmacologic treatment of arrhythmias, and catheter ablation if accessory pathways are present. Surgical treatment by systemic-to-pulmonary shunt, Glenn shunt, or Fontan procedures may be considered.

3. Management of Anesthesia. Hazards during anesthesia in patients with Ebstein's anomaly include accentuation of arterial hypoxemia due to increases in the magnitude of the right-to-left intracardiac shunt and the development of supraventricular tachydysrhythmias.

D. Tricuspid Atresia Tricuspid atresia is characterized by arterial hypoxemia, a small right ventricle, a large left ventricle, and marked decreases in pulmonary blood flow.

1. Treatment is anastomosis of the right atrial appendage to the right pulmonary artery to bypass the right ventricle and provide direct atriopulmonary communication (Fontan procedure).

2. Management of Anesthesia for patients undergoing Fontan procedures has been successfully achieved with opioids or volatile anesthetics. Immediately after cardiopulmonary bypass and continuing into the early postoperative period, it is important to maintain increased right atrial pressures (16–20 mm Hg) to facilitate pulmonary blood flow, and avoid increases in pulmonary vascular resistance (acidosis, hypothermia, peak airway pressures higher than 15 cm H_2O, or reactions to the tracheal tube), which may cause right-sided heart failure. Early tracheal extubation and spontaneous ventilation are desirable. Subsequent management of anesthesia in patients who have undergone Fontan procedures is facilitated by monitoring the central venous pressure (which equals the pulmonary artery pressure in these patients) to assess the intravascular fluid volume and to detect sudden impairment of left ventricular function and increased pulmonary vascular resistance.

E. Transposition of the Great Arteries results in complete separation of the pulmonary and systemic circulations. Survival is possible only if there is communication between the two circulations (VSD, ASD, or PDA).

1. Signs and Symptoms. Persistent cyanosis and tachypnea at birth may be the first clues, and congestive heart failure is often present.

2. Treatment. Immediate management involves creating intracardiac mixing such as prostaglandin E to maintain patency of the ductus arteriosus and/or balloon atrial septostomy (Rashkind procedure). Ultimately, correction involves an "arterial switch" operation in which the pulmonary artery and ascending aorta are reanastomosed with the "correct" ventricles, and coronary arteries are reimplanted, so that the aorta is connected to the left ventricle and the pulmonary artery is connected to the right ventricle.

3. Management of Anesthesia is often accomplished with ketamine combined with or without opioids or benzodiazepines for maintenance of anesthesia. The use of nitrous oxide is limited, as it is important to administer high inspired oxygen concentrations. Dehydration must be avoided during the perioperative period because these patients may have hematocrits in excess of 70%, predisposing them to cerebral venous thrombosis.

F. Mixing of Blood between the Pulmonary and Systemic Circulations. Rare congenital heart defects that result in mixing of blood from the pulmonary and systemic circulations manifest as cyanosis and arterial hypoxemia of varying severity depending on the magnitude of the pulmonary blood flow (**Table 3-12**).

TABLE 3-12	Congenital Heart Defects Resulting in Mixing of Blood from the Pulmonary and Systemic Circulations
Defect	**Considerations**
Truncus arteriosus (single arterial trunk is the origin of both the aorta and pulmonary artery)	• Presents as cyanosis, arterial hypoxemia, failure to thrive, and CHF. • Surgical treatment consists of banding of the right and left pulmonary arteries to decrease pulmonary blood flow. • Positive end-expiratory pressure (PEEP) may decrease pulmonary blood flow and decrease symptoms of CHF.
Partial anomalous pulmonary venous return (pulmonary vein empties into the right atrium instead of the left)	• Presents as fatigue, exertional dyspnea, CHF. • Angiography is useful for diagnosis.
Total anomalous pulmonary venous return (all four veins drain into the systemic venous circulation)	• Presents as CHF. • PEEP may decrease pulmonary blood flow. • IV infusions can increase right atrial pressure and cause pulmonary edema. • Surgical manipulation of the right atrium can cause obstruction.

TABLE 3-12	Congenital Heart Defects Resulting in Mixing of Blood from the Pulmonary and Systemic Circulations—cont'd
Defect	**Considerations**
Hypoplastic left-sided heart syndrome	• Treatment is initial reconstruction of the ascending aorta using the proximal pulmonary artery, followed by a Fontan procedure. • Coronary blood flow is compromised, and ventricular fibrillation is a high risk. • Anesthetic management is with high-dose opioids and muscle relaxation. • High PaO_2 implies excessive pulmonary blood flow at the expense of systemic blood flow—treatments are maneuvers to increase pulmonary vascular resistance.

III. MECHANICAL OBSTRUCTION OF THE TRACHEA

The trachea can be obstructed by circulatory anomalies that produce a vascular ring or by dilation of the pulmonary artery secondary to absence of the pulmonic valve and can present as stridor or other upper airway obstruction (**Table 3-13**).

TABLE 3-13	Mechanical Obstruction of the Trachea
Defect	**Considerations**
Double aortic arch	• Vascular ring presses on the trachea and esophagus. • Presents as inspiratory stridor, difficulty managing secretions, and dysphagia. • Treatment is surgical resection. • Endotracheal tube should be inserted beyond the level of tracheal compression if possible. • Gastric tube can cause occlusion of the trachea if the endotracheal tube is above the level of compression.
Aberrant left pulmonary artery	• Presents as expiratory stridor or wheezing. • Esophageal obstruction is rare. • Surgical division of the aberrant pulmonary artery is the treatment of choice.
Absent pulmonary valve	• Results in dilation of the pulmonary artery, which can compress the trachea and left main-stem bronchus. • Tracheal intubation and continuous airway pressure of 4–6 mm Hg can keep the trachea distended. • Treatment is surgical insertion of a tubular graft with artificial pulmonic valve.

CHAPTER 4

Abnormalities of Cardiac Conduction and Cardiac Rhythm

The clinical significance of cardiac dysrhythmias for the anesthesiologist depends on the effect they have on vital signs and the potential for deterioration into a life-threatening rhythm. The electrical impulse in the heart moves along the cardiac conduction system, propagating a wave of depolarization and causing progressive contraction of cardiac muscle cells. The depolarization and repolarization events correspond to electrical waves recorded on an electrocardiogram (ECG) (**Fig. 4-1**).

I. MECHANISMS OF TACHYDYSRHYTHMIAS

A. Reentry Pathways Dysrhythmias. Reentry pathways account for most premature beats and tachydysrhythmias. Reentry requires two pathways over which electrical impulses can be conducted at different velocities. Pharmacologic or physiologic events (hypoxemia, electrolyte disturbance, acid-base changes, autonomic nervous system changes, myocardial ischemia, drugs) may alter the balance between conduction velocities and refractory periods of the dual pathways, resulting in the initiation or termination of reentrant dysrhythmias.

B. Automaticity is affected by the slope of phase 4 depolarization and or the resting membrane potential. Sympathetic stimulation increases heart rate by increasing the slope of phase 4 depolarization and decreasing the resting membrane potential. Parasympathetic stimulation decreases heart rate by decreasing the slope of phase 4 depolarization and increasing the resting membrane potential.

C. Afterdepolarizations are oscillations in membrane potential that occur during or after repolarization. Under special circumstances these afterdepolarizations can trigger a complete depolarization that can be self-sustaining and result in a triggered dysrhythmia.

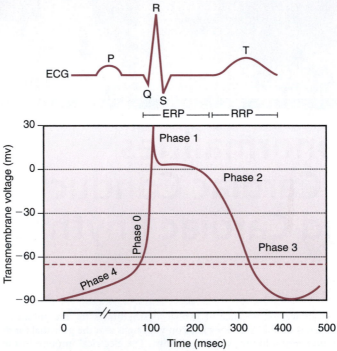

Figure 4-1 · Transmembrane action potential generated by an automatic cardiac cell and the relationship of this action potential to events depicted on the electrocardiogram.

II. SUPRAVENTRICULAR TACHYDYSRHYTHMIAS

A. Sinus Dysrhythmia is a normal variant in sinus rhythm caused by changes in intrathoracic pressure during inspiration and expiration (Bainbridge reflex).
B. Sinus Tachycardia (Table 4-1) is characterized by a gradual change of heart rate to 100 to 160 bpm. The ECG shows a normal P wave before each QRS complex and normal PR unless a coexisting conduction block is present. Treatment is correction of the underlying cause (e.g., hypovolemia, pain, anxiety, hypoxemia, hypotension, fever, heart failure). Administration of a β-blocker may lower the heart rate and decrease myocardial oxygen demand. Prognosis is related to the physiologic or pathologic process causing the acceleration of sinus node activity.
C. Premature Atrial Beats (PACs) are common in patients with and without heart disease. Noncardiac precipitating factors include caffeine, emotional stress, alcohol, nicotine, recreational drugs, and hyperthyroidism. PACs, unlike ventricular premature beats (VPBs), are not followed by a compensatory pause on the ECG. PACs do not require acute therapy unless they are associated with initiation of a tachydysrhythmia, when treatment is directed at controlling or converting the secondary dysrhythmia.

TABLE 4-1	Perioperative Causes of Sinus Tachycardia

I. Physiologic Increase in Sympathetic Tone
  Pain
  Anxiety/fear
  Light anesthesia
  Hypovolemia/anemia
  Arterial hypoxemia
  Hypotension
  Hypoglycemia
  Fever/infection
II. Pathologic Increase in Sympathetic Tone
  Myocardial ischemia/infarction
  Congestive heart failure
  Pulmonary embolus
  Hyperthyroidism
  Pericarditis
  Pericardial tamponade
  Malignant hyperthermia
  Ethanol withdrawal
III. Drug-Induced Increase in Heart Rate
  Atropine/glycopyrrolate
  Sympathomimetic drugs
  Caffeine
  Nicotine
  Cocaine/amphetamines

D. Supraventricular Tachycardia (SVT) is any tachydysrhythmia (average heart rate of 160–180 bpm) initiated and sustained by tissue at or above the atrioventricular (AV) node. AV nodal reentrant tachycardia (AVNRT) is the most common type of SVT and accounts for 50% of diagnosed SVTs. AVNRT is most commonly due to a reentry circuit in which there is anterograde conduction over the slower AV nodal pathway and retrograde conduction over a faster accessory pathway. Atrial fibrillation and atrial flutter are SVTs, but their electrophysiology and treatment are distinctly different from other forms of SVT and they are discussed separately.

    1. Treatment is often initially a vagal maneuver such as carotid sinus massage or a Valsalva maneuver. If this is not effective, pharmacologic treatment directed at blocking AV nodal conduction is indicated. Adenosine, calcium channel blockers, and β-blockers may be used to terminate SVT. Intravenous digoxin is not clinically useful in acute control of SVT because of a delayed peak effect and narrow therapeutic index. Electrical cardioversion is indicated for SVT unresponsive to drug therapy or SVT associated with hemodynamic instability. Radiofrequency catheter ablation may be used to treat recurrent AVNRT.

2. Anesthetic Management of patients with a history of SVT focuses on avoiding precipitating events, such as increased sympathetic tone, electrolyte imbalances, and acid-base disturbances.

E. Multifocal Atrial Tachycardia is an irregular rhythm in which the ECG shows three or more P wave morphologies with variable PR intervals. Treatment consists of treating the underlying abnormality (exacerbation of pulmonary disease, methylxanthine toxicity, congestive heart failure [CHF], sepsis, electrolyte abnormalities). Pharmacologic treatment has limited success and is considered secondary, and cardioversion is generally ineffective. Anesthetic management consists of avoidance of medications or procedures that worsen the pulmonary status and treatment of hypoxemia.

F. Atrial Flutter is an organized atrial rhythm with an atrial rate of 250 to 350 bpm and varying degrees of AV block. Flutter waves are usually seen on the ECG, with an associated ventricular rate of 120 to 160 bpm. If atrial flutter is hemodynamically significant, the treatment of choice is cardioversion. Patients with atrial flutter lasting longer than 48 hours should be anticoagulated and evaluated by transesophageal echocardiography for the presence of atrial thrombus prior to any attempt at cardioversion. Pharmacologic control of the ventricular response with intravenous amiodarone, diltiazem, or verapamil may be attempted if vital signs are stable. Elective anesthesia should be postponed until control of the rhythm has been achieved.

G. Atrial Fibrillation is the most common sustained cardiac dysrhythmia in the U.S. population (0.4% incidence). Postoperative atrial fibrillation is common in elderly patients undergoing cardiothoracic surgery. Predisposing factors for atrial fibrillation include rheumatic heart disease (especially mitral valve disease), hypertension, thyrotoxicosis, ischemic heart disease, chronic obstructive pulmonary disease, acute alcohol intoxication, pericarditis, pulmonary embolus, and atrial septal defect. The most important clinical consequence of atrial fibrillation is a thromboembolic event causing a stroke due to the presence of atrial thrombi.

1. Sign and Symptoms may include palpitations, angina pectoris, CHF, pulmonary edema, hypotension, fatigue, and generalized weakness.

2. Diagnosis. The ECG shows chaotic atrial activity and no discernible P waves. Ventricular rate is about 180 bpm in patients with normal AV nodes.

3. Treatment goals are control of ventricular rate and conversion to sinus rhythm. Cardioversion is indicated when hemodynamic compromise is present. The preferred drug for conversion of patients with significant heart disease is amiodarone. Other choices are propafenone, ibutilide, and sotalol. Control of the ventricular response in patients with atrial fibrillation is typically achieved with drugs that slow AV nodal conduction, such as β-blockers, calcium channel blockers, and digoxin.

4. Anticoagulation. Individuals with atrial fibrillation are at increased risk of stroke and are usually treated with anticoagulants. IV heparin is the most commonly used anticoagulant for acute treatment. For chronic anticoagulation, warfarin is most often used, but aspirin therapy may be sufficient for individuals considered to be at low risk of thromboembolic complications.

5. Anesthetic Management. If new-onset atrial fibrillation occurs prior to induction of anesthesia, surgery should be postponed if possible until control of the dysrhythmia has been achieved. Hemodynamically significant atrial fibrillation should be treated with cardioversion. Pharmacologic control may be attempted if vital signs allow. Patients with chronic atrial fibrillation should be maintained on their antidysrhythmic drugs perioperatively with close attention paid to serum magnesium and potassium levels, particularly if the patient is on digoxin.

III. VENTRICULAR RHYTHMS

A. Ventricular Ectopy (or ventricular premature beats) arises from single (unifocal) or multiple (multifocal) foci located below the AV node. Characteristic ECG findings include a premature and wide QRS complex, no preceding P wave, ST segment and T-wave deflection opposite to the QRS deflection, and a compensatory pause before the next sinus beat. A "vulnerable" period occurs in the middle third of the T wave, during which a VPB may initiate repetitive beats, including ventricular tachycardia or ventricular fibrillation. This is known as the R-on-T phenomenon. Symptoms of VPBs include palpitations, near syncope, and syncope.

    1. Treatment. VPBs should be treated when they are frequent, polymorphic, occurring in runs of three or more, or taking place during the vulnerable period because these characteristics are associated with an increased incidence of ventricular tachycardia and ventricular fibrillation. The first step is to eliminate or correct the underlying cause (**Table 4-2**). Amiodarone, lidocaine, and other antidysrhythmics are not indicated unless VPBs progress to ventricular tachycardia or are frequent enough to cause hemodynamic instability. Drug therapy is not at all effective in suppression of ventricular dysrhythmias caused by mechanical irritation of the heart.

    2. Prognosis. Benign VPBs occur at rest and disappear with exercise. An increased frequency of VPBs with exercise may be an indication of

TABLE 4-2   Factors Associated with Ventricular Premature Beats
Normal heart
Arterial hypoxemia
Myocardial ischemia
Myocardial infarction
Myocarditis
Sympathetic nervous system activation
Hypokalemia
Hypomagnesemia
Digitalis toxicity
Caffeine
Cocaine
Alcohol
Mechanical irritation (central venous or pulmonary artery catheter)

underlying heart disease. In the absence of structural heart disease, asymptomatic ventricular ectopy is associated with increased risk of sudden death. The most common pathologic conditions associated with VPBs are myocardial ischemia, valvular heart disease, cardiomyopathy, QT interval prolongation, and the presence of electrolyte abnormalities, especially hypokalemia and hypomagnesemia.

3. Anesthetic Management. When receiving anesthetic, if a patient exhibits six or more VPBs per minute and repetitive or multifocal forms of ventricular ectopy, there is an increased risk of developing a life-threatening dysrhythmia. Treatment should be directed at correcting underlying causes, including repositioning of intracardiac catheters. β-Blockers may be helpful. Amiodarone, lidocaine, and other dysrhythmics are indicated only if the VPBs progress to ventricular tachycardia or are frequent enough to cause hemodynamic instability.

B. Ventricular Tachycardia (VT) is present when three or more consecutive VPBs occur at a calculated heart rate of greater than 120 bpm (usually 150–200 bpm). The rhythm is regular with wide QRS complexes and no discernible P waves. Palpitations, presyncope, and syncope are the three most common symptoms. VT is common after an acute myocardial infarction and in the presence of inflammatory or infectious diseases of the heart. Digitalis toxicity may manifest as VT. Torsade de pointes (TdP) is a distinct form of VT initiated by a VPB in the setting of a prolonged QT interval.

1. Treatment. Symptomatic or unstable VT should be cardioverted immediately. If vital signs are stable and the VT is persistent or recurrent after cardioversion, amiodarone is recommended. Alternative drugs include procainamide, sotalol, and lidocaine. Catheter ablation or implantation of a cardioverter/defibrillator are options for drug-refractory VT.

C. Ventricular Fibrillation (VF) is a rapid, grossly irregular ventricular rhythm with marked variability in QRS cycle length, morphology, and amplitude. A pulse or blood pressure *never* accompanies VF.

1. Treatment is electrical defibrillation as soon as possible. The best chance for survival is when defibrillation occurs within 3 to 5 minutes of cardiac arrest. For refractory VF, administration of epinephrine or vasopressin may improve response to electrical defibrillation. After three defibrillation attempts, amiodarone, lidocaine, or, in the case of TdP, magnesium is indicated. Contributing factors should be sought and treated (hypoxia, hypovolemia, acidosis, hypokalemia, hyperkalemia, hypoglycemia, hypothermia, drug or environmental toxins, cardiac tamponade, tension pneumothorax, coronary ischemia, pulmonary embolus, and hemorrhage). Long-term treatment for recurrent VF is placement of a permanent automatic implantable cardioverter/defibrillator (ICD).

2. Anesthetic Management. Cardiopulmonary resuscitation (CPR) must be initiated immediately, followed as soon as possible with defibrillation. Underlying causes should be sought and corrected.

IV. VENTRICULAR PRE-EXCITATION SYNDROMES

Congenital alternate (accessory) pathways can conduct electrical impulses in the heart, with the potential for reentrant tachycardias.

A. Wolff-Parkinson-White (WPW) Syndrome

1. Signs and Symptoms (Table 4-3)

2. Treatment (Table 4-4). Although antidysrhythmics can provide therapeutic management of the dysrhythmias associated with WPW syndrome, catheter ablation is considered the best treatment for symptomatic WPW syndrome.

3. Anesthetic Management. Patients with known WPW syndrome should continue to receive their antidysrhythmic drugs. The goal of management is to avoid any event (e.g., increased sympathetic nervous system activity due to pain, anxiety, or hypovolemia) or drug (digoxin, verapamil) that could enhance anterograde conduction of cardiac impulses through an accessory pathway. Equipment for electrical cardioversion must be available.

V. PROLONGED QT SYNDROME (LQTS)

Prolonged QT syndrome can be congenital or acquired. Several genetically determined syndromes usually present as syncope in late childhood. Episodes may be precipitated by stress, exercise, or other events that stimulate the sympathetic nervous system. Acquired LQTS may be caused by many prescription medications, such as antibiotics, antidysrhythmics, antidepressants, and antiemetics.

TABLE 4-3	Manifestations of Wolff-Parkinson-White Syndrome

- Symptomatic tachyarrhythmia is typically first seen in early adulthood.
- It may first be seen perioperatively.
- Symptoms may include palpitations with or without dizziness, syncope, dyspnea, or angina.
- Sudden death may be the first sign (presumable due to VF).
- ECG findings include delta wave and AV tachycardia that is most commonly orthodromic (narrow QRS) but may be antidromic (wide QRS).
- Atrial fibrillation and/or atrial flutter may be present, which can result in very rapid ventricular response rates and/or VF.

TABLE 4-4	Treatment of Wolff-Parkinson-White Syndrome

Orthodromic (narrow QRS) tachycardia	• Vagal maneuvers • Adenosine • Verapamil • β−Blockers • Amiodarone
Antidromic (wide QRS) tachycardia	• Procainamide if systolic BP >90 mm Hg • Cardioversion if systolic BP <90 mm Hg
Atrial fibrillation	• Procainamide • Cardioversion if hemodynamically unstable

A. Diagnosis. LQTS is associated with prolongation of the QTc (>460–480 ms). During a syncopal episode, the most common finding on the ECG is polymorphic ventricular tachycardia, or torsade de pointes.

B. Treatment of LQTS includes correction of electrolyte abnormalities and discontinuance of drugs associated with QT. Additional treatment options include β-blocker therapy, cardiac pacing, and AICD implantation.

C. Anesthetic Management (Table 4-5)

VI. MECHANISMS OF BRADYDYSRHYTHMIAS

Bradydysrhythmias (heart rate <60 bpm) are most commonly caused by sinoatrial (SA) node dysfunction or a conduction block.

A. Sinus Bradycardia

1. Diagnosis. Sinus bradycardia occurs at a heart rate of less than 60 bpm. The ECG shows a regular rhythm with a normal-appearing P wave before each QRS complex.

2. Treatment. Atropine, epinephrine, or dopamine may be used to treat severely symptomatic patients, but cardiac pacing is the long-term treatment of choice.

3. Anesthetic Management. Sinus bradycardia in asymptomatic patients requires no treatment. If severely symptomatic, immediate transcutaneous or transvenous pacing is indicated, with or without pharmacologic support.

4. Bradycardia Associated with Spinal and Epidural Anesthesia. Bradycardia or asystole may develop suddenly (within seconds or minutes) in a patient with a previously normal or even increased heart rate, or the heart rate slowing may be progressive. It most often occurs approximately an hour after the anesthetic is initiated, during normal arterial oxygen saturation. Approximately half of patients complain of shortness of breath, nausea, restlessness, light-headedness, or tingling fingers and manifest a

TABLE 4-5	Anesthesia Management in Patients with Prolonged QT Syndrome

- Perform preoperative ECG to exclude LQTS in a patient with a family history of sudden death.
- Consider preoperative β−blockade or left stellate ganglion block.
- Consider the effects of volatile agents on the QT interval (isoflurane and sevoflurane prolong QT).
- Avoid events that lead to sympathetic activation and prolongation of the QT interval.
- Treat hypokalemia and hypomagnesemia.
- Administer esmolol to treat acute arrhythmias.
- A defibrillator should be immediately available.
- Consider treating with phenytoin in the postoperative period.

deterioration in mental status prior to arrest. The risk of bradycardia and asystole may persist into the postoperative period. Proposed mechanisms include reflex-induced bradycardia resulting from decreased venous return and activation of vagal reflex arcs. Another possibility is unopposed parasympathetic nervous system activity resulting from the anesthetic-induced sympathectomy. Bradydysrhythmias associated with spinal or epidural anesthesia should be treated aggressively.

5. Bradycardia Associated with Sinus Node. Dysfunction of the SA node, also referred to as sick sinus syndrome, is a common cause of bradycardia and accounts for more than 50% of the indications for placement of a permanent cardiac pacemaker.

B. Junctional Rhythm. Junctional (nodal) rhythm is due to activity of a cardiac pacemaker in the tissues surrounding the AV node. Junctional pacemakers usually have an intrinsic rate of 40 to 60 bpm. The ECG shows a P wave preceding the QRS with shortened PR interval or no P wave. Atropine can be used to treat hemodynamically significant junctional rhythms.

VII. CONDUCTION DISTURBANCES

Abnormalities of the conduction system can lead to heart block (**Table 4-6**).

TABLE 4-6 Conduction Disturbances of the Heart	
Conduction Disturbance	**Characteristics**
First-Degree AV block	• PR interval >0.2 sec • Usually asymptomatic • Atropine is usually effective treatment
Second-Degree AV block: Mobitz I (Wenckebach)	• Progressive prolongation of the PR interval until a beat is dropped • Usually transient and asymptomatic
Second-Degree AV Block: Mobitz II	• Complete interruption of cardiac conduction with dropped beats • Usually symptomatic with palpitations and near syncope • Higher risk to progress to third-degree heart block than Mobitz I • Treatment is cardiac pacing (atropine usually not effective)
Right Bundle Branch Block (RBBB)	• QRS ≥0.12 sec and rSR in V_1 and V_2 • Usually benign
Left Bundle Branch Block (LBBB)	• QRS >0.12 sec and absence of Q waves in leads 1 and V_6 • Often associated with ischemic heart disease
Third-Degree Heart Block (Complete Heart Block)	• If block is nodal, heart rate 45–55 bpm • If block is infranodal, heart rate 30–40 bpm • Treatment is pacing—IV isoproterenol may temporize

VIII. TREATMENT OF CARDIAC DYSRHYTHMIAS

A. Antidysrhythmic Drugs (Table 4-7)
B. Electrical Cardioversion
1. **Synchronized Cardioversion** entails delivery of an electrical discharge synchronized to the R wave of the ECG so that the current is delivered during the QRS complex. It is used to treat acute unstable supraventricular

TABLE 4-7	Cardiac Antidysrhythmia Drugs
Indication	**Side Effects**
Adenosine: supraventricular tachyarrhythmias, atrial fibrillation, atrial flutter	Peripheral vasodilation, flushing Dyspnea Bronchospasm Angina Denervation hypersensitivity in heart transplant patients
Amiodarone: supraventricular tachyarrhythmias, VT, prevention of recurrent atrial fibrillation, improved response to defibrillation	Prolonged elimination half-life Bradycardia Hypotension Pulmonary fibrosis Postoperative ventilatory failure Skeletal muscle weakness Peripheral neuropathy Hepatitis Cyanotic facial discoloration Corneal deposits Thyroid dysfunction
β–Adrenergic blockers: ventricular rate control in atrial fibrillation, atrial flutter, and narrow-complex tachycardias. **Sotalol:** ventricular tachycardia, atrial fibrillation or flutter in WPW syndrome	Bradycardia AV conduction delay Hypotension Bronchospasm Lethargy Myocardial depression
Calcium channel blockers: SVT, atrial fibrillation, atrial flutter. *Contraindicated* in WPW syndrome	Second- or third-degree heart block Myocardial depression Peripheral vasodilation Bradycardia
Digoxin: atrial tachyarrhythmias, atrial fibrillation, atrial flutter	Toxicity, especially in renal failure and/or hypokalemia Possible enhanced conduction through accessory pathways
Lidocaine: VPBs, ventricular tachyarrhythmias, recurrent ventricular fibrillation	Accumulation and toxicity with decreased hepatic blood flow Central nervous system toxicity Direct myocardial depressant Peripheral vasodilation
Magnesium: may be useful for torsade de pointes	Muscle relaxation

TABLE 4-7	Cardiac Antidysrhythmia Drugs—cont'd	
Indication		**Side Effects**
Procainamide: ventricular tachycardia with pulse, atrial flutter or fibrillation, atrial fibrillation in WPW syndrome, SVT resistant to vagal maneuvers or adenosine		Prolongs QT Hypotension Lupuslike syndrome Myocardial depression Potentiation of neuromuscular blockade Accumulation in patients with renal failure
Epinephrine: to improve circulation during cardiopulmonary resuscitation, cardiac arrest due to β-blocker or calcium channel blocker overdose		Hypertension Tachycardia
Vasopressin: to support circulation during cardiopulmonary resuscitation		Vasoconstriction
Atropine: asystole, pulseless electrical activity, bradycardia		Tachycardia
Isoproterenol: symptomatic bradycardia, complete heart block, cardiac transplantation patients		Bronchodilator Tachycardia Peripheral vasodilation
Dopamine: symptomatic bradycardia unresponsive to atropine		Tachycardia Hypertension Peripheral vasoconstriction

tachycardias (such as SVT, atrial flutter, and atrial fibrillation) and to convert chronic stable rate-controlled atrial flutter or atrial fibrillation to sinus rhythm. Propofol and short-acting benzodiazepines are commonly used for sedation.

C. Defibrillation is the delivery of an electrical discharge that is not synchronized, because it is usually used to treat ventricular fibrillation, where there is no R wave. Modern defibrillators are classified as either monophasic or biphasic.

D. Radiofrequency Catheter Ablation. Cardiac dysrhythmias amenable to radiofrequency catheter ablation include reentrant supraventricular dysrhythmias and some ventricular dysrhythmias. The procedure is usually performed under conscious sedation.

E. Artificial Cardiac Pacemakers

    1. Transcutaneous Cardiac Pacing. Patients with symptomatic bradycardia or severe conduction block require immediate pacing. Transcutaneous pacing should be considered a temporizing measure until transvenous cardiac pacing can be instituted.

    2. Permanently Implanted Cardiac Pacemakers. Cardiac pacing is the only long-term treatment for symptomatic bradycardia regardless of cause. An artificial cardiac pacemaker can be inserted intravenously (endocardial lead) or via a subcostal approach (epicardial or myocardial lead).

    3. Pacing Modes. A five-letter generic code is used to describe the various characteristics of cardiac pacemakers. (1) the cardiac chamber(s) being paced (*A*, atrial; *V*, ventricular; *D*, dual chamber); (2) the cardiac chamber(s) that detects (senses) electrical signals (*A*, atrial; *V*, ventricular; *D*, dual); (3) the response to sensed signals (*I*, inhibition; *T*, triggering; *D*, dual: inhibition and triggering); (4) *R*, denotes activation of rate response features, and (5) for multisite pacing, the chamber(s) in which multisite pacing is delivered. The most common pacing modes are AAI, VVI, and DDD (**Table 4-8**).

a. DDD Pacing. The pacemaker responds to increases in sinus node discharge rate, such as during exercise. DDD pacing minimizes the incidence of pacemaker syndrome (syncope, weakness, orthopnea, paroxysmal nocturnal dyspnea, hypotension, pulmonary edema) that is a result of the loss of AV synchrony and the subsequent decrease in cardiac output.

b. DDI Pacing. Sensing occurs in both the atrium and ventricle, but the only response to a sensed event is inhibition. DDI pacing is useful in the presence of atrial tachydysrhythmias.

c. Rate-Adaptive Pacemakers are used in patients who lack an appropriate heart rate response to exercise.

TABLE 4-8 Types of Pacing Pulse Generators: *A* (Atrium), *V* (Ventricle), *O* (None-Asynchronous), *I* (Inhibited), *T* (Triggering), *R* (Rate-Adaptive)

Letter Code	Description
Single-Chamber Pacing Modes	
AOO	Asynchronous (fixed) atrial pacing
VOO	Asynchronous ventricular pacing
AAI	"Demand" atrial pacing: pacemaker senses and is inhibited by intrinsic atrial depolarization (P wave)
VVI	"Demand" ventricular pacing: pacemaker senses and is inhibited by intrinsic ventricular depolarization (R wave)
AAT	Triggered atrial pacing; pacer is triggered by intrinsic atrial depolarization (P wave)
VVT	Triggered ventricular pacing; pacer is triggered by intrinsic ventricular depolarization (R wave)
Dual-Chamber Pacing Modes	
DDD	Paces and senses in atrium and ventricle
DDI	Senses in both the atrium and ventricle and is inhibited
Rate-Adaptive Pacing Modes	
AAIR	Single chamber
VVIR	Single chamber
DDIR	Dual chamber
DDDR	Dual chamber

4. Choice of Pacing Mode depends on the primary indication for the artificial pacemaker. (Sinus node disease requires an atrial pacemaker; AV node disease calls for a dual-chamber pacemaker; the need for a rate response to exercise requires a rate-adaptive pacemaker.)

5. Complications of Permanent Cardiac Pacing. Early complications related to insertion (e.g., pneumothorax, hemothorax, air embolism) occur in about 5% of patients, and late complications in 2% to 7%. Early pacemaker failure is usually due to electrode displacement or breakage. Pacemaker failure that occurs more than 6 months after implantation is usually due to premature battery depletion.

F. Implanted Cardioverter-Defibrillator Therapy. ICDs were approved for use by the U.S. Food and Drug Administration in 1985 for patients at risk of ventricular fibrillation (VF). The ICD senses VF, the capacitor charges, and, prior to shock delivery, a confirmatory algorithm is fulfilled by signal analysis. This process prevents inappropriate shocks for self-terminating events or spurious signals. Approximately half of patients with ICDs will have an adverse event related to the device within the first year after implantation, such as failure to sense or pace, inappropriate therapy, and dislodgment.

G. Surgery in Patients with Cardiac Devices

1. Preoperative Evaluation includes determining the reason for the device and assessment of its current function. A preoperative history of vertigo, presyncope, or syncope in a patient with a pacemaker or a decrease in heart rate from the initial heart rate setting could reflect pacemaker dysfunction. The ECG is not a diagnostic aid if the intrinsic heart rate is greater than the preset pacemaker rate. In such cases, proper function of a ventricular synchronous or sequential artificial cardiac pacemaker is best confirmed by electronic evaluation. ICDs are often switched off preoperatively and reinstituted postoperatively.

2. Management of Anesthesia in patients with artificial cardiac pacemakers includes (1) monitoring the ECG to confirm proper functioning of the pulse generator and (2) ensuring the availability of equipment (external defibrillator/pacer, external converter magnet) and drugs (atropine, isoproterenol) to maintain an acceptable intrinsic heart rate should the artificial cardiac pacemaker unexpectedly fail. Pulmonary artery catheters may become entangled in, or dislodge, a recently placed transvenous (endocardial) electrode but are unlikely to dislodge electrodes more than 4 weeks after implantation. Improved shielding of cardiac pacemakers has reduced the problems associated with electromagnetic interference from electrocautery, which can either cause a device to revert to asynchronous functioning or be completely inhibited. The grounding pad for electrocautery should be as far as possible from the pulse generator; the electrocautery current should be kept as low as possible and applied in short bursts. The presence of a temporary transvenous cardiac pacemaker presents a special risk of ventricular fibrillation due to microshock currents conducted by the pacing electrodes.

3. Anesthesia for Cardiac Pacemaker Insertion. Most pacemakers are inserted using conscious sedation and routine monitoring. Drugs such as atropine or isoproterenol should be available in the event that a decrease in heart rate compromises hemodynamics before the new pacemaker is functional.

CHAPTER 5

Systemic and Pulmonary Arterial Hypertension

I. SYSTEMIC HYPERTENSION

Systemic hypertension (blood pressure [BP] ≥140/90) affects approximately 25% of adults in the United States. Hypertension (HTN) is defined in adults as a systemic blood pressure of 140/90 mm Hg or more on at least two occasions measured at least 1 to 2 weeks apart (**Table 5-1**). HTN is a significant risk factor for the development of ischemic heart disease and a major cause of congestive heart failure (CHF), stroke, arterial aneurysm, and end-stage renal disease.

   A. Pathophysiology. Systemic HTN is termed *essential* or *primary* when a cause cannot be identified and as *secondary* when an identifiable cause is present.

   1. Essential HTN accounts for more than 95% of all cases of HTN and is characterized by a familial incidence and inherited biochemical abnormalities (**Table 5-2**).

   2. Secondary HTN accounts for less than 5% of all cases of systemic HTN and is most commonly due to renal artery stenosis (**Table 5-3**).

B. Treatment of Essential HTN. The standard goal of therapy is to decrease systemic blood pressure to lower than 140/90 mm Hg, or, in the presence of diabetes mellitus or renal disease, to lower than 130/80 mm Hg. Treatment resulting in normalization of blood lowers the incidence of cerebrovascular accidents, risks of progression to CHF, and renal failure.

   1. Lifestyle Modification. Lifestyle modifications of proven value for lowering blood pressure include weight reduction, moderation of alcohol intake, smoking cessation, increased physical activity, maintenance of recommended levels of dietary calcium and potassium, and moderation in dietary salt intake.

TABLE 5-1	Classification of Systemic Hypertension	
Category	Systolic Blood Pressure (mm Hg)	Diastolic Blood Pressure (mm Hg)
Normal	<120	<80
Prehypertension	120–139	80–89
Stage 1 hypertension	140–159	90–99
Stage 2 hypertension	≥160	≥100

Reprinted with permission from Chobanian AV, Bakris G, Black H, et al: Seventh Report of the Joint National Committee on Prevention, Detection, Evaluation and Treatment of High Blood Pressure. Hypertension 2003;42:1206–1252.

2. Pharmacologic Therapy. Thiazide diuretics are recommended as initial therapy for uncomplicated HTN. The hypertensive patient may have co-morbid conditions that provide indications for antihypertensive therapy with drugs of a particular class (**Table 5-4**).

C. Treatment of Secondary HTN. Treatment of secondary HTN is usually surgical, and pharmacologic therapy is reserved for patients in whom surgery is not possible.

D. Hypertensive Crises. A hypertensive crisis typically presents with a blood pressure higher than 180/120 and is categorized as either a hypertensive urgency or emergency, based on the presence or absence of impending or progressive target organ damage.

    1. Hypertensive Emergency. Patients with evidence of acute or ongoing target organ damage (encephalopathy, intracerebral hemorrhage,

TABLE 5-2	Conditions Associated with Essential Hypertension

- Increased sympathetic nervous system activity
- Sodium and water retention
- Hypercholesterolemia
- Insulin resistance
- Obesity
- Alcohol and tobacco use
- Obstructive sleep apnea
- Glucose intolerance
- Ischemic heart disease and angina pectoris
- Left ventricular hypertrophy
- Congestive heart failure
- Cerebrovascular disease
- Peripheral vascular disease
- Renal insufficiency

TABLE 5-3 Common Causes of Secondary Hypertension

Causes	Clinical Findings	Laboratory Evaluation
Renovascular disease	Epigastric or abdominal bruit Severe hypertension in young patient	MRI angiography Aortography Duplex ultrasonography CT angiography
Hyperaldosteronism	Fatigue Weakness Headache Paresthesia Nocturnal polyuria and polydipsia	Urinary potassium Serum potassium Plasma renin Plasma aldosterone
Aortic coarctation	Elevated blood pressure in upper limbs relative to lower limbs Weak femoral pulses Systolic bruit	Aortography Echocardiography MRI or CT
Pheochromocytoma	Episodic headache, palpitations, and diaphoresis Paroxysmal hypertension	Plasma metanephrines Urinary catecholamines Spot urine metanephrines Adrenal CT/MRI scan
Cushing's syndrome	Truncal obesity Proximal muscle weakness Purple striae "Moon facies" Hirsutism	Dexamethasone suppression test Urinary cortisol Adrenal CT scan Glucose tolerance test
Renal parenchymal disease	Nocturia Edema	Urinary glucose, protein and casts Serum creatinine Renal ultrasonography Renal biopsy
Pregnancy-induced hypertension	Peripheral and pulmonary edema Headache Seizures Right upper quadrant pain	Urinary protein Uric acid Cardiac output Platelet count

CT, computed tomography; MRI, magnetic resonance imaging.

acute left ventricular failure, pulmonary edema, unstable angina, dissecting aortic aneurysm, acute myocardial infarction, eclampsia, microangiopathic hemolytic anemia, renal insufficiency) require prompt treatment. The treatment goal is to decrease the diastolic blood pressure by about 20% within the first 60 minutes, and then more gradually.

2. Hypertensive Urgency occurs when BP is severely elevated, without evidence of target organ damage. Patients can present with headache, epistaxis, or anxiety. Some benefit from oral antihypertensive therapy

TABLE 5-4	Common Antihypertensive Drugs		
Class	**Subclass**	**Generic Name**	**Trade Name**
Diuretics	Thiazides	Chlorothiazide	Diuril
		Hydrochlorothiazide	Hydrodiuril,
		Indapamide	Microzide
		Metolazone	Lozol
			Zaroxolyn,
			Mykrox
	Loop	Bumetanide	Bumex
		Furosemide	Lasix
		Torsemide	Demadex
	Potassium-sparing	Amiloride	Midamor
		Spironolactone	Aldactone
		Triamterene	Dyrenium
Adrenergic antagonists	β-Blockers	Atenolol	Tenormin
		Bisoprolol	Zebeta
		Metoprolol	Lopressor
		Nadolol	Corgard
		Propranolol	Inderal
		Timolol	Blocadren
	α_1-Blockers	Doxazosin	Cardura
		Prazosin	Minipress
		Terazosin	Hytrin
	Combined α- and β-blockers	Carvedilol	Coreg
		Labetalol	Normodyne,
			Trandate
	Centrally acting	Clonidine	Catapres
		Methyldopa	Aldomet
Vasodilators		Hydralazine	Apresoline
ACEIs		Benazepril	Lotensin
		Captopril	Capoten
		Enalapril	Vasotec
		Fosinopril	Monopril
		Lisinopril	Prinivil, Zestril
		Moexipril	Univasc
		Quinipril	Accupril
		Ramipril	Altace
		Trandolapril	Mavik
Angiotensin receptor blockers		Candesartan	Atacand
		Eprosartan	Teveten
		Irbesartan	Avapro
		Losartan	Cozaar
		Olmesartan	Benicar
		Telmisartan	Micardis
		Valsartan	Diovan

TABLE 5-4	Common Antihypertensive Drugs—cont'd		
Class	**Subclass**	**Generic Name**	**Trade Name**
Calcium channel blockers	Dihydropyridine	Amlodipine	Norvasc
		Felodipine	Plendil
		Israpidine	DynaCirc
		Nicardipine	Cardene
		Nifedipine	Adalat, Procardia
		Nisoldipine	Sular
	Nondihydropyridine	Diltiazem	Cardizem, Dilacor, Tiazac
		Verapamil	Calan, Isoptin, Coer, Covera

ACE, angiotensin-converting enzyme.

because noncompliance with or unavailability of prescribed medications is often responsible for this problem.

3. Pharmacologic Therapy (Table 5-5) depends on the patient's comorbidities and symptoms and signs at presentation.

E. Management of Anesthesia in Patients with Essential HTN (Table 5-6). For most patients, there is no evidence that postoperative complications are increased when hypertensive patients (diastolic blood pressure as high as 110 mm Hg) undergo elective surgery (**Table 5-7**). However, coexisting HTN may increase the incidence of postoperative myocardial reinfarction in patients with prior myocardial infarction and the incidence of neurologic complications in patients undergoing carotid endarterectomy.

  1. Preoperative Evaluation. Evaluate for the presence of end-organ damage (angina pectoris, left ventricular hypertrophy, CHF, cerebrovascular disease, stroke, peripheral vascular disease, renal insufficiency). Elective surgery should be postponed if end-organ damage can be improved or further evaluation would alter the anesthetic plan. Most antihypertensive drugs should be continued throughout the perioperative period to ensure optimal control of blood pressure.

   a. Angiotensin-Converting Enzyme Inhibitors (ACEIs) and Angiotensin Receptor Blockers (ARBs). Surgical procedures involving major fluid shifts in patients treated with ACEIs have been associated with hypotension that is responsive to fluid infusion and administration of sympathomimetic drugs. It may be prudent to discontinue ACEIs 24 to 48 hours preoperatively in patients at high risk of intraoperative hypovolemia and hypotension. The hypotension experienced by patients treated with ARBs can be refractory to conventional vasoconstrictors such as ephedrine and phenylephrine, necessitating use of vasopressin or one of its analogues. ARBs should be discontinued on the day before surgery.

2. Induction of Anesthesia can produce an exaggerated decrease in blood pressure due to peripheral vasodilation in the presence of decreased intravascular fluid volume.

TABLE 5-5 Treatment of Hypertensive Emergencies

Etiology/Manifestation	Primary Agents	Cautions	Comments
Encephalopathy and intracranial hypertension	Nitroprusside, labetalol, fenoldopam, nicardipine	Cerebral ischemia may result from lower blood pressure due to altered autoregulation. Risk of cyanide toxicity Nitroprusside increases intracranial pressure.	Lower blood pressure may lessen bleeding in intracerebral hemorrhage. Elevated BP often resolves spontaneously.
Myocardial ischemia	Nitroglycerin	Avoid β-blockers in acute congestive heart failure.	Include morphine and oxygen therapy.
Acute pulmonary edema	Nitroglycerin, nitroprusside, fenoldopam	Avoid β-blockers in acute congestive heart failure.	Include morphine, loop diuretic, and oxygen therapy.
Aortic dissection	Esmolol, vasodilators Trimethaphan	Vasodilators may cause reflex tachycardia.	Goal: lessening of pulsatile force of left ventricular contraction.
Renal insufficiency	Fenoldopam, nicardipine	Tachyphylaxis occurs with fenoldopam.	May require emergent hemodialysis. Avoid ACE inhibitors and ARBs.

TABLE 5-5 Treatment of Hypertensive Emergencies—cont'd

Etiology/Manifestation	Primary Agents	Cautions	Comments
Preeclampsia and eclampsia	Methyldopa, hydralazine Magnesium sulfate Labetalol, nicardipine	Hydralazine can cause lupuslike syndrome. Patients have risk of flash pulmonary edema. Calcium channel blockers may reduce uterine blood flow and inhibit labor.	Definitive therapy is delivery. ACE inhibitors and ARBs are contraindicated during pregnancy due to teratogenicity.
Pheochromocytoma	Phentolamine, phenoxybenzamine, propranolol	Unopposed α-adrenergic stimulation following β-blockade worsens hypertension.	
Cocaine intoxication	Nitroglycerin, nitroprusside, phentolamine	Unopposed α-adrenergic stimulation following β-blockade worsens hypertension.	

ACEIs, angiotensin-converting enzyme inhibitors; ARBs, angiotensin receptor blockers.

TABLE 5-6	Management of Anesthesia for Patients with Hypertension
Preoperative Evaluation	
Determine adequacy of blood pressure control.	
Review pharmacology of drugs being administered to control blood pressure.	
Evaluate for evidence of end-organ damage.	
Continue drugs used for control of blood pressure.	
Induction and Maintenance of Anesthesia	
Anticipate exaggerated blood pressure response to anesthetic drugs.	
Limit duration of direct laryngoscopy.	
Administer a balanced anesthetic to blunt hypertensive responses.	
Consider placement of invasive hemodynamic monitors.	
Monitor for myocardial ischemia.	
Postoperative Management	
Anticipate periods of systemic hypertension.	
Maintain monitoring of end-organ function.	

a. Direct Laryngoscopy and tracheal intubation can produce significant HTN in patients with essential HTN, even if these patients are normotensive preoperatively. Myocardial ischemia is more likely to occur in association with the HTN and tachycardia that accompany laryngoscopy and intubation. These patients may benefit from maneuvers that suppress tracheal reflexes and blunt the autonomic responses to tracheal manipulation (deep inhalation anesthesia; injection of an opioid, lidocaine, β-blocker, or vasodilator; limiting duration of direct laryngoscopy to ≤15 sec).

3. Maintenance of Anesthesia. Management of intraoperative blood pressure lability is as important as preoperative control of HTN in these patients. Regional anesthesia can certainly be used in hypertensive patients. However, a high sensory level of anesthesia with its associated sympathetic denervation can unmask unsuspected hypovolemia.

a. Intraoperative HTN in response to painful stimuli is likely, even in patients whose blood pressure is controlled preoperatively. Volatile anesthetics are useful in attenuating sympathetic nervous system activity responsible for pressor responses. Volatile anesthetics attenuate systemic nervous system activity. Alternatively, antihypertensive medication can be administered by bolus or by continuous infusion.

b. Intraoperative Hypotension may be treated by decreasing the depth of anesthesia, increasing fluid infusion rates, and/or administering sympathomimetic drugs such as ephedrine or phenylephrine. Intraoperative hypotension in patients being treated with ACE inhibitors or ARBs is responsive to administration of intravenous fluids, sympathomimetic drugs, and/or vasopressin.

TABLE 5-7	Risk of General Anesthesia and Elective Surgery in Hypertensive Patients	
Preoperative Systemic Blood Pressure Status	Incidence of Perioperative Hypertensive Episodes (%)	Incidence of Postoperative Cardiac Complications (%)
Normotensive	8*	11
Treated and rendered normotensive	27	24
Treated but remain hypertensive	25	7
Untreated and hypertensive	20	12

* $P < .05$ compared with other groups in the same column.
Reprinted with permission from Goldman L, Caldera DL: Risk of general anesthesia and elective operation in the hypertensive patient. Anesthesiology 1979;50:285–292.

c. Intraoperative Monitoring. Invasive monitoring with an intra-arterial catheter and a central venous or pulmonary artery catheter may be useful if extensive surgery is planned and there is evidence of left ventricular dysfunction or other significant end-organ damage.

4. Postoperative Management. Postoperative HTN is common and requires prompt treatment to decrease the risk of myocardial ischemia, cardiac dysrhythmias, CHF, stroke, and bleeding.

II. IDIOPATHIC PULMONARY ARTERIAL HYPERTENSION (PAH)

Idiopathic PAH is defined as a mean pulmonary artery pressure greater than 25 mm Hg at rest or greater than 30 mm Hg with exercise, without evidence of left-sided heart disease, myocardial disease, congenital heart disease, and any clinically significant respiratory, connective tissue, or chronic thromboembolic disease. Pulmonary artery occlusion pressure is 15 mm Hg or less, and pulmonary vascular resistance (PVR) is higher than 3 Wood units (mm Hg/L/min) (**Table 5-8**). For classification of PAH, see **Table 5-9**.

A. Clinical Presentation and Evaluation. Common symptoms are breathlessness, weakness, fatigue, abdominal distension, syncope, and angina pectoris. Physical findings may include a parasternal lift, murmur of pulmonic insufficiency (Graham-Steel murmur) and/or tricuspid regurgitation, a pronounced pulmonic component of S2, an S3 gallop, jugular venous distension, peripheral edema, hepatomegaly, and ascites. The laboratory evaluation and diagnostic studies used in the workup of PAH of any cause are listed in **Table 5-10**. Right-sided heart catheterization can aid in evaluating disease severity and determining potential response to vasodilator therapy.

TABLE 5-8	Calculation of Pulmonary Vascular Resistance	
$\dfrac{(\overline{PAP} - PAOP) \times 80}{CO}$	PVR is expressed in dynes /sec/cm^{-5}, with normal PVR = 50–150 dynes/sec/cm^{-5}	
$\dfrac{(\overline{PAP} - PAOP)}{CO}$	PVR is expressed in Wood units (mm Hg/L/min), with normal PVR = 1 Wood unit	

CO, cardiac output (L/min); PAOP, pulmonary artery occlusion pressure (mm Hg); $\overline{PAP}$ mean pulmonary artery pressure (mm Hg);

B. Physiology and Pathophysiology. PAH develops in response to pulmonary vasoconstriction, vascular wall remodeling, and thrombosis in situ. Right ventricular (RV) wall stress increases in response to PAH. RV stroke volume and left ventricular filling are reduced, leading to low cardiac output and systemic hypotension. RV dilation results in annular dilation of right-sided heart valves producing tricuspid regurgitation and/or pulmonic insufficiency. RV myocardial perfusion is limited as the RV wall stress increases. Hypoxemia can occur by three mechanisms: (1) right-to-left shunting through a patent foramen ovale; (2) increased oxygen extraction associated with exertion in the face of a fixed cardiac output; and (3) ventilation/perfusion (V/Q) mismatch.

C. Treatment of PAH (Fig. 5-1)

1. Oxygen, Anticoagulation, and Diuretics. Oxygen therapy improves survival and reduces progression of PAH. Anticoagulation may reduce risk of thrombosis and thromboembolism due to sluggish pulmonary blood flow, dilation of the right side of the heart, venous stasis, and the limitation in physical activity imposed by this disease. Diuretics can decrease preload in patients with right-sided heart failure.

2. Calcium Channel Blockers. Nifedipine, diltiazem, and amlodipine are the most commonly used calcium channel blockers for this purpose and have been shown to improve 5-year survival in patients who are responsive to vasodilators.

3. Phosphodiesterase Inhibitors dilate pulmonary blood vessels and improve cardiac output. Sildenafil (Viagra) administration has been associated with improved exercise capacity and reduction in RV mass.

4. Inhaled Nitric Oxide (NO) improves ventilation/perfusion matching and improves oxygenation by relaxing pulmonary vascular smooth muscle. Problems associated with NO administration include PAH, platelet inhibition, methemoglobinemia, formation of toxic nitrate metabolites, and the technical requirements for its application.

5. Prostacyclins (epoprostenol, treprostinil, iloprost) are systemic and pulmonary vasodilators that also have antiplatelet activity. Prostacyclins reduce PVR and improve cardiac output and exercise tolerance; they can be administered by continuous infusion, by inhalation, and by intermittent subcutaneous injection. All demonstrate short-term improvements in

TABLE 5-9 **Classification of Pulmonary Hypertension**

1. Pulmonary arterial hypertension
   1.1 Idiopathic
   1.2 Familial
   1.3 Associated with…
      1.3.1 Collagen vascular disease
      1.3.2 Congenital systemic-to-pulmonary shunts
      1.3.3 Portal hypertension
      1.3.4 HIV infection
      1.3.5 Drugs and toxins
      1.3.6 Other (thyroid disorders, glycogen storage disease, Gaucher's disease, hereditary hemorrhagic telangiectasia, hemoglobinopathies, myeloproliferative disorders, splenectomy)
   1.4 Associated with significant venous or capillary involvement
      1.4.1 Pulmonary veno-occlusive disease
      1.4.2 Pulmonary capillary hemangiomatosis
   1.5 Persistent pulmonary hypertension of the newborn
2. Pulmonary hypertension with left heart disease
   2.1 Left-sided atrial or ventricular heart disease
   2.2 Left-sided valvular disease
3. Pulmonary hypertension associated with lung diseases and/or hypoxemia
   3.1 Chronic obstructive pulmonary disease
   3.2 Interstitial lung disease
   3.3 Sleep-disordered breathing
   3.4 Alveolar hypoventilation disorders
   3.5 Chronic exposure to high altitude
   3.6 Developmental abnormalities
4. Pulmonary hypertension due to chronic thrombotic and/or embolic disease
   4.1 Thromboembolic obstruction of proximal pulmonary arteries
   4.2 Thromboembolic obstruction of distal pulmonary arteries
   4.3 Nonthrombotic pulmonary embolism (tumor, parasites, foreign material)
5. Miscellaneous (sarcoidosis, histiocytosis X, lymphangiomatosis, compression of pulmonary vessels [adenopathy, tumor, fibrosing mediastinitis])

HIV, human immunodeficiency virus.
Reprinted with permission from Simonneau G, Galiè N, Rubin LJ, et al: Clinical classification of pulmonary hypertension. J Am Coll Cardiol 2004;43(12 Suppl):5S–12S. Copyright 2004, the American College of Cardiology Foundation.

TABLE 5-10	Clinical Findings in Pulmonary Hypertension
Diagnostic Modality	**Key Findings**
Chest radiograph	Prominent pulmonary arteries Right atrial and right ventricular enlargement Parenchymal lung disease
Electrocardiography	P pulmonale Right axis deviation Right ventricular strain or hypertrophy Complete or incomplete right bundle branch block
Two-dimensional echocardiography	Right atrial enlargement Right ventricular hypertrophy, dilation, or volume overload Tricuspid regurgitation Elevated estimated pulmonary artery pressures Congenital heart disease
Pulmonary function tests	Obstructive or restrictive pattern Low diffusing capacity
V/Q scan	Ventilation/perfusion mismatching
Pulmonary angiography	Vascular filling defects
Chest CT scan	Main pulmonary artery size >30 mm Vascular filling defects Mosaic perfusion defects
Abdominal ultrasound or CT scan	Cirrhosis Portal hypertension
Blood tests	Antinuclear antibody Rheumatoid factor Complete blood count Coagulation profile HIV titers Thyroid-stimulating hormone
Sleep study	High respiratory disturbance index

CT, computed tomography; HIV, human immunodeficiency virus; V/Q, ventilation/perfusion.
Reprinted with permission from Dincer HE, Presberg KW: Current management of pulmonary hypertension. Clin Pulm Med 2004;11: 40–53.

hemodynamics but have not been associated with sustained improvement or decreased mortality.

6. Endothelin Receptor Antagonists. Endothelin interacts with two receptors: endothelin A (pulmonary vasoconstriction and smooth muscle proliferation) and endothelin B (vasodilation, enhanced endothelin clearance, increased production of NO and prostacyclin). Endothelin receptor antagonists lower pulmonary arterial pressure and PVR and improve RV function, exercise tolerance, quality of life, and mortality.

7. Surgical Treatment. RV assist devices can be used in severe PAH and right-sided heart failure. Balloon atrial septostomy is a procedure that

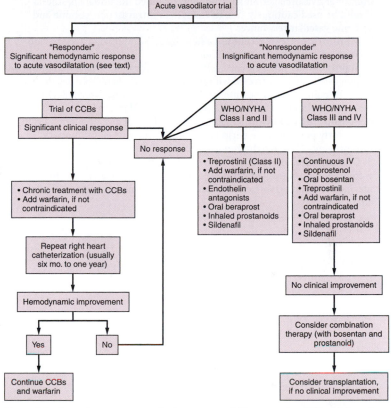

Figure 5-1 • Outpatient treatment of pulmonary arterial hypertension. CCBs, calcium channel blockers; NYHA, New York Heart Association; WHO, World Health Organization. (Reprinted with permission from Dincer HE, Presberg KW: Current management of pulmonary hypertension. Clin Pulm Med 2004;11:40–53.)

allows right-to-left shunting of blood to decompress the right heart. Lung transplantation is the only curative therapy for many types of PAH.

D. Anesthetic Management. Increased RV afterload, hypoxemia, hypotension, and inadequate RV preload contribute to elevated risk of RV failure. Hypoxia, hypercarbia, and acidosis must be aggressively controlled because they cause increased PVR. Reduction in systemic vascular resistance by inhalational anesthetics or sedatives may be dangerous because of the relatively fixed cardiac output. Maintenance of sinus rhythm is crucial.

   1. Preoperative Preparation and Induction. In a PAH patient who is not yet on long-term therapy, administration of sildenafil or L-arginine preoperatively may be helpful. Pulmonary vasodilator therapy must be continued in the preoperative period. Ketamine and etomidate may inhibit pulmonary vasorelaxation and should be avoided. Regional anesthesia should be used cautiously, due to changes in intravascular volume and systemic vascular resistance.

2. Monitoring. Central venous catheterization and intra-arterial blood pressure monitoring is recommended.

3. Maintenance. Inhalational agents are useful for maintenance of anesthesia. Hypotension can be corrected with norepinephrine, phenylephrine, or fluids. A potent pulmonary vasodilator such as milrinone, nitroglycerin, NO, or prostacyclin should be available to treat PAH should it develop.

4. Postoperative Period. Patients with PAH are at risk of sudden death in the early postoperative period due to worsening PAH, pulmonary thromboembolism, dysrhythmias, and fluid shifts.

5. Obstetric Population. Delivery methods that decrease patient effort are recommended. Nitroglycerin should be immediately available at the time of uterine involution to offset the effects of uterine blood return to the central circulation.

6

Heart Failure
and Cardiomyopathies

I. HEART FAILURE (HF)

HF is defined by the inability of the heart to fill with or eject blood at a rate appropriate to meet tissue requirements. HF affects about 1% of adults over age 65 in the United States. Systolic heart failure (SHF) is more common among middle-aged men, and diastolic heart failure (DHF) is usually seen in elderly women. HF is most often due to (1) ischemic heart disease or cardiomyopathy; (2) cardiac valve abnormalities; (3) systemic hypertension; (4) diseases of the pericardium; or (5) pulmonary hypertension (cor pulmonale).

A. Forms of Ventricular Dysfunction

1. Systolic and Diastolic Heart Failure. Decreased ventricular systolic wall motion reflects systolic dysfunction, whereas diastolic dysfunction is characterized by abnormal ventricular relaxation and reduced compliance.

   a. Systolic Heart Failure. Causes of SHF include coronary artery disease (CAD), dilated cardiomyopathy (DCM), chronic pressure overload (aortic stenosis and chronic hypertension), and chronic volume overload (regurgitant valvular lesions and high output cardiac failure). Patients with left bundle branch block and SHF are at high risk of sudden death.

   b. Diastolic Heart Failure occurs in patients with normal or near-normal left ventricular (LV) systolic function. DHF can be classified into four stages. Class I DHF is characterized by an abnormal LV relaxation pattern with normal left atrial pressure. Classes II, III, and IV include abnormal relaxation and reduced LV compliance resulting with increased LV end-diastolic pressure (LVEDP). Ischemic heart disease, essential hypertension (HTN), and aortic stenosis are the most common causes of DHF. The major differences between SHF and DHF are presented in **Table 6-1**.

   c. Acute and Chronic Heart Failure. Acute HF is defined as a change in the signs and symptoms of HF requiring emergency therapy. Chronic HF occurs in patients with long-standing cardiac disease and is associated

75

TABLE 6-1	Characteristics of Patients with Diastolic Versus Systolic Heart Failure	
Characteristic	**Diastolic Heart Failure**	**Systolic Heart Failure**
Age	Often elderly	Typically 50–70 years old
Sex	Often female	More often male
Left ventricular ejection fraction	Preserved, ≥ 40%	Depressed, ≤40%
Left ventricular cavity size	Usually normal, often with concentric left ventricular hypertrophy	Usually dilated
Chest radiography	Congestion ± cardiomegaly	Congestion and cardiomegaly
Gallop rhythm present	Fourth heart sound	Third heart sound
Hypertension	+++	++
Diabetes mellitus	+++	++
Previous myocardial infarction	+	+++
Obesity	+++	+
Chronic lung disease	++	0
Sleep apnea	++	++
Dialysis	++	0
Atrial fibrillation	+ Usually paroxysmal	+ Usually persistent

+, occasionally associated with; ++, often associated with; +++, usually associated with; 0, no association.

with signs and symptoms of venous congestion. In patients with acute HF, systemic hypotension is often present without peripheral edema.

d. Left-Sided and Right-Sided Heart Failure. In patients with left-sided HF, high LVEDP leads to pulmonary venous congestion with symptoms of dyspnea, orthopnea, paroxysmal nocturnal dyspnea, and pulmonary edema. Right-sided HF causes systemic venous congestion, with peripheral edema and hepatomegaly. The most common cause of right-sided HF is left-sided HF.

e. Low-Output and High-Output Heart Failure. The most common causes of low-output HF are CAD, cardiomyopathy, HTN, valvular disease, and pericardial disease. Causes of high cardiac output HF include anemia, pregnancy, arteriovenous fistulas, hyperthyroidism, beriberi, and Paget's disease. In high-output HF, ventricular failure is due to an increased hemodynamic burden; to myocardial toxicity in thyrotoxicosis and beriberi; and to myocardial anoxia in severe, prolonged anemia.

B. Pathophysiology of Heart Failure. The initiating mechanisms of heart failure are pressure overload (aortic stenosis, essential HTN), volume overload (mitral or aortic regurgitation), myocardial ischemia/infarction, myocardial inflammatory disease, and restricted diastolic filling (constrictive pericarditis, restrictive myocarditis).

1. **The Frank-Starling Relationship** refers to an increase in stroke volume (SV) that accompanies an increase in LV end-diastolic volume and pressure. When myocardial contractility is decreased (as in HF), a smaller increase in SV occurs with any given increase in LV end-diastolic pressure. Constriction of venous capacitance vessel shifts blood centrally, increases preload, and helps maintain cardiac output (CO).

2. **Activation of the Sympathetic Nervous System (SNS)** promotes arteriolar and venous constriction that maintains systemic blood pressure and shifts blood to the central circulation. Blood is redistributed from the kidneys, splanchnic organs, skeletal muscles, and skin to the coronary and cerebral circulations, resulting in activation of the renin-angiotensin-aldosterone system (RAAS) and increased renal sodium and water retention. Down-regulation of β-adrenergic receptors occurs during HF, and plasma catecholamines are increased. High norepinephrine levels promote myocyte necrosis and cell death and ventricular remodeling. β-Blocker therapy may decrease the deleterious effects of catecholamines on the heart.

3. **Alterations in the Inotropic State, Heart Rate, and Afterload.** The maximum velocity of contraction of cardiac muscle is referred to as V_{max}. V_{max} is increased in increased inotropic states (increased catecholamines) and decreased in HF. Afterload is the tension the ventricular muscle must develop to open the aortic or pulmonic valve and is increased in the presence of systemic HTN. Forward SV can be increased patients with HF by administering vasodilating drugs and decreasing afterload. In the presence of SHF, the SV is relatively fixed and CO is dependent on heart rate. In SHF, increased heart rate maintains CO. In DHF, tachycardia reduces ventricular filling time and reduces CO. Heart rate control is a target for therapy of DHF.

4. **Humoral-Mediated Responses and Biochemical Pathways.** During HF, vasoconstriction is initiated via increased activity of the SNS and RAAS, parasympathetic withdrawal, high levels of circulating vasopressin, endothelial dysfunction, and release of inflammatory mediators. B-type natriuretic peptide (BNP), which promotes diuresis, natriuresis, vasodilation, antihypertrophy, anti-inflammation, and inhibition of the RAAS and SNS, is secreted by both atrial and ventricular myocardium. In HF, the ventricle becomes the principal site for BNP production.

5. **Myocardial Remodeling** is the process by which mechanical, neurohormonal, and genetic factors change the LV size, shape, and function to maintain CO. Angiotensin-converting enzyme inhibitors (ACEIs) have been shown to promote a "reverse-remodeling" process and are first-line therapy for HF.

C. Signs and Symptoms of Heart Failure (Table 6-2)
D. Diagnosis of Heart Failure

1. **Laboratory Diagnosis.** Plasma BNP levels below 100 pg/mL indicate that HF is unlikely (90% negative predictive value) and levels above 500 pg/mL are consistent with the diagnosis of HF (90% positive predictive value). Abnormal renal function tests may indicate decreased renal perfusion,

TABLE 6-2	Signs and Symptoms of Congestive Heart Failure
Signs and Symptoms of Pulmonary Vascular Congestion	
Left ventricular failure	• Dyspnea and/or tachypnea (increased lung stiffness due to interstitial pulmonary edema) • Orthopnea (inability of the ventricle to tolerate increased venous return when recumbent) • Paroxysmal nocturnal dyspnea (shortness of breath that awakens the patient from sleep) • Nocturia • Pulmonary rales • S3 gallop • Acute pulmonary edema • Decreased cerebral blood flow (confusion, insomnia, anxiety, memory deficits) • Systemic hypotension and cool extremities (severe HF)
Signs and Symptoms of Systemic Venous Congestion	
Right ventricular failure	• Jugular venous distension • Organomegaly (e.g., hepatic congestion) • Right upper quadrant tenderness • Ascites • Peripheral edema

and abnormal liver function tests may occur if liver congestion occurs. Hyponatremia, hypomagnesemia, and hypokalemia may be present.

   a. Electrocardiography is usually abnormal and has a low predictive value for the diagnosis of HF.

   b. Chest Radiography may reveal cardiomegaly, pulmonary venous congestion, interstitial or alveolar pulmonary edema, Kerley lines, pleural effusions, or pericardial effusion. Radiographic evidence of pulmonary edema may lag behind the clinical evidence of pulmonary edema by up to 12 hours.

   c. Echocardiography can assess ejection fraction, LV structure and functionality, the presence of other structural abnormalities such as valvular and pericardial disease, the presence and degree of diastolic dysfunction, and right ventricular (RV) function.

E. Classification of Heart Failure

1. The New York Heart Association Functional Classification correlates with survival and quality of life. It groups patients into four classes:
Class I: Ordinary physical activity does not cause symptoms.
Class II: Symptoms occur with ordinary exertion.
Class III: Symptoms occur with less than ordinary exertion.
Class IV: Inability to carry on any physical activity without discomfort. Symptoms present at rest.

2. The American College of Cardiology and American Heart Association classifies patients according to disease progression:
Stage A: Patients at high risk of heart failure but without structural heart disease or symptoms of HF
Stage B: Patients with structural heart disease but without symptoms of HF

Stage C: Patients with structural heart disease with previous or current symptoms of HF
Stage D: Patients with refractory heart failure requiring specialized interventions

F. Management of Heart Failure

1. Management of Chronic Heart Failure. Treatment options include lifestyle modification, patient and family education, medical therapy, corrective surgery, implantable devices, and cardiac transplantation (**Fig. 6-1**).

2. Management of Systolic Heart Failure

a. Inhibitors of the Renin-Angiotensin-Aldosterone System

1.) *ACEIs* are the first line of treatment for HF. ACEIs have been proven to decrease ventricular remodeling, potentiate reverse remodeling, and reduce morbidity and mortality of patients in any stage of HF. These benefits appear to be less in African Americans than in white patients.

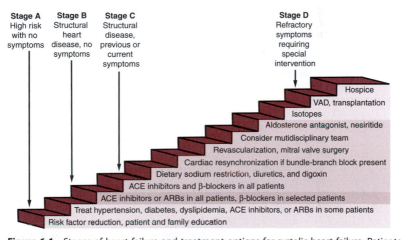

Figure 6-1 • Stages of heart failure and treatment options for systolic heart failure. Patients with stage A heart failure are at high risk of heart failure but do not yet have structural heart disease or symptoms of heart failure. This group includes patients with hypertension, diabetes, coronary artery disease, previous exposure to cardiotoxic drugs, or a family history of cardiomyopathy. Patients with stage B heart failure have structural heart disease but no symptoms of heart failure. This group includes patients with left ventricular hypertrophy, previous myocardial infarction, left ventricular systolic dysfunction, or valvular heart disease, all of whom would be considered to have New York Heart Association (NYHA) class I symptoms. Patients with stage C heart failure have known structural heart disease and current or previous symptoms of heart failure. Their current symptoms may be classified as NYHA class I, II, III, or IV. Patients with stage D heart failure have refractory symptoms of heart failure at rest despite maximal medical therapy, are hospitalized, and require specialized interventions or hospice care. All such patients would be considered to have NYHA class IV symptoms. ACE, angiotensin-converting enzyme; ARB, angiotensin receptor blocker; VAD, ventricular assist device. (Reproduced with permission from Jessup M, Brozena S: Heart failure. N Engl J Med 2003;348:2007–2018. Copyright © 2003 Massachusetts Medical Society. All rights reserved.)

2.) *Angiotensin II Receptor Blockers* have similar but not superior efficacies compared with ACEIs and are recommended for patients who cannot tolerate ACEIs.

3.) *Aldosterone Antagonists* may reduce sodium and water retention, hypokalemia, and ventricular remodeling, as well as reduce mortality and hospitalization rates in New York Heart Association class III and IV patients.

4.) β-*Blockers* reduce morbidity and hospitalizations; improve quality of life, survival, and ejection fraction; and decrease ventricular remodeling.

5.) *Diuretics* decrease ventricular diastolic pressure and decrease diastolic ventricular wall stress, preventing the cardiac distension that interferes with subendocardial perfusion and negatively affects myocardial metabolism and function.

6.) *Digitalis* improves cardiac inotropy and decreases activation of the SNS and the RAAS. It is not clear that digitalis treatment improves survival. Digitalis can be added to therapy in patients who are symptomatic despite treatment with diuretics, ACEIs, and β-blockers. Patients with atrial fibrillation and HF may particularly benefit from digoxin. Elderly patients or those with impaired renal function are at risk for digitalis toxicity, which may be manifested by anorexia, nausea, blurred vision, and cardiac dysrhythmias. Treatment of toxicity includes reversing hypokalemia, treating cardiac dysrhythmias, administering antidigoxin antibodies, and/or implementing temporary cardiac pacing.

7.) *Vasodilators.* In patients with dilated left ventricles, vasodilators increase SV and decrease ventricular filling pressures. African-American patients show improved clinical outcomes when treated with a combination of hydralazine and nitrates.

8.) *Statins* decrease morbidity and mortality in patients with SHF, via anti-inflammatory and lipid-lowering effects.

3. Management of Diastolic Heart Failure (Table 6-3)

4. Surgical Management of Heart Failure. Treatments that target the cause of HF include coronary revascularization by percutaneous interventions or coronary artery bypass surgery, postinfarction ventricular aneurysmectomy, and heart transplantation. Ventricular assist devices may facilitate recovery of heart function in some patients or provide a bridge to transplantation. Cardiac resynchronization therapy (CRT, also known as biventricular pacing) allows the heart to contract more efficiently and promotes reverse remodeling. Implanted cardioverter/defibrillators (ICDs) prevent sudden death in certain patients with advanced heart failure (**Table 6-4**).

5. Management of Acute Heart Failure (Table 6-5). The hemodynamic profile of acute HF is characterized by high ventricular filling pressures, low cardiac output, and hypertension or hypotension.

6. Prognosis. The mortality rate during the first 4 years following the diagnosis of HF approaches 40%. Factors associated with a poor prognosis include increased urea and creatinine levels, hyponatremia, hypokalemia, severely depressed ejection fraction, high levels of endogenous BNP, very limited exercise tolerance, and the presence of multifocal premature ventricular contractions.

TABLE 6-3	Management of Diastolic Heart Failure
Goals	**Management Strategies**
Prevent development of diastolic heart failure by decreasing risk factors	Treat coronary artery disease Treat hypertension Control weight gain Treat diabetes mellitus
Allow adequate filling time of left ventricle by decreasing heart rate	Administer β-blockers, calcium channel blockers, digoxin
Control volume overload	Treat with diuretics, long-acting nitrates Prescribe low-sodium diet
Restore and maintain sinus rhythm	Treat with cardioversion, amiodarone, digoxin
Decrease ventricular remodeling	Administer ACEIs, statins
Correct precipitating factors	Perform aortic valve replacement, coronary revascularization

II. MANAGEMENT OF ANESTHESIA IN PATIENTS WITH HEART FAILURE (Table 6-6)

III. CARDIOMYOPATHIES

According to the American Heart Association, "Cardiomyopathies are a heterogeneous group of diseases of the myocardium associated with mechanical and/or electrical dysfunction that usually (but not invariably) exhibit inappropriate ventricular hypertrophy or dilation and are due to a variety of causes that frequently are genetic." Cardiomyopathies either are confined to the heart (primary [**Table 6-7**]) or are part of generalized systemic disorders (secondary [**Table 6-8**]), often leading to cardiovascular death or progressive heart failure–related disability.

IV. HYPERTROPHIC CARDIOMYOPATHY

Hypertrophic cardiomyopathy (HCM) is the most common genetic cardiovascular disease (1:500), affects all ages, and has autosomal dominant (AD) inheritance. HCM is characterized by LV hypertrophy in the absence of other causes (e.g., HTN).

TABLE 6-4	Indications for Implantable Cardioverter-Defibrillator Devices	
Cause of Heart Failure	**Condition**	
Coronary artery disease	Ejection fraction <30% Ejection fraction <40% if electrophysiologic study demonstrates inducible ventricular dysrhythmias	
All other causes	After first episode of syncope or aborted ventricular tachycardia/ventricular fibrillation	

TABLE 6-5 Management of Acute Heart Failure	
Therapeutic Modality	**Effects**
Diuretics (furosemide, hydrochlorothiazide)	May improve symptoms rapidly, but high doses can adversely affect clinical outcomes.
Vasodilators (nitroglycerin, nitroprusside)	Reduce LV filling pressure, and systemic vascular resistance; increase SV.
Inotropes • Catecholamines (epinephrine, norepinephrine, dopamine, dobutamine) • Phosphodiesterase inhibitors (amrinone, milrinone)	Catecholamines improve excitation-contraction coupling by direct adrenergic−receptor stimulation. Phosphodiesterase inhibitors block degradation of cyclic adenosine monophosphate.
Calcium sensitizers (levosimendan)	A new class of inotropes that increase contractility without increasing myocardial oxygen consumption, heart rate, or dysrhythmias.
Exogenous B-type natriuretic peptides (nesiritide)	Bind to both A- and B-type natriuretic receptors. Promote arterial, venous, and coronary vasodilation. Decrease LVEDP. Improve dyspnea, and induce diuresis and natriuresis.
Nitric oxide synthase inhibitors	Large amount of inflammation-related nitric oxide produced by the heart and endothelium in HF has negative inotropic and profound vasodilatory effect, leading to shock and vascular collapse. NO synthase inhibitors are currently investigational.
Intra-aortic balloon pump	Balloon placed via femoral artery into descending aorta inflates during diastole, promoting coronary perfusion, and deflates during systole, creating "suction" that enhances LV ejection.
LV and RV assist devices	Can improve survival in patients with severe cardiogenic shock and allow some myocardial recovery. May bridge to transplant.

A. Pathophysiology. Vigorous contraction of the hypertrophied septum results in the following: accelerated blood flow through a narrow left ventricular outflow tract (LVOT); a Venturi effect on the anterior leaflet of the mitral valve moves the leaflet into the LVOT (systolic anterior movement, or SAM), leading to increased LVOT obstruction and mitral regurgitation. Situations that worsen LVOT obstruction are presented in **Table 6-9**. Diastolic dysfunction is common. Myocardial ischemia may be present in the absence of CAD. Dysrhythmias result from the disorganized cellular architecture, myocardial scarring, and expanded interstitial matrix and are associated with risk of sudden death.

B. Signs and Symptoms vary widely, with most patients remaining asymptomatic throughout life. Symptoms may include angina pectoris (often relieved by lying down), fatigue or syncope, tachydysrhythmias, and HF. Cardiac examination may reveal a double apical impulse, gallop rhythm, and cardiac murmurs (increased by Valsalva's maneuver, nitroglycerin, and standing versus lying down). Sudden death is most likely between the ages of 10 and 30 years.

TABLE 6-6 Management of Anesthesia in Patients with Heart Failure

Preoperative medications	• Continue β-blockers and digoxin. • Consider holding ACEIs. • Discontinue ARBs.
Electrolytes	Correct hypokalemia.
Anesthetic induction	• All types of general anesthesia have been used successfully. • Opioids may be beneficial.
Monitoring	• Provide intra-arterial pressure monitoring, CVP, and PA monitoring according to surgery and patient condition. • Transesophageal echocardiography may be helpful.
Regional anesthesia	Decreased systemic vascular resistance may benefit CO but can be difficult to control.
Patients after heart transplant	• Patients have high risk of infection due to immunosuppression. • Heart rate is not responsive to indirect adrenergic-agonists or anticholinergic agents; use isoproterenol or epinephrine. • Blunted response to beta-adrenergic agents may occur. • Heart is very preload dependent.
Postoperative management	• HF during surgery requires postoperative ICU care and monitoring. • Treat pain aggressively.

CVP, central venous pressure; ICU, intensive care unit; PA, pulmonary artery.

TABLE 6-7 Classification of Primary Cardiomyopathies

Genetic	Hypertrophic cardiomyopathy Arrhythmogenic right ventricular cardiomyopathy Left ventricular noncompaction Glycogen storage disease Conduction system disease (Lenègre's disease) Ion channelopathies: long QT syndrome, Brugada syndrome, short QT syndrome,
Mixed	Dilated cardiomyopathy Primary restrictive nonhypertrophied cardiomyopathy
Acquired	Myocarditis (inflammatory cardiomyopathy): viral, bacterial, rickettsial, fungal, parasitic (Chagas disease) Stress cardiomyopathy Peripartum cardiomyopathy

TABLE 6-8	Classification of Secondary Cardiomyopathies
Infiltrative	Amyloidosis Gaucher's disease Hunter's syndrome
Storage	Hemochromatosis Glycogen storage disease Niemann-Pick disease
Toxic	Drugs: cocaine, alcohol Chemotherapy drugs: doxorubicin, daunorubicin, cyclophosphamide Heavy metals: lead, mercury Radiation therapy
Inflammatory	Sarcoidosis
Endomyocardial	Hypereosinophilic (Löffler's) syndrome Endomyocardial fibrosis
Endocrine	Diabetes mellitus Hyperthyroidism or hypothyroidism Pheochromocytoma Acromegaly
Neuromuscular	Duchenne-Becker dystrophy Neurofibromatosis Tuberous sclerosis
Autoimmune	Lupus erythematosus Rheumatoid arthritis Scleroderma Dermatomyositis Polyarteritis nodosa

C. Diagnosis. Electrocardiogram (ECG) results are abnormal in 75% to 90% of patients (e.g., LVH, ST- and T-wave abnormalities, Q waves, left atrial enlargement) and may be the only sign of the disease in asymptomatic patients. Echocardiography can demonstrate the presence of myocardial hypertrophy and assess EF (usually >80%), systolic anterior motion, and diastolic dysfunction. Cardiac catheterization allows direct measurement of the increased LVEDP and LVOT pressure gradient. Endomyocardial biopsy and DNA analysis are reserved for patients in whom the diagnosis cannot be otherwise established.

D. Treatment. HCM is associated with high risk of sudden death in some patients and must be treated aggressively.

1. Medical Therapy. β-Blockers and calcium channel blockers have been used extensively to treat HCM. Patients at high risk of sudden death may require amiodarone therapy or placement of an internal cardioverter/defibrillator. Atrial fibrillation (AF) is associated with an increased risk of thromboembolism, congestive HF, and sudden death. Amiodarone is the most effective antidysrhythmic drug for prevention of paroxysms of AF in these patients. β-Blockers and calcium channel blockers can control the heart rate. Long-term anticoagulation is indicated in those with recurrent or chronic AF.

2. Surgical Therapy. The small subgroup of patients with HCM who have both large outflow tract gradients (≥50 mm Hg) and severe symptoms despite

TABLE 6-9	Factors Influencing LVOT Obstruction in Patients with HCM

Events That Increase Outflow Obstruction

Increased myocardial contractility
  β-Adrenergic stimulation (catecholamines)
  Digitalis
Decreased preload
  Hypovolemia
  Vasodilators
  Tachycardia
  Positive pressure ventilation
Decreased afterload
  Hypotension
  Vasodilators

Events That Decrease Outflow Obstruction

Decreased myocardial contractility
  β-Adrenergic blockade
  Volatile anesthetics
  Calcium entry blockers
Increased preload
  Hypervolemia
  Bradycardia
Increased afterload
  Hypertension
  α-Adrenergic stimulation

medical therapy benefit from surgical removal of a small amount of cardiac muscle from the ventricular septum (septal myomectomy). The procedure abolishes or greatly reduces the LVOT gradient in most patients, with subsequent reduction in intraventricular systolic and end-diastolic pressures.

E. Prognosis. Annual mortality is approximately 1%. However, the subset of patients at high risk of sudden death (family history of sudden death or history of malignant ventricular dysrhythmias) has a mortality rate of 5% per year.

F. Management of Anesthesia (Table 6-10). Management of anesthesia in patients with HCM is directed toward minimizing LVOT obstruction (decreasing myocardial contractility, increasing preload and afterload).

V. DILATED CARDIOMYOPATHY (DCM)

DCM is characterized by LV or biventricular dilation, systolic dysfunction, and normal LV wall thickness. African-American men have an increased risk of developing DCM. DCM is the most common type of cardiomyopathy, the

TABLE 6-10	Anesthetic Considerations in Patients with HCM
Preoperative evaluation/ management	• Obtain ECG and updated echocardiogram • Continue β-blockers and/or calcium channel blockers • Premedicate to reduce anxiety • Correct hypovolemia • Turn off ICD, have external defibrillator immediately available
Intraoperative management	• All induction agents are acceptable if used cautiously • Avoid sudden decreases in SVR and tachycardia • During positive pressure ventilation, use small tidal volumes, avoid PEEP • Maintain preload aggressively • Volatile agents may be helpful in decreasing contractility • Treat hypotension with pure $\tilde{\alpha}$ agonist (phenylephrine) • Treat arrhythmias aggressively; cardiovert early
Monitors	• Transesophageal echocardiography is very useful • CVP and PA catheters are not accurate in assessing LV filling in patients with HCM
Parturients	• Regional anesthesia may be used safely. • Phenylephrine for hypotension, not ephedrine. • Use oxytocin with caution. • *AVOID* diuretics, digoxin, and nitrates in pulmonary edema, because they provoke LVOT obstruction.
Postoperative management	• Monitor closely throughout recovery • Treat pain, shivering, anxiety aggressively to avoid/reduce SNS activation • Treat hypovolemia promptly

third most common cause of HF, and the most common indication for cardiac transplantation.

A. Signs and Symptoms. Symptoms include those of HF, exertional chest pain that mimics angina pectoris. Ventricular dilation causes functional mitral and/or tricuspid regurgitation. Supraventricular and ventricular dysrhythmias, conduction system abnormalities, and sudden death are common. Systemic embolization is also common.

B. Diagnosis

1. The ECG often shows ST segment and T-wave abnormalities and LBBB. Cardiac dysrhythmias are common.

2. Chest Radiograph may show LV dilation.

3. Echocardiography reveals dilation of all four chambers, especially the left ventricle, and global hypokinesis. Other findings can include regional wall motion abnormalities (in the absence of CAD), mural thrombi, and valvular regurgitation secondary to annular dilation.

4. Laboratory Testing should eliminate other causes of cardiac dilation such as hyperthyroidism.

5. Endomyocardial Biopsy is not recommended.

C. Treatment (Table 6-11)

TABLE 6-11	Treatment of Dilated Cardiomyopathy
Supportive measures	• Weight control, low-sodium diet, fluid restriction, smoking and alcohol cessation
Medical management	• Similar to that for chronic HF • Anticoagulation to prevent systemic embolization • ICD implantation in patients who have had a cardiac arrest
Surgical management	• Cardiac transplantation

D. Prognosis. The 5-year mortality rate is 50%. Factors that predict a poor prognosis include an ejection fraction less than 25%, pulmonary capillary wedge pressure greater than 20 mm Hg, cardiac index less than 2.5 $L/min/m^2$, hypotension, pulmonary hypertension, and increased central venous pressure.
E. Management of Anesthesia. Because DCM is a cause of heart failure, the anesthetic management of these patients is the same as described in the heart failure section of this chapter.

VI. PERIPARTUM CARDIOMYOPATHY (PPCM)

PPCM is a rare, dilated form of cardiomyopathy of unknown cause that occurs anywhere from the third trimester of pregnancy until 5 months after delivery in women with no history of heart disease (1:3000–1:4000 live births). Risk factors include obesity, multiparity, advanced maternal age (>30 years of age), multifetal pregnancy, preeclampsia, and African-American ethnicity.
A. Signs and Symptoms are nonspecific and include dyspnea, fatigue, and peripheral edema.
B. Diagnosis is based on the echocardiographic documentation of a new finding of dilated cardiac chambers and LV systolic dysfunction during the period surrounding parturition.
C. Treatment goals are to alleviate the symptoms of HF. Diuretics, vasodilators (hydralazine, nitrates), and digoxin can be used. ACEIs are teratogenic but can be useful following delivery. Anticoagulation is recommended. Heart transplantation is considered in patients who do not improve.
D. Prognosis. Mortality ranges from 25% to 50%, with most deaths occurring within 3 months after delivery. Prognosis is correlated with the degree of normalization of left ventricle size and function within 6 months of delivery.
E. Management of Anesthesia requires assessment of cardiac status and careful planning of the analgesia and/or anesthesia required for delivery. Regional anesthesia may provide a desirable decrease in afterload.

VII. SECONDARY CARDIOMYOPATHIES WITH RESTRICTIVE PHYSIOLOGY

Secondary cardiomyopathies with restrictive physiology are caused by systemic diseases that produce myocardial infiltration and severe diastolic dysfunction (e.g., amyloidosis, hemochromatosis, sarcoidosis, carcinoid). Although there is impaired diastolic function and reduced ventricular compliance, systolic function is usually normal. Cardiomyopathies with restrictive physiology must be differentiated from constrictive pericarditis, which has a similar physiology but is more likely if there is a clinical history of pericarditis.

A. Signs and Symptoms of left ventricular and/or RV failure may be present, but cardiomegaly is absent. Atrial fibrillation and thromboembolic events are common. Cardiac conduction disturbances are particularly common in amyloidosis and sarcoidosis.

B. Diagnosis

   1. General Findings. The ECG may demonstrate conduction abnormalities. The chest radiograph may show signs of pulmonary congestion and/or pleural effusion, but cardiomegaly is absent. Chemical laboratory tests should be directed toward diagnosis of the systemic disease responsible for the cardiac infiltration.

   2. Echocardiography will demonstrate diastolic dysfunction and normal systolic function, enlarged atria, and normal ventricular size. In cardiac amyloidosis, the ventricular mass appears characteristically large.

   3. Endomyocardial Biopsy can elucidate the exact etiology of the infiltrative cardiomyopathy.

C. Treatment. Symptomatic treatment is similar to that for DHF. Maintenance of normal sinus rhythm is extremely important. SV is relatively fixed, and the onset of bradycardia may precipitate acute HF. With cardiac sarcoidosis, malignant ventricular dysrhythmias are common and may necessitate insertion of an ICD. Anticoagulation is recommended in patients with atrial fibrillation or low output states. Cardiac transplantation is not a treatment option because myocardial infiltration will recur in the transplanted heart.

D. Prognosis is very poor.

E. Management of Anesthesia. Management of anesthesia for patients with restrictive cardiomyopathy uses the same principles as for patients with cardiac tamponade (see Chapter 7).

VIII. COR PULMONALE

Cor pulmonale is RV enlargement (hypertrophy and/or dilation) that may progress to right HF, caused by diseases that induce pulmonary hypertension (chronic obstructive pulmonary disease, restrictive lung disease, respiratory insufficiency of central origin, obesity-hypoventilation syndrome, idiopathic pulmonary hypertension).

A. Pathophysiology. Chronic or acute alveolar hypoxia (PaO_2 <55 mm Hg) causes pulmonary vasoconstriction. Long-standing chronic hypoxia promotes pulmonary vasculature remodeling and an increase in pulmonary vascular resistance. The right ventricle has an increased workload and hypertrophies. Eventually, RV dysfunction occurs, leading to RV failure.

B. Signs and Symptoms occur late in the course of the disease and include peripheral edema, dyspnea, and effort-related syncope. Accentuation of the pulmonic component of the second heart sound, a diastolic murmur of pulmonic regurgitation, and a systolic murmur caused by tricuspid regurgitation indicate severe pulmonary hypertension. Signs of overt right ventricular failure include increased jugular venous pressure and hepatosplenomegaly.

C. Diagnosis. The ECG may show signs of right atrial and right ventricular hypertrophy (peaked P waves in leads II, III, and aVF—"p pulmonale,"), right axis deviation, and a partial or complete right bundle branch block. Echocardiography can assist in estimating pulmonary artery pressure, assessing the size and function of the right atrium and ventricle, and evaluating the presence and severity of tricuspid or pulmonic regurgitation.

D. Treatment (Table 6-12)

E. Prognosis depends on the underlying cause.

F. Management of Anesthesia

1. Preoperative Management. Preoperative preparation is directed toward (1) eliminating and controlling acute and chronic pulmonary infection, (2) reversing bronchospasm, (3) improving clearance of airway secretions, (4) expanding collapsed or poorly ventilated alveoli, (5) hydration, and (6) correcting any electrolyte imbalances.

2. Intraoperative Management (Table 6-13)

3. Postoperative Management. Avoid factors that exacerbate pulmonary HTN and maintain oxygen therapy as needed.

TABLE 6-12 Treatment of Cor Pulmonale

Reduce RV workload by promoting pulmonary vasodilation

- Maintain PaO_2 >60 mm Hg (SpO_2 >90%) with supplemental oxygen
- Correct PCO_2 and pH abnormalities
- Diuretics (use with caution—resulting alkalosis can cause CO_2 retention)
- Digitalis for RV failure

Treat atrial fibrillation (digitalis)

Lung transplantation (single or double) or heart-lung transplantation may be considered in cases unresponsive to medical therapy.

TABLE 6-13 Intraoperative Management of Cor Pulmonale

- Induction of anesthesia can be safely accomplished with any method
- Adequate depth of anesthesia for intubation to avoid precipitating bronchospasm
- Volatile agents can promote bronchodilation
- Avoid large opioid dosing due to respiratory depression and CO_2 retention
- Humidification of gases can maintain mucociliary function
- Intra-arterial catheter allows frequent sampling of arterial blood gases
- CVP and PA monitoring according to invasiveness of surgery
- Transesophageal echocardiography may be an alternative monitor of RV function
- Use regional anesthesia with caution: high motor block can interfere with muscles of respiration and decreased systemic vascular resistance is deleterious in the presence of fixed pulmonary HTN.

Pericardial Diseases and Cardiac Trauma

The three most common responses to pericardial injury are characterized as acute pericarditis, pericardial effusion, and constrictive pericarditis. Cardiac tamponade is a possibility whenever pericardial fluid accumulates under pressure.

I. ACUTE PERICARDITIS (Table 7-1)

A. Diagnosis of acute pericarditis is based on the presence of chest pain, pericardial friction rub, and changes on the electrocardiogram (ECG). ECG changes evolve through four stages: stage I, diffuse ST segment elevation and PR segment depression; stage II, normalization of the ST and PR segments; stage III, widespread T-wave inversions; and stage IV, normalization of the T waves.
B. Treatment. Salicylates or nonsteroidal anti-inflammatory drugs may be useful in decreasing pericardial inflammation, and symptomatic pain relief can be provided by oral analgesics such as codeine. Corticosteroids can relieve symptoms of acute pericarditis but may be associated with an increased incidence of relapse and is reserved for patients who do not respond to conventional therapy.
C. Relapsing Pericarditis may follow acute pericarditis of any cause but is rarely life threatening. Treatment may include standard treatments for acute pericarditis and/or corticosteroids (prednisone) or immunosuppressive drugs such as azathioprine.
D. Pericarditis may be infective or autoimmune and can follow cardiac surgery, blunt or penetrating trauma, hemopericardium, or epicardial pacemaker implantation.

II. PERICARDIAL EFFUSION AND CARDIAC TAMPONADE

Cardiac tamponade occurs when buildup of the fluid in the pericardial space impairs cardiac filling.

TABLE 7-1	Causes of Acute Pericarditis and Pericardial Effusion

Infectious
- Viral
- Bacterial
- Fungal
- Tuberculous

Postmyocardial infarction (Dressler's syndrome)

Posttraumatic/postcardiotomy

Metastatic disease

Drug induced

Mediastinal radiation

Systemic disease
- Rheumatoid arthritis
- Systemic lupus erythematosus
- Scleroderma

A. Signs and Symptoms of a pericardial effusion depend on its size and duration. Acute changes in pericardial volume as small as 100 mL may result in cardiac tamponade. Larger volumes can accumulate if the effusion develops gradually. Right atrial pressure increases as pericardial fluid pressure increases.

  1. Cardiac Tamponade.
   a. Clinical Signs and Symptoms (Table 7-2)
      1.) Cardiac output is maintained as long as central venous pressure exceeds right ventricular end-diastolic pressure.
      2.) Loculated pericardial effusion may selectively compress one or more cardiac chambers, producing localized cardiac tamponade.

B. Diagnosis. Echocardiography is the most accurate and practical method for diagnosing pericardial effusion and cardiac tamponade. Computed tomography (CT) and magnetic resonance imaging (MRI) are also useful in detecting both pericardial effusion and pericardial thickening.

TABLE 7-2	Signs and Symptoms of Cardiac Tamponade

- Large effusions—compression of adjacent structures; dyspnea, cough, chest pain, hoarseness, hiccups, dysphagia
- Elevation of jugular venous pressure (distension of the jugular vein during inspiration is called Kussmaul's sign)
- Pulsus paradoxus (decrease in systolic blood pressure >10 mm Hg during inspiration)
- Hypotension
- Low voltage on ECG
- Equalization of right and left atrial pressures and right ventricular pressures
- Activation of the sympathetic nervous system

C. Treatment. Removal of fluid is required for definitive treatment and should be performed when central venous pressure is increased.

D. Temporizing Measures to maintain stroke volume until definitive treatment of cardiac tamponade can be instituted include expanding intravascular volume, administering catecholamines to increase myocardial contractility, and correcting metabolic acidosis resulting from low cardiac output.

E. Management of Anesthesia. General anesthesia and positive-pressure ventilation in the presence of hemodynamically significant cardiac tamponade can result in life-threatening hypotension due to anesthesia-induced peripheral vasodilation, direct myocardial depression, or decreased venous return from the increased intrathoracic pressure associated with positive-pressure ventilation.

    1. Pericardiocentesis under local anesthesia is the preferred initial management of hypotensive patients with cardiac tamponade.

    2. If it is not possible to relieve cardiac tamponade before induction of anesthesia, the principal goals of anesthetic induction are to maintain adequate cardiac output and blood pressure (**Table 7-3**).

III. CONSTRICTIVE PERICARDITIS

Chronic constrictive pericarditis is characterized by fibrous scarring and adhesions that obliterate the pericardial cavity, creating a "rigid shell" around the heart. Subacute constrictive pericarditis is fibroelastic.

A. Signs and Symptoms (Table 7-4)

B. Diagnosis of constrictive pericarditis depends on the confirmation of an increased central venous pressure without other signs or symptoms of heart disease. Features of constrictive pericarditis may also be present in patients with restrictive cardiomyopathy, but several features help to distinguish these two entities (**Table 7-5**).

C. Treatment of constrictive pericarditis consists of surgical stripping and removal of the adherent constricting pericardium. This procedure may result in considerable bleeding from the epicardial surface of the heart.

TABLE 7-3 Management of Anesthesia in Patients with Cardiac Tamponade
• Avoid or mitigate decreases in myocardial contractility, heart rate, and systemic vascular resistance during induction (ketamine, combined nitrous-narcotic technique with pancuronium).
• Avoid increases in intrathoracic pressure (coughing, straining).
• Minimize time of initiation of positive-pressure ventilation to incision whenever possible.
• Administer intravenous fluids to maintain preload.
• Administer catecholamines to maintain cardiac output.
• Monitor central venous pressure, intra-arterial pressure.
• Anticipate hypertensive response after surgical relief of tamponade.

TABLE 7-4 Signs and Symptoms of Constrictive Pericarditis

- Decreased exercise tolerance and fatigue
- Venous congestion signs that mimic right-sided heart failure: jugular venous distension, hepatic congestion, ascites, peripheral edema
- Equalization of intracardiac pressures
- Atrial arrhythmias
- Pulsus paradoxus usually *not* seen (seen in tamponade)
- Kussmaul's sign *more commonly* seen than in tamponade
- Early diastolic sound heard "pericardial knock" (not usually seen in tamponade)

TABLE 7-5 Differentiation of Constrictive Pericarditis from Restrictive Cardiomyopathy

Feature	Constrictive Pericarditis	Restrictive Cardiomyopathy
Medical history	Previous pericarditis, cardiac surgery, trauma, radiotherapy, connective tissue disease	No such history
Mitral or tricuspid regurgitation	Usually absent	Often present
Ventricular septal movement with respiration	Movement toward left ventricle on inspiration	Little movement toward left ventricle
Respiratory variation in mitral and tricuspid flow velocity	Greater than 25% in most cases	Less than 15% in most cases
Equilibration of diastolic pressures in all cardiac chambers	Within 5 mm Hg in nearly all cases	In only a small proportion of cases
Respiratory variation of ventricular peak systolic pressures	Right and left ventricular peak systolic pressures are out of phase (discordant)	Right and left ventricular peak systolic pressures are in phase
MRI/CT	Show pericardial thickening in most cases	Rarely shows pericardial thickening
Endomyocardial biopsy	Normal or nonspecific	Shows amyloid in some cases

Adapted from Hancock EW: Differential diagnosis of restrictive cardiomyopathy and constrictive pericarditis. Heart 2001;86:343–349.

D. Management of Anesthesia. Anesthetic drugs and techniques should be chosen that minimize changes in heart rate, systemic vascular resistance, venous return, and myocardial contractility. Optimization of intravascular volume is essential. When hemodynamic compromise (hypotension) is present prior to surgery, management of anesthesia is as described for cardiac tamponade. Invasive monitoring of arterial and central venous pressure is useful because removal of adherent pericardium may result in significant fluid/blood losses. Cardiac dysrhythmias are common.

IV. PERICARDIAL AND CARDIAC TRAUMA

A. Pericardial Trauma

1. Diagnosis. Suspicion of pericardial trauma/pericardial rupture could be raised when unexplained alterations in pulse and blood pressure occur after initial resuscitation, especially if a sternal fracture and/or multiple rib fractures are present. Other indications may be mediastinal air on a chest radiograph or radiographic evidence of cardiac herniation.

2. Treatment. Severe lacerations associated with hemodynamic instability and cardiac herniation require emergency thoracotomy.

B. Myocardial Contusion

1. Signs and Symptoms typically include chest pain and palpitations in the setting of recent chest trauma. Cardiac failure is uncommon.

2. Diagnosis. ECG changes are nonspecific. Serum troponin I and T may be elevated. Echocardiography may demonstrate impaired ventricular wall motion, valvular regurgitation, or pericardial effusion.

3. Treatment of myocardial contusion is supportive, consisting of hemodynamic support and management of dysrhythmias. When anesthesia and surgery are anticipated in patients with suspected myocardial contusion, invasive hemodynamic monitoring is recommended. Anesthetic drugs that depress myocardial function should be avoided. A cardioverter/defibrillator and drugs for dysrhythmia treatment should be immediately available.

CHAPTER 8

Vascular Disease

The incidence of perioperative cardiac complications is higher in patients undergoing vascular surgery than the general population. Vascular surgery patients are at a particularly high risk of perioperative myocardial infarction, but the risk differs based on the type of vascular surgery performed.

I. DISEASES OF THE THORACIC AND ABDOMINAL AORTA

Diseases of the aorta are most often aneurysmal. Occlusive disease is more likely to occur in peripheral arteries. The aorta and its major branches are affected by two entities that may be present simultaneously or may occur at different stages of the same disease process. An aneurysm is a dilation of all three layers of the aorta. An aortic dissection occurs when a tear in the intima allows blood to create an extraluminal channel called the false lumen, potentially compromising blood flow to the aortic branch arteries. Aneurysms and dissections can both rupture, with rapid exsanguination.

II. ANEURYSMS AND DISSECTION OF THE THORACIC AORTA

A. Etiology (**Table 8-1**)
B. Classification (**Fig. 8-1**)
C. Signs and Symptoms (**Table 8-2**)
D. Diagnosis. Widening of the mediastinum on chest radiograph or computed tomography (CT) and magnetic resonance imaging (MRI) may identify thoracic aortic disease. In acute aortic dissection, transesophageal echocardiography with color Doppler imaging is most useful. Angiography of the aorta may be required for patients undergoing elective surgery on the thoracic aorta to define relevant anatomy.

TABLE 8-1	Etiology of Thoracic Aortic Aneurysm and Dissection
Systemic hypertension	
Congenital disorders of connective tissue (e.g., Marfan syndrome, Ehlers-Danlos syndrome, bicuspid aortic valve)	
Deceleration injury	
Blunt trauma	
Surgical manipulation of the aorta	
Pregnancy	

E. Preoperative Evaluation. Myocardial ischemia/infarction, respiratory failure, renal failure, and stroke are the principal causes of morbidity and mortality associated with thoracic aortic surgery; preoperative assessment of the function of these organ systems is needed. Cigarette smoking and chronic obstructive pulmonary disease (COPD) are important predictors of respiratory failure after thoracic aortic surgery. Patients with severe stenosis of one or both common or internal carotid arteries should be considered for carotid endarterectomy before elective surgery on the thoracic aorta.

F. Indications for Surgery. Thoracic aortic aneurysm repair is indicated when aneurysm size exceeds a diameter of 5 cm. Ascending and aortic arch

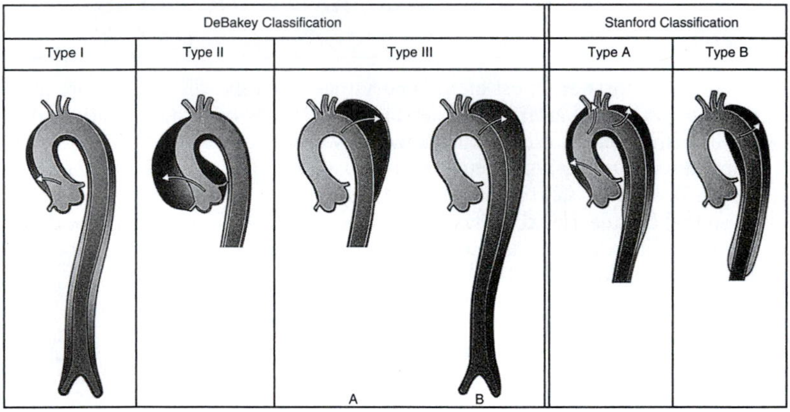

Figure 8-1 • The two most widely used classifications of aortic dissection. The DeBakey classification includes three types: Type I, the intimal tear usually originates in the proximal ascending aorta and the dissection involves the ascending aorta and variable lengths of the aortic arch and descending and abdominal aorta; type II, the dissection is confined to the ascending aorta; type III, the dissection is confined to the descending thoracic aorta (type IIIa) or extends into the abdominal aorta and iliac arteries (type IIIb). The Stanford classification has two types: Type A, all cases in which the ascending aorta is involved by the dissection, with or without involvement of the arch or the descending aorta; type B, cases in which the ascending aorta is not involved. (From Kouchoukos NT, Dougenis D: Surgery of the thoracic aorta. N Engl J Med 1997;336:1876–1888. Copyright 1997 Massachusetts Medical Society with permission.)

TABLE 8-2 Signs and Symptoms of Aneurysms and Dissections of the Thoracic Aorta

- Often symptomatic
- Signs and symptoms due to local compression of adjacent structures; hoarseness, stridor, dysphagia, dyspnea, plethora, and facial edema due to superior vena cava obstruction
- Congestive heart failure due to aortic regurgitation
- Excruciating tearing chest pain of chest, neck, or between the shoulder blades
- Diminished peripheral pulses
- Stroke
- Paraplegia
- Hypertension
- Peripheral vasoconstriction
- Myocardial infarction
- Cardiac tamponade

dissection requires emergent or urgent surgery. Descending thoracic aortic dissection is generally associated with better survival compared with dissection of the ascending aorta and is rarely treated with urgent surgery.

1. Type A Dissection. In hospital mortality is approx 27% in surgically treated patients and 56% in those treated medically. Long-term survival rates are 90% to 96% versus 69% to 89%, respectively.

2. Ascending Aorta. All patients with acute dissection involving the ascending aorta should be considered candidates for surgery.

3. Aortic Arch. Resection of the aortic arch requires cardiopulmonary bypass, profound hypothermia, and a period of circulatory arrest. Neurologic deficits are the major complications, occurring in 3% to 18% of patients.

4. Descending Thoracic Aorta. Elective resection is advisable if the aneurysm exceeds 5 to 6 cm in diameter or if symptoms are present. Patients with an uncomplicated acute type B aortic dissection can be treated with medical therapy consisting of intra-arterial monitoring of systemic blood pressure and urinary output and administration of drugs to control blood pressure and the force of left ventricular contraction (β-blockers, nitroprusside). Surgery is indicated for patients with type B aortic dissection with signs of impending rupture, ischemia of the legs, abdominal viscera, or spinal cord and/or renal failure.

5. Endovascular Repair by placement of intraluminal stent grafts to treat patients with aneurysms of the descending thoracic aorta may be particularly useful in the elderly and in those with coexisting medical conditions, such as hypertension, chronic obstructive pulmonary disease, and renal insufficiency.

G. Unique Risks of Surgery. Surgical resection of thoracic aortic aneurysms can be associated with spinal cord ischemia (anterior spinal artery syndrome), the potential for adverse hemodynamic responses such as myocardial ischemia and heart failure, and renal insufficiency.

1. Anterior Spinal Artery Syndrome presents as flaccid paralysis of the lower extremities and bowel and bladder dysfunction. Sensation and proprioception are spared.

   a. Spinal Cord Blood Supply. The spinal cord is supplied by one anterior spinal artery and two posterior spinal arteries. The anterior spinal artery begins at the fusion of branches of both vertebral arteries and is reinforced by 6 to 8 radicular arteries, the largest of which is the artery of Adamkiewicz. Damage can result from surgical resection of the artery of Adamkiewicz or exclusion of the origin of the artery by the cross-clamp. Anterior spinal artery blood flow is then reduced directly, and collateral blood flow is also reduced because aortic pressure distal to the cross-clamp is very low.

   b. Risk Factors. A major risk factor for paraplegia is a duration of aortic cross-clamping longer than 30 minutes. Prolonged cross-clamp (X-clamp) time warrants additional protective techniques for spinal cord protection, such as partial circulatory assistance (left atrium–to–femoral artery shunt); reimplantation of critical intercostal arteries when possible; cerebrospinal fluid drainage; maintenance of proximal hypertension during cross-clamping; reduction of spinal cord metabolism by moderate hypothermia (30° to 32°C); avoidance of hyperglycemia; and the use of mannitol, corticosteroids, and/or calcium channel blockers.

2. Hemodynamic Responses to Aortic Cross-Clamping. Thoracic aortic clamping and unclamping are associated with severe hemodynamic and homeostatic disturbances in virtually all organ systems due to decrease in blood flow distal to the X-clamp and substantial increase in blood flow above the level of aortic occlusion. Increased systemic vascular resistance (SVR), decreased cardiac output (CO), and no change in heart rate (HR) are common. The level of X-clamp is critical to the nature of hemodynamic change: minimal with infrarenal X-clamp, and dramatic with intrathoracic X-clamp.

   a. Vasodilators (nitroprusside, nitroglycerin) may reduce clamp-induced decreases in CO and EF.

   b. Perfusion Pressures Distal to the X-Clamp are decreased and may be adversely affected by vasodilator therapy, compromising perfusion of distal organs. Drugs and volume replacement must be adjusted to maintain distal aortic perfusion pressure even if that results in an increase in blood pressure proximal to the clamp.

   c. Increase in Cerebrospinal Fluid (CSF) Pressure and decrease in anterior spinal artery pressure occurs with X-clamping the thoracic aorta. CSF drainage might increase spinal cord blood flow and decrease the incidence of neurologic complications.

3. Hemodynamic Responses to Aortic Unclamping include substantial decreases in SVR and systemic blood pressure. Gradual release of the aortic clamp is recommended to allow time for volume replacement and to slow the washout of the vasoactive and cardiodepressant mediators from ischemic tissues. Correction of metabolic acidosis does not significantly influence the degree of hypotension following aortic declamping.

H. Management of Anesthesia

1. Proper Monitoring is more important than the selection of specific anesthetic drugs (**Table 8-3**).

TABLE 8-3 Anesthesia Management: Monitoring During Thoracic Aortic Surgery

System Monitored	Management Considerations
Systemic blood pressure	Place arterial catheter in right upper extremity and femoral artery. • X-clamp proximal to the left subclavian artery will prevent monitoring of blood pressure if catheter is in the left upper extremity. • Loss of pressure tracing warns of innominate artery occlusion. • Simultaneous blood pressure monitoring allows assessment of cerebral perfusion pressure and distal organ perfusion pressure. • Common recommendation: Maintain upper extremity mean arterial pressure (MAP) $\geq$ 100 mm Hg, and lower extremity MAP $\geq$ 50 mm Hg during X-clamp.
Neurologic function	• Somatosensory evoked potentials are not helpful. • Motor evoked potentials may reflect anterior spinal cord function but are not useful in the presence of muscle relaxants.
Cardiac function	Perform transesophageal echocardiography. Insert pulmonary artery catheter.
Intravascular volume	Maintain urine flow; consider diuretics, mannitol.
Induction and maintenance of anesthesia	Selective endobronchial intubation facilitates surgical exposure. Volatile agents and opioids are commonly used.

2. Temporary Shunts (proximal aorta–to–femoral artery or left atrium–to–femoral artery shunts) or partial cardiopulmonary bypass may be considered when attempting to maintain renal and spinal cord perfusion.

I. **Postoperative Management.** Amelioration of pain is essential for patient comfort and to facilitate coughing and maneuvers designed to prevent atelectasis. If neuraxial analgesia is used during the immediate postoperative period, opioids are preferred over local anesthetics to prevent masking of anterior spinal artery syndrome. Patients recovering from thoracic aortic aneurysm resection are at risk of developing cardiac, pulmonary, and renal failure during the immediate postoperative period. Systemic hypertension may require treatment with drugs such as nitroglycerin, nitroprusside, hydralazine, and labetalol.

II. ANEURYSMS OF THE ABDOMINAL AORTA

A. **Diagnosis.** Abdominal aortic aneurysms are usually detected as asymptomatic, pulsatile abdominal masses. Abdominal ultrasonography, CT, and MRI are useful for accurate measurement of aneurysm size and evaluation of relevant vascular anatomy.

B. Treatment. Surgery is usually recommended for abdominal aortic aneurysms larger than 5 cm in diameter. Endovascular aneurysm repair is an alternative to surgical repair.

C. Preoperative Evaluation. Coexisting medical conditions, especially coronary artery disease, chronic obstructive pulmonary disease, and renal dysfunction, are important to identify preoperatively. Myocardial ischemia/infarction is responsible for most postoperative deaths following elective abdominal aortic aneurysm resection. Preoperative evaluation of cardiac function might include stress testing with or without echocardiography or radionuclide imaging. Severe reductions in vital capacity and forced expiratory volume in 1 second and abnormal renal function significantly increase the risk of elective aneurysm repair.

D. Rupture of an Abdominal Aortic Aneurysm. The classic triad of hypotension, back pain, and a pulsatile abdominal mass is present in only about half of patients.

   1. Stable Patients. Exsanguination may be prevented by clotting and the tamponade effect of the retroperitoneum. Euvolemic resuscitation is deferred until the aortic rupture is surgically controlled in the operating room, because euvolemic resuscitation and increase in blood pressure without surgical control of bleeding may lead to loss of retroperitoneal tamponade, further bleeding, hypotension, and death.

   2. Unstable Patients with a suspected ruptured abdominal aortic aneurysm require immediate operation and control of the proximal aorta without preoperative confirmatory testing or optimal volume resuscitation.

E. Management of Anesthesia (Table 8-4). Management of anesthesia for resection of an abdominal aortic aneurysm requires consideration of commonly associated medical conditions of ischemic heart disease, hypertension, chronic obstructive pulmonary disease, diabetes mellitus, and renal dysfunction.

F. Postoperative Management

   1. Adequate Analgesia either with neuraxial opioids or patient-controlled analgesia is very important in facilitating early tracheal extubation.

   2. Systemic Hypertension is common during the postoperative period and may be more likely in patients with preoperative hypertension.

TABLE 8-4	Anesthesia Considerations in Abdominal Aortic Aneurysm Resection
Monitoring	• Intra-arterial pressure monitoring • PA catheter, particularly in patients with history of LV dysfunction or history of previous MI and when suprarenal X-clamping is anticipated • Consider echocardiography • Urine output monitoring
Anesthetic maintenance	• Volatile agents and opioids • Consider combined GA/epidural anesthesia
Fluid management	• Administration of crystalloid and colloid prior to unclamping to minimize declamping hypotension

GA, general anesthetic; LV, left ventricular; MI, myocardial infarction.

G. Endovascular Aortic Aneurysm Repair involves percutaneous placement of stents via small incisions over the femoral vessels, under general or regional anesthesia. Monitoring consists of at least intravascular blood pressure and urine output monitoring. The potential for conversion to an open aneurysm repair must be considered.

III. PERIPHERAL VASCULAR DISEASE

Peripheral arterial disease results in compromised blood flow to the extremities. Chronic impairment of blood flow to the extremities is most often due to atherosclerosis, whereas arterial embolism is most likely to be responsible for acute arterial occlusion. Vasculitis may also be responsible for compromised peripheral blood flow (**Table 8-5**). An ankle-brachial index (ratio of systolic blood pressure at the ankle to the systolic blood pressure in the brachial artery) of less than 0.90 correlates extremely well with angiogram-positive disease.

A. Risk Factors associated with development of peripheral atherosclerosis are similar to those that cause ischemic heart disease: diabetes mellitus, hypertension, tobacco use, dyslipidemia, hyperhomocysteinemia, and a family history of premature atherosclerosis.

B. Signs and Symptoms. Intermittent claudication and rest pain are the principal symptoms of peripheral arterial disease. Decreased or absent arterial pulses are the most reliable physical findings associated with peripheral arterial disease. Bruits, subcutaneous atrophy, hair loss, coolness, pallor, cyanosis, and dependent rubor in the extremities may be additional findings.

C. Diagnostic Tests. Doppler ultrasonography and the resulting pulse volume waveform are used to identify arterial vessels with stenotic lesions.

TABLE 8-5 Peripheral Vascular Diseases
Chronic peripheral arterial occlusive disease (atherosclerosis)
Distal abdominal aorta or iliac arteries
Femoral arteries
Subclavian steal syndrome
Coronary-subclavian steal syndrome
Acute peripheral arterial occlusive disease (embolism)
Systemic vasculitis
Takayasu's arteritis
Thromboangiitis obliterans
Wegener's granulomatosis
Temporal arteritis
Polyarteritis nodosa
Other vascular syndromes
Raynaud's phenomenon
Kawasaki syndrome

D. Treatment

1. Medical Therapy includes exercise programs and identification and treatment or modification of risk factors for atherosclerosis, such as smoking cessation, lipid-lowering therapy, and treatment of hypertension.

2. Revascularization procedures are indicated in patients with disabling claudication, ischemic rest pain, or impending limb loss.

a. Percutaneous Transluminal Angioplasty of iliac arteries has a high initial success rate that may be further improved by stent placement. Femoral and popliteal artery percutaneous transluminal angioplasty has a lower success rate than iliac artery percutaneous transluminal angioplasty.

b. Surgical Procedures used for vascular reconstruction include aortobifemoral bypass, axillobifemoral bypass, femoral-femoral bypass, femoropopliteal and tibioperoneal reconstruction. Amputation is necessary for patients with advanced limb ischemia in whom revascularization is not possible or has failed.

1.) *Operative* risk of reconstructive peripheral arterial surgery is primarily related to the presence of associated atherosclerotic vascular disease, particularly ischemic heart disease and cerebrovascular disease.

2.) *Mortality* is usually a result of myocardial infarction in patients with preoperative evidence of ischemic heart disease, a history of coronary artery bypass grafting, or congestive heart failure. In patients with severe or unstable ischemic heart disease, percutaneous coronary intervention or coronary artery bypass grafting might be considered before performing revascularization surgery. In patients with stable coronary artery disease, outcomes are not improved by prior coronary revascularization.

E. Management of Anesthesia.

Management of anesthesia for surgical revascularization of the lower extremities incorporates principles similar to those described for the management of patients for abdominal aortic aneurysm repair.

1. Perioperative β-Blockade. The American College of Cardiology/American Heart Association identify the following patients as candidates for perioperative β-blockade: (1) patients undergoing vascular surgery with or without evidence of preoperative ischemia and with or without high or intermediate risk factors, (2) patients receiving long-term β-blocker therapy, and (3) patients undergoing vascular surgery even if they have only low risk factors.

2. Regional (Epidural or Spinal) Anesthesia promotes increased graft blood flow, postoperative analgesia, less activation of the coagulation system, and fewer postoperative respiratory complications. Placement of an epidural catheter at least 1 hour before intraoperative heparinization is not associated with an increased incidence of untoward neurologic events.

3. Infrarenal Aortic Cross-Clamping and Unclamping is associated with fewer hemodynamic derangements than occur in patients undergoing resection of an abdominal aortic aneurysm.

4. Monitoring. Central venous catheter or echocardiography may be useful.

F. Postoperative Management

includes provision of analgesia, treatment of fluid and electrolyte derangements, and control of heart rate and blood pressure to reduce the incidence of myocardial ischemia/infarction.

Dexmedetomidine, an α_2-agonist, can attenuate the increase in heart rate and plasma catecholamine concentrations.

G. Subclavian Steal Syndrome. Occlusion of the subclavian or innominate artery proximal to the origin of the vertebral artery results in diversion of blood flow from the ipsilateral vertebral artery to the distal subclavian artery. Central nervous system symptoms (syncope, vertigo, ataxia, hemiplegia) and/or arm ischemia are usually present and accentuated by exercise of the ipsilateral arm. Pulse is absent or diminished in the ipsilateral arm, and systolic blood pressure is likely to be at least 20 mm Hg lower in that arm. Subclavian endarterectomy may be curative.

H. Coronary-Subclavian Steal Syndrome is a rare complication of using the internal mammary artery (IMA) for coronary revascularization. Proximal stenosis in the left subclavian artery leads to reversal of blood flow through the patent IMA graft. Symptoms include angina pectoris, central nervous system ischemia, and a 20-mm Hg or more decrease in systolic blood pressure in the ipsilateral arm.

IV. ACUTE ARTERIAL OCCLUSION

Acute arterial occlusion differs from the gradual development of arterial occlusion caused by atherosclerosis and is usually a result of cardiogenic embolism.

A. Signs and Symptoms include intense pain, paresthesias, motor weakness distal to the site of arterial occlusion, loss of a palpable peripheral pulse, cool skin, and sharply demarcated skin color changes (pallor or cyanosis) distal to the arterial occlusion.

B. Diagnosis is confirmed by arteriography.

C. Treatment is surgical embolectomy and anticoagulation. Intra-arterial thrombolysis may be effective.

D. Management of Anesthesia is similar to that for patients with chronic peripheral arterial disease.

V. SYSTEMIC VASCULITIS

Peripheral vascular disease may manifest as part of a systemic vasculitis due to a connective tissue disease, sepsis, or malignancy.

A. Takayasu's Arteritis is an idiopathic, progressive occlusive vasculitis that causes narrowing, thrombosis, or aneurysms of systemic and pulmonary arteries. It is diagnosed definitively based on contrast angiography.

    1. Signs and Symptoms (Table 8-6)

    2. Treatment is Corticosteroids. Anticoagulation may be indicated in some patients.

    3. Management of Anesthesia (Table 8-7)

B. Thromboangiitis Obliterans (Buerger's Disease) is an inflammatory vasculitis leading to occlusion of small- and medium-sized arteries and veins in the extremities. The diagnosis is confirmed by biopsy of active vascular lesions.

    1. Signs and Symptoms include claudication of the upper or lower extremities. Raynaud's phenomenon is common.

    2. Treatment is smoking cessation. Surgical revascularization is not usually feasible because of the involvement of small distal blood vessels.

TABLE 8-6	Signs and Symptoms of Takayasu's Arteritis
Central Nervous System	
Vertigo	
Visual disturbances	
Syncope	
Seizures	
Cerebral ischemia or infarction	
Cardiovascular System	
Multiple occlusions of peripheral arteries	
Ischemic heart disease	
Cardiac valve dysfunction	
Cardiac conduction defects	
Lungs	
Pulmonary hypertension	
Ventilation-perfusion mismatch	
Kidneys	
Renal artery stenosis	
Musculoskeletal System	
Ankylosing spondylitis	
Rheumatoid arthritis	

TABLE 8-7	Anesthesia Considerations in Takayasu's Arteritis
Preoperative considerations	• Monitor for adrenal suppression due to chronic corticosteroid use. • In laryngoscopy and intubation, consider that neck hyperextension can compromise blood flow through the carotid arteries.
Choice of anesthetic technique	• Regional may not be possible due to anticoagulation. • Hypotension can compromise perfusion to vital organs. • Adequate arterial pressure must be maintained.
Monitoring	• Noninvasive blood pressure measurement may be difficult due to subclavian and brachial artery stenosis. • EEG monitoring may be helpful for detecting cerebral ischemia.

3. Management of Anesthesia requires avoidance of events that might damage already ischemic extremities. Positioning and padding of pressure and maintenance of normothermia are critical. Systemic blood pressure should be measured noninvasively. If regional anesthetic techniques are selected, epinephrine should be omitted from the local anesthetic solution to avoid the possibility of accentuating vasospasm.

C. Wegener's Granulomatosis is characterized by formation of necrotizing granulomas in inflamed blood vessels in multiple organ systems (**Table 8-8**).

1. Treatment with cyclophosphamide can produce remissions in approximately 90% of patients.

2. Management of Anesthesia in patients with Wegener's granulomatosis requires an appreciation of the widespread organ system involvement of this disease. Immunosuppression results from cyclophosphamide treatment. Avoidance of trauma during laryngoscopy is important because bleeding from granulomas and dislodgment of friable ulcerated tissue can occur. A smaller than expected endotracheal tube may be required if the glottic opening is narrowed by granulomatous changes. Arteritis involving peripheral vessels may interfere with placement of an indwelling arterial catheter to monitor blood pressure or limit the frequency of arterial punctures to obtain samples for blood gas analysis.

TABLE 8-8 Signs and Symptoms of Wegener's Granulomatosis
Central Nervous System
Cerebral aneurysms
Peripheral neuropathy
Respiratory Tract and Lungs
Sinusitis
Laryngeal stenosis
Epiglottic destruction
Ventilation-perfusion mismatch
Pneumonia
Hemoptysis
Bronchial destruction
Cardiovascular System
Cardiac valve destruction
Disturbances of cardiac conduction
Myocardial ischemia
Kidneys
Hematuria
Azotemia
Renal failure

D. Temporal Arteritis is inflammation of the arteries of the head and neck, manifesting as headache, scalp tenderness, or jaw claudication. Prompt initiation of treatment with corticosteroids is indicated in patients with visual symptoms to prevent blindness. Evidence of arteritis on a biopsy specimen of the temporal artery is present in approximately 90% of patients.

E. Polyarteritis Nodosa most often occurs in women, often in association with hepatitis B antigenemia and allergic reactions to drugs. Renal failure is the most common cause of death.

> **1. Diagnosis** depends on histologic evidence of vasculitis on biopsy and demonstration of characteristic aneurysms on arteriography.
>
> **2. Treatment** usually includes corticosteroids and cyclophosphamide, removal of offending drugs, and treatment of underlying diseases such as cancer.
>
> **3. Management of Anesthesia** in patients with polyarteritis nodosa should take into consideration the likelihood of co-existing renal disease, cardiac disease, and systemic hypertension. Supplemental corticosteroids may be indicated.

F. Kawasaki Syndrome (mucocutaneous lymph node syndrome) occurs primarily in children and manifests as fever, conjunctivitis, inflammation of the mucous membranes, swollen erythematous hands and feet, truncal rash, and cervical lymphadenopathy and vasculitis.

> **1. Treatment** consists of γ-globulin and aspirin.
>
> **2. Management of Anesthesia** must consider the possibility of intraoperative myocardial ischemia.

G. Raynaud's Phenomenon is episodic vasospastic ischemia of the digits. It affects women more often than men.

> **1. Classification.** Raynaud's phenomenon is categorized as primary (Raynaud's disease) or secondary when it is associated with other diseases such as scleroderma or systemic lupus erythematosus.
>
> **2. Etiology.** Mechanisms postulated to cause Raynaud's phenomenon include increased sympathetic nervous system activity, digital vascular hyperreactivity to vasoconstrictive stimuli, circulating vasoactive hormones, and decreased intravascular pressure.
>
> **3. Diagnosis.** Noninvasive tests that can be used to evaluate patients with Raynaud's phenomenon include digital pulse volume recording and measurement of digital systolic blood pressure and digital blood flow. Raynaud's phenomenon is the initial complaint in most patients who present with a limited form of scleroderma called CREST syndrome. CREST is an acronym for subcutaneous calcinosis, Raynaud's phenomenon, esophageal dysmotility, sclerodactyly (scleroderma limited to the fingers), and telangiectasia.
>
> **4. Treatment** includes protecting the hands and feet from exposure to cold. Calcium channel blockers such as nifedipine and sympathetic nervous system antagonists such as prazosin can be used to treat Raynaud's phenomenon. In rare instances, surgical sympathectomy might be considered for treatment of persistent, severe digital ischemia.
>
> **5. Management of Anesthesia.** Increasing the ambient temperature of the operating room and maintaining normothermia are basic considerations. Systemic blood pressure is usually monitored via a noninvasive technique. Regional anesthesia is acceptable for peripheral operations in patients with

Raynaud's phenomenon, but it may be prudent not to include epinephrine in the anesthetic solution because the catecholamine could provoke undesirable vasoconstriction.

VI. CAROTID ARTERY DISEASE

Cerebrovascular accidents (strokes) are characterized by sudden neurologic deficits due to ischemic, hemorrhagic, or thrombotic events. Hemorrhagic stroke is classified as intracerebral or subarachnoid. A transient ischemic attack is a sudden vascular-related focal neurologic deficit that resolves within 24 hours.

A. **Cerebrovascular Anatomy.** The blood supply to the brain (20% of cardiac output) is brought via two pairs of blood vessels: the internal carotid arteries and the vertebral arteries. These vessels join to form the major intracranial blood vessels (anterior cerebral arteries, middle cerebral arteries, posterior cerebral arteries) and the circle of Willis.

1. **Etiology of Acute Ischemic Stroke** is usually cardioembolism, large-vessel atherothromboembolism (such as from disease at the carotid bifurcation), or small-vessel occlusive disease (lacunar infarction). Echocardiography is very useful in evaluating the source of cardioembolism.

2. **Risk Factors for Ischemic Stroke** include hypertension, cigarette smoking, hyperlipidemia, diabetes mellitus, excessive alcohol consumption (more than six drinks daily), and increased homocysteine levels.

B. **Carotid Endarterectomy.** Surgical treatment of symptomatic carotid artery stenosis greatly decreases the risk of stroke, especially in men with severe carotid stenosis. Surgical treatment for asymptomatic disease is still controversial. Carotid angioplasty and stenting may become alternatives to carotid endarterectomy.

1. **Preoperative Evaluation.** Patients should be examined for co-existing cardiovascular and renal disease. Ischemic heart disease is a major cause of morbidity and mortality following carotid endarterectomy. Patients with severe coronary artery disease and severe carotid occlusive disease present a dilemma. No randomized studies have determined the benefit of combined versus staged procedures. It is useful to establish the usual range of blood pressure for each patient preoperatively to provide a guide for acceptable perfusion pressures during anesthesia and surgery. The effect of a change in head position on cerebral function should also be ascertained, to avoid positions that further impede cerebral blood flow.

2. **Management of Anesthesia** for carotid endarterectomy must meet two goals: maintenance of hemodynamic stability and prompt emergence allowing immediate assessment of neurologic status in the operating room. Carotid endarterectomy can be performed under general anesthesia or under regional (cervical plexus) block, allowing the patient to remain awake to facilitate neurologic assessment during carotid artery cross-clamping. Maintenance of an adequate blood pressure and normocarbia is important because cerebral autoregulation may be abnormal in these patients. Monitoring usually includes an intra-arterial catheter. Patients with poor left ventricular function and/or severe coronary artery disease might require a central venous or pulmonary artery catheter or transesophageal echocardiography. The utility of electroencephalographic (EEG) monitoring

during carotid endarterectomy is limited because EEG may not detect subcortical or small cortical infarcts, false-negative results are not uncommon, and the EEG can be affected by changes in temperature, blood pressure, and depth of anesthesia. Transcranial Doppler ultrasonography allows continuous monitoring of blood flow velocity and the presence of microembolic events.

3. Postoperative Management and Complications include hypertension or hypotension, myocardial ischemia/infarction, development of significant soft-tissue edema or a hematoma in the neck, and the onset of neurologic signs and symptoms of a new stroke or thrombosis at the endarterectomy site. Hypertension is common, and infusion of nitroprusside or nitroglycerin and/or the use of longer-acting drugs such as hydralazine or labetalol are treatment options. Hypotension due to carotid sinus hypersensitivity is usually treated with vasopressors such as phenylephrine.

4. Endovascular Treatment of Carotid Disease may become the leading alternative to carotid endarterectomy. The major complication of carotid stenting is microembolization of atherosclerotic material into the cerebral circulation during the procedure.

VII. PERIPHERAL VENOUS DISEASE

Deep vein thrombosis (usually involving a leg vein) and subsequent pulmonary embolism are a leading cause of postoperative morbidity and mortality. Factors that predispose to thromboembolism are multiple and include events associated with anesthesia and surgery (**Table 8-9**).

TABLE 8-9	Factors Predisposing to Thromboembolism

Venous stasis
- Recent surgery
- Trauma
- Lack of ambulation
- Pregnancy
- Low cardiac output (congestive heart failure, myocardial infarction)
- Stroke

Abnormality of the venous wall
- Varicose veins
- Drug-induced irritation

Hypercoagulable state
- Surgery
- Estrogen therapy (oral contraceptives)
- Cancer
- Deficiencies of endogenous anticoagulants (antithrombin III, protein C, protein S)
- Stress response associated with surgery
- Inflammatory bowel disease

History of previous thromboembolism
- Morbid obesity
- Advanced age

A. Deep Vein Thrombosis (DVT)

1. Diagnosis of DVT by clinical signs is unreliable. Compression ultrasonography, venography, and impedance plethysmography are all used (**Fig. 8-2**). Inherited abnormalities associated with initial and recurrent venous thrombosis/embolism include congenital deficiencies of antithrombin III, protein C, protein S, or plasminogen.

2. Treatment. Anticoagulation is the first-line treatment. Therapy is initiated with heparin (unfractionated or low-molecular-weight heparin) followed by an oral vitamin K antagonist (warfarin), dose-adjusted to achieve a prothrombin time with an international normalized ratio between 2.0 and 3.0. Inferior vena cava filters may be used in patients with recurrent pulmonary embolism despite adequate anticoagulant therapy or in whom anticoagulation is contraindicated.

3. Complications of Anticoagulation include bleeding and immune-mediated thrombocytopenia associated with heparin.

B. Prevention of Venous Thromboembolism

1. Clinical Risk Factors and Recommended Prophylaxis (Table 8-10)

2. Regional Anesthesia is associated with reduced risk (20%–40%) of deep venous thromboembolism and pulmonary embolism following total knee or total hip arthroplasty.

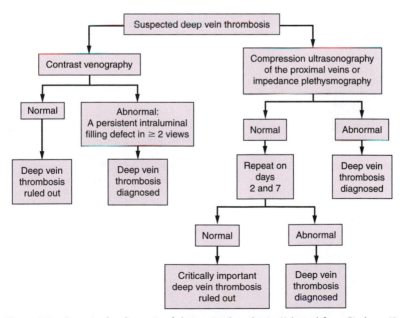

Figure 8-2 • Steps in the diagnosis of deep vein thrombosis. (Adapted from Ginsberg JS: Management of venous thromboembolism. N Engl J Med 1996; 335:1816–1828. Copyright 1996 Massachusetts Medical Society.)

111

TABLE 8-10	Risk and Predisposing Factors for Development of Deep Venous Thrombosis After Surgery or Trauma		
Event	**Low Risk**	**Moderate Risk**	**High Risk**
General surgery	<40 years old Operation < 60 minutes	>40 years old Operation > 60 minutes	>40 years old Operation > 60 minutes Previous deep vein thrombosis Previous pulmonary embolism Extensive trauma Major fractures
Orthopedic surgery			Knee or hip replacement
Trauma			Extensive soft-tissue injury Major fractures Multiple trauma sites
Medical conditions	Pregnancy	Postpartum period Myocardial infarction Congestive heart failure	Stroke
Incidence of deep vein thrombosis without prophylaxis	2%	10%–40%	40%–80%
Symptomatic pulmonary embolism	0.2%	1%–8%	5%–10%
Fatal pulmonary embolism	0.002%	0.1%–0.4%	1%–5%
Recommended steps to minimize deep vein thrombosis	Graduated compression stockings Early ambulation	External pneumatic compression Subcutaneous heparin Intravenous dextran	External pneumatic compression Subcutaneous heparin Intravenous Dextran Vena caval filter Warfarin

Adapted from Weinmann EE, Salzman EW: Deep-vein thrombosis. N Engl J Med 1994;331:1630–1642.

CHAPTER 9

Respiratory Diseases

Pulmonary complications also play an important part in determining long-term mortality after surgery. Preoperative modification of disease severity and patient optimization decrease the incidence of these complications. Respiratory diseases can be divided into the following categories: acute upper respiratory tract infection (URI), asthma, chronic obstructive pulmonary disease (COPD), acute respiratory failure, restrictive lung disease, pulmonary embolism (PE), and lung transplantation.

I. ACUTE UPPER RESPIRATORY TRACT INFECTION

Infectious (viral or bacterial) nasopharyngitis accounts for approximately 95% of all URIs. Noninfectious nasopharyngitis is allergic and vasomotor in origin.

A. Signs and Symptoms of acute URI include sneezing and runny nose. A history of allergies may indicate an allergic etiology rather than infection. With infectious etiologies, there is usually fever, purulent nasal discharge, productive cough, fever, and malaise. The patient may be tachypneic, wheezing, or appear toxic.

B. Diagnosis is usually based on clinical signs and symptoms. Viral cultures and laboratory tests lack sensitivity and are impractical in a busy clinical setting.

C. Management of Anesthesia

　1. Preoperative Considerations. Most studies regarding URIs and postoperative complications have been done in pediatric patients. Patients with systemic signs of infection (fever, purulent rhinitis, productive cough, rhonchi) undergoing elective surgery, particularly airway surgery, are at risk of adverse events, and delaying surgery should be considered. Patients who have had a URI for days or weeks and are stable to improving can be safely managed without postponing surgery. Delaying surgery does not reduce the incidence of adverse respiratory events if anesthesia is administered within 4 weeks of the URI. Airway hyperreactivity may require 6 weeks or more to resolve.

　2. Intraoperative Management of patients with a URI includes adequate hydration, focus on reducing secretions, and limited manipulation of a potentially sensitive airway. The laryngeal mask airway (vs. endotracheal intubation) may reduce the risk of bronchospasm. It has not been proven that prophylactic bronchodilators reduce the incidence of perioperative bronchospasm.

3. Postoperative adverse respiratory events include bronchospasm, laryngospasm, airway obstruction, postintubation croup, desaturation, and atelectasis. Intraoperative and immediate postoperative hypoxemia is common and amenable to treatment with supplemental oxygen.

II. ASTHMA

Asthma is characterized by chronic airway inflammation, reversible expiratory airflow obstruction in response to various stimuli, and bronchial hyperreactivity. It is estimated that asthma affects 4% to 5% of the U.S. population. Bronchial asthma typically appears early in life. Approximately one half of cases develop before age 10 and another third occur before age 40.

A. Signs and Symptoms include wheezing, productive or nonproductive cough, dyspnea, chest discomfort or tightness that may lead to "air hunger," and eosinophilia.

B. Pathogenesis: Allergen-Induced versus Abnormal Autonomic Regulation

1. Evidence for Allergen-Induced Immunologic Model: (1) Atopy is the single greatest risk factor for the development of asthma. (2) A personal and/or family history of allergic diseases is often present. (3) There is usually a positive wheal-and-flare skin reaction to intradermal injection of extracts of airborne antigens. (4) Serum immunoglobulin E levels are increased and/or there is a positive response to provocative tests involving the inhalation of specific antigens. (5) Evidence of genetic linkage of high total serum IgE levels and atopy has been observed.

2. Model of Abnormal Autonomic Nervous System Regulation of Neural Function. Chemical mediators released from mast cells probably interact with the autonomic nervous system. Some chemical mediators can stimulate airway receptors and trigger bronchoconstriction, while other mediators sensitize bronchial smooth muscle to the effects of acetylcholine. Stimulation of muscarinic receptors can facilitate mediator release from mast cells, providing a positive feedback loop for sustained inflammation and bronchoconstriction.

C. Diagnosis

1. Forced Expiratory Volume in 1 second (FEV_1) and maximum mid-expiratory flow rate are direct measures of the severity of expiratory airflow obstruction (**Fig. 9-1** and **Table 9-1**).

2. Flow-Volume Loops show characteristic downward scooping of the expiratory limb of the loop. (**Fig. 9-2**).

3. Mild Asthma is Usually Accompanied by a Normal PaO_2 and $PaCO_2$. Hypocarbia and respiratory alkalosis are the most common arterial blood gas findings in the presence of asthma. Hypercarbia may indicate failure of the skeletal muscles necessary for breathing.

4. The Differential Diagnosis includes viral tracheobronchitis, sarcoidosis, rheumatoid arthritis with bronchiolitis, and extrinsic compression (thoracic aneurysm, mediastinal neoplasm) or intrinsic compression (epiglottitis, croup) of the upper airway, congestive heart failure, pulmonary embolism, and pulmonary edema.

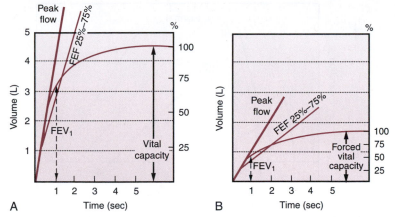

Figure 9-1 • Spirographic changes of a normal subject **(A)** and a patient in bronchospasm **(B)**. The FEV_1 is typically less than 80% of the vital capacity in the presence of obstructive airway disease. Peak flow and maximum mid-expiratory flow rate ($FEF_{25\%-75\%}$) are also decreased in these patients **(B)**. (Adapted from Kingston HGG, Hirshman CA: Perioperative management of the patient with asthma. Anesth Analg 1984;63:844–855).

D. Treatment (Table 9-2). Asthma treatment has two components: (1) "controller" treatments, which modify the airway environment such that acute airway narrowing occurs less frequently (e.g., inhaled and systemic corticosteroids, theophylline, and antileukotrienes) and (2) "reliever" or rescue agents for acute bronchospasm (e.g., β-adrenergic agonists and anticholinergic drugs).
E. Status Asthmaticus is defined as unresolving bronchospasm that, despite treatment, is considered life threatening. Treatment is summarized in **Table 9-3**.

TABLE 9-1	Classification of Asthma Based on Severity of Expiratory Airflow Obstruction			
Severity	**FEV_1 (% Predicted)**	**$FEF_{25\%-75\%}$ (% Predicted)**	**PaO_2 (mm Hg)**	**$PaCO_2$ (mm Hg)**
Mild (asymptomatic)	65–80	60–75	>60	<40
Moderate	50–64	45–59	>60	<45
Marked	35–49	30–44	<60	>50
Severe (status asthmaticus)	<35	<30	<60	>50

$FEF_{25\%-75\%}$ forced exhaled flow at 25% to 75% of forced vital capacity.
Adapted from Kingston HGG, Hirshman CA: Perioperative management of the patient with asthma. Anesth Analg 1984;63:844–855.

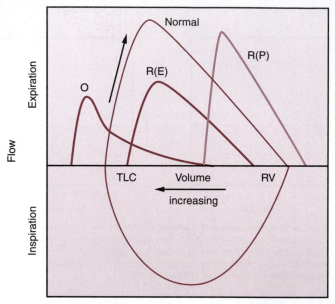

Figure 9-2 • Flow-volume curves in different conditions: O, obstructive disease; R(E), extraparenchymal restrictive disease with limitation in inspiration and expiration; R(P), parenchymal restrictive disease. Forced expiration is plotted in all conditions; forced inspiration is shown only for the normal curve. RV, residual volume; TLC, total lung capacity. By convention, lung volume increases to the left on the abscissa. The *arrow* alongside the normal curve indicates the direction of expiration from TLC to RV. (Adapted from Weinberger SE: Disturbances of respiratory function. In Fauci B, Braunwald E, Isselbacher KJ, et al [eds]: Harrison's Principles of Internal Medicine, 14th ed. New York, McGraw-Hill, 1998.).

F. Management of Anesthesia

1. Preoperative Evaluation requires assessment of disease severity, effectiveness of current therapy, and the potential need for additional therapy prior to surgery. Preoperative evaluation begins with a clinical history to elicit the severity and characteristics of the patient's asthma (**Table 9-4**). Auscultation of the chest to detect wheezing or crepitations is important. Pulmonary function tests (especially FEV_1) before and after bronchodilator therapy may be indicated in patients scheduled for major elective surgery. Measurement of arterial blood gases is indicated if there is any question about the adequacy of ventilation or oxygenation.

a. Preoperative Medication. Anti-inflammatory and bronchodilator therapy should be continued until the time of anesthesia induction. Supplementation with "stress dose" corticosteroids may be indicated before major surgery. Patients should be free of wheezing and have a peak expiratory flow greater than 80% of predicted or at the level of the patient's personal best value prior to surgery.

116

TABLE 9-2 Pharmacologic Agents Used in the Treatment of Asthma

Class	Drug	Actions	Adverse Effects
Anti-inflammatory drugs	Corticosteroids: beclomethasone, triamcinolone, flunisolide, fluticasone, budesonide	Decrease airway inflammation, reduce airway hyperresponsiveness	Dysphonia, myopathy of laryngeal muscles, oropharyngeal candidiasis
	Cromolyn	Inhibit mediator release from mast cells, membrane stabilization	
	Leukotriene modifiers: zafirlukast (Accolate), pranlukast (Ultair), montelukast (Singulair), zileuton (Zyflo)	Reduce synthesis of leukotrienes by inhibiting 5-lipoxygenase enzyme	Increased hepatic enzyme levels
Bronchodilators	β-adrenergic agonists: albuterol, metaproterenol, salmeterol	Stimulate β₂-receptors of tracheobronchial tree	Tachycardia, tremors, dysrhythmias, hypokalemia
	Anticholinergics: ipratropium, atropine, glycopyrrolate	Decrease vagal tone by blocking muscarinic receptors in airway smooth muscle	
Methylxanthines	Theophylline	Increase cAMP by inhibiting phosphodiesterase, block adenosine receptors, release endogenous catecholamines	Disrupted sleep cycle, nervousness, nausea, vomiting, anorexia, headache, dysrhythmias

cAMP, cyclic adenosine monophosphate.

TABLE 9-3	Treatment of Status Asthmaticus

β_2-Agonists by metered-dose inhaled every 15–20 minutes

Intravenous corticosteroids (cortisol 2 mg/kg followed by 0.5 mg/kg/hr or methylprednisolone 60–125 mg every 6 hours)

Supplemental oxygen

Tracheal intubation and mechanical ventilation (when $PaCO_2$ >50 mm Hg)

Empirical broad-spectrum antibiotics

General anesthesia with volatile agents to produce bronchodilation

2. Induction and Maintenance of Anesthesia should aim to suppress airway reflexes to avoid bronchoconstriction in response to mechanical stimulation of the airways.

a. Regional Anesthesia may avoid instrumentation of the airway and tracheal intubation when the operative site is suitable for this.

b. General Anesthesia. Induction of anesthesia with propofol is preferable to thiopental, which is associated with a higher incidence of wheezing. Ketamine may produce smooth muscle relaxation and contribute to decreased airway resistance.

1.) After unconsciousness is produced, the lungs are ventilated with a volatile anesthetic agent to establish a depth of anesthesia sufficient to permit tracheal intubation without precipitating bronchospasm. Intravenous or intratracheal injection of lidocaine 1 to 3 minutes before tracheal intubation can be helpful.

2.) After endotracheal intubation, it may be difficult to differentiate light anesthesia from bronchospasm as the cause of a decrease in pulmonary compliance. Administration of neuromuscular-blocking drugs relieves the difficulty of ventilation due to light anesthesia but has no effect on bronchospasm.

TABLE 9-4	Characteristics of Asthma to Evaluate Preoperatively

Age at onset

Triggering events

  Hospitalization for asthma

  Frequency of emergency department visits

Need for intubation and mechanical ventilation

Allergies

Cough

Sputum characteristics

Current medications

Anesthetic history

3.) Drugs with limited ability to evoke the release of histamine should be selected.

4.) Theoretically, antagonism of neuromuscular blockade with anticholinesterase drugs could precipitate bronchospasm secondary to stimulation of postganglionic cholinergic receptors in airway smooth muscle. Bronchospasm does not predictably occur after administration of anticholinesterase drugs, probably because of the protective bronchodilating effects provided by the simultaneous administration of anticholinergic drugs.

5.) During mechanical ventilation in asthmatic patients, a slow inspiratory flow rate provides optimal distribution of ventilation relative to perfusion. Sufficient time for exhalation is necessary to prevent air trapping. Humidification and warming of inspired gases may be especially helpful.

6.) Maintenance of adequate hydration ensures less viscous airway.

7.) If possible, extubation should occur while anesthesia is still sufficient to suppress hyperreactive airway reflexes. When it is unwise to extubate the trachea before the patient is fully awake, suppressing airway reflexes and/or the risk of bronchospasm by administration of intravenous lidocaine or pretreatment with inhaled bronchodilators should be considered.

3. Intraoperative Bronchospasm is often due to factors other than asthma (**Table 9-5**).

III. CHRONIC OBSTRUCTIVE PULMONARY DISEASE

COPD is characterized by the progressive development of airflow limitation that is not fully reversible. It includes chronic bronchitis with obstruction of small airways and emphysema with enlargement of air sacs, destruction of lung parenchyma, loss of elasticity, and closure of small airways. Risk factors for COPD are (1) cigarette smoking; (2) respiratory infection; (3) occupational exposure to dust especially in coal mining, gold mining, and the textile industry; and (4) genetic factors such as α_1-antitrypsin deficiency.

A. Signs and Symptoms. Physical findings vary with severity of COPD. As expiratory airflow obstruction increases in severity, tachypnea and a prolonged expiratory phase are evident. Breath sounds are decreased, and expiratory wheezes are common.

B. Diagnosis. A chronic productive cough and progressive exercise limitation are the hallmarks of the persistent expiratory airflow obstruction characteristic of COPD (**Tables 9-6** and **9-7**). Patients with predominant chronic bronchitis present with a chronic productive cough, whereas patients with predominant emphysema complain of dyspnea. Wheezing is common with mucus accumulation in the airways and may mimic asthma.

1. Pulmonary Function Tests reveal decreases in the FEV_1/forced vital capacity (FVC) ratio and even greater decreases in the forced expiratory flow between 25% and 75% of vital capacity ($FEF_{25\%-75\%}$). Lung volumes show an increased residual volume and normal to increased functional residual capacity (FRC) and total lung capacity (TLC) (**Fig. 9-3**).

TABLE 9-5	Differential Diagnosis of Intraoperative Bronchospasm and Wheezing

Mechanical obstruction of endotracheal tube

Kinking

Secretions

Overinflation of the tracheal tube cuff

Inadequate depth of anesthesia

Active expiratory efforts

Decreased functional residual capacity

Endobronchial intubation

Pulmonary aspiration

Pulmonary edema

Pulmonary embolus

Pneumothorax

Acute asthmatic attack

2. Chest Radiography. Abnormalities may be minimal, even with severe COPD. Hyperlucency and hyperinflation (flattening of the diaphragm with loss of its normal domed appearance and a very vertical cardiac silhouette) suggest the diagnosis of emphysema.

3. Arterial Blood Gases can be used to categorize patients with COPD as "pink puffers" (PaO_2 usually higher than 60 mm Hg and $PaCO_2$ normal) or

TABLE 9-6	Comparative Features of Chronic Obstructive Pulmonary Disease	
Feature	**Chronic Bronchitis**	**Pulmonary Emphysema**
Mechanism of airway obstruction	Decreased airway lumen due to mucus and inflammation	Loss of elastic recoil
Dyspnea	Moderate	Severe
FEV_1	Decreased	Decreased
PaO_2	Marked decrease ("blue bloater")	Modest decrease ("pink puffer")
$PaCO_2$	Increased	Normal to decreased
Diffusing capacity	Normal	Decreased
Hematocrit	Increased	Normal
Cor pulmonale	Marked	Mild
Prognosis	Poor	Good

Stage	Characteristics
TABLE 9-7	**Spirometric Classification of the Severity of COPD Based on Postbronchodilator FEV_1 Measurements**
0: At risk	Normal spirometry Chronic symptoms (cough, sputum production)
I: Mild COPD	FEV_1/FVC <70% FEV_1 ≥80% predicted, with or without chronic symptoms (cough, sputum production)
II: Moderate COPD	FEV_1/FVC <70% 50% ≤FEV_1, <80% predicted, with or without chronic symptoms (cough, sputum production)
III: Severe COPD	FEV_1/FVC <70% 30% ≤FEV_1, <50% predicted, with or without chronic symptoms (cough, sputum production)
IV: Very severe COPD	FEV_1/FVC <70% FEV_1 <30% predicted or FEV_1 <50% predicted plus chronic respiratory failure, i.e., PaO_2 <60 mm Hg and/or PCO_2 >50 mm Hg

FVC, forced vital capacity.
Adapted from the Global Initiative for Chronic Obstructive Lung Disease: Global strategy for the diagnosis, management and prevention of COPD: Update 2005. At www.goldcopd.com.

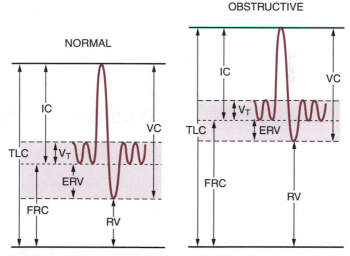

Figure 9-3 • Lung volumes in chronic obstructive pulmonary disease compared with normal values. In the presence of obstructive lung disease, vital capacity (VC) is normal to decreased, residual volume (RV) and FRC are increased, TLC is normal to increased, and the RV/TLC ratio is increased. ERV, expiratory reserve volume; IC, inspiratory capacity; V_T, tidal volume.

"blue bloaters" (PaO_2 usually less than 60 mm Hg and $PaCO_2$ chronically increased to more than 45 mm Hg). "Blue bloaters" typically exhibit cough and sputum production, frequent respiratory tract infection, and recurrent episodes of cor pulmonale (because pulmonary hypertension and right-sided heart failure result from chronic arterial hypoxemia and respiratory acidosis). Pink puffers are typically thin and free of signs of right-sided heart failure (because PaO_2 is usually only mildly depressed and pulmonary vasoconstriction does not occur).

C. Treatment

1. Drug Therapy (Table 9-8)

2. Lung Volume Reduction Surgery may be considered in selected patients with emphysema who have regions of overdistended, poorly functioning lung tissue. Surgical removal of the overdistended areas allows more normal areas of the lung to expand and improves not only lung function but quality of life.

a. Management of Anesthesia for Lung Volume Reduction Surgery includes use of a double-lumen endobronchial tube to permit lung separation, avoidance of nitrous oxide, and avoidance of excessive positive airway pressure.

b. CVP Monitoring is unreliable in these patients.

D. Management of Anesthesia

1. Preoperative

a. Pulmonary Function Testing. Pulmonary function tests and arterial blood gases can be useful for predicting pulmonary function following lung resection but do not reliably predict the risk of postoperative pulmonary complications after nonthoracic surgery. Indications for a preoperative pulmonary evaluation include (1) hypoxemia on room air or the need for home oxygen therapy without a known cause, (2) bicarbonate more than 33 mEq/L or PCO_2 more than 50 mm Hg in a patient whose pulmonary disease has not been previously evaluated, (3) a history of respiratory failure due to a problem that still exists, (4) severe shortness of breath attributed to respiratory disease, (5) planned pneumonectomy, (6) difficulty assessing pulmonary

TABLE 9-8 Treatment of Patients with COPD
Cessation of cigarette smoking
Supplemental oxygen if PaO_2 is <55 mm Hg, hematocrit is >55%, or evidence of cor pulmonale
β_2-Agonists (even small improvements in airway resistance decrease symptoms and may decrease infective exacerbations)
Anticholinergic drugs (most effective in patients with COPD)
Inhaled corticosteroids
Intermittent broad-spectrum antibiotics
Annual vaccination against influenza and pneumococci
Diuretics in patients with cor pulmonale and right-sided heart failure with peripheral edema

function by clinical signs, (7) distinguishing among potential causes of significant respiratory compromise, (8) determining the response to bronchodilators, and (9) suspected pulmonary hypertension. Right ventricular function should be carefully assessed by clinical examination and echocardiography in patients with advanced pulmonary disease.

> **1.) *Flow Volume Loops.*** Patients with COPD experience a decrease in the expiratory flow rate at any given lung volume. The expiratory curve is concave upward, and the residual volume is increased. Patients with restrictive lung disease will show a decrease in all lung volumes (**Fig. 9-2**).

b. Risk Reduction Strategies (Table 9-9)

> **1.) *Smoking Cessation.*** Within 12 hours after cessation of smoking, the PaO_2 at which hemoglobin is 50% saturated with oxygen (P_{50}) increases from 22.9 to 26.4 mm Hg and plasma levels of carboxyhemoglobin decrease from 6.5% to approximately 1%. The effects of nicotine on the heart are transient, lasting only 20 to 30 minutes. It likely takes 6 weeks for hepatic enzyme activity to return to normal following cessation of smoking.

2. Intraoperative

a. Regional Anesthesia. Peripheral nerve block carries a lower risk of pulmonary complications than either spinal or general anesthesia. Regional anesthesia is a useful choice in patients with COPD only if

TABLE 9-9	Anesthesia Management Strategies to Reduce Risks of Postoperative Pulmonary Complications in Patients with COPD
Preoperative	
Encourage cessation of smoking for at least 6 weeks.	
Treat evidence of expiratory airflow obstruction.	
Treat respiratory infection with antibiotics.	
Initiate patient education regarding lung volume expansion maneuvers.	
Intraoperative	
Use minimally invasive surgery (endoscopic) techniques when possible.	
Consider use of regional anesthesia.	
Avoid surgical procedures likely to require more than 3 hours.	
Postoperative	
Institute lung volume expansion maneuvers (voluntary deep breathing, incentive spirometry, continuous positive airway pressure).	
Maximize analgesia (neuraxial opioids, intercostal nerve blocks, patient-controlled analgesia).	

Adapted from Smetana GW: Preoperative pulmonary evaluation. N Engl J Med 1999;340:937–944, copyright 1999 Massachusetts Medical Society.

large doses of sedative and anxiolytic drugs will not be needed. Small doses of a benzodiazepine (e.g., midazolam, in increments of 1–2 mg IV) can be administered without producing unacceptable ventilatory depression. Regional anesthetic techniques that produce sensory anesthesia above T6 can impair ventilatory functions.

b. General Anesthesia. Volatile anesthetics are rapidly eliminated through the lungs and cause bronchodilation. Nitrous oxide should be used with caution due to the possibility of enlargement or rupture of the bullae resulting in development of a tension pneumothorax. Inhaled anesthetics may attenuate regional hypoxic pulmonary vasoconstriction and cause more intrapulmonary shunting, and increased FiO_2 may be necessary. Humidification of inspired gases and low gas flows can help to keep airway secretions moist. Mechanical ventilation with large tidal volumes (10–15 mL/kg) combined with slow inspiratory flow rates minimize the likelihood of turbulent airflow and help maintain optimal ventilation-to-perfusion matching. Slow respiratory rates (6–10 breaths per minute) provide sufficient time for complete exhalation to occur and for venous return and are less likely to be associated with undesirable degrees of hyperventilation.

3. Postoperative. Prevention of pulmonary complications is based on maintaining adequate lung volumes, especially FRC, and facilitating an effective cough.

a. Lung Expansion Maneuvers (deep breathing exercises, incentive spirometry, chest physiotherapy, positive-pressure breathing techniques) are of proven benefit for preventing postoperative pulmonary complications in high-risk patients.

b. Postoperative Neuraxial Analgesia with opioids may permit early tracheal extubation and early ambulation with increased FRC and improved oxygenation. Neuraxial opioids may be especially useful after intrathoracic and upper abdominal surgery. Sedation and delayed respiratory depression can be seen, especially when poorly lipid-soluble opioids such as morphine have been used. Neuraxial analgesia has not been proven to decrease the incidence of clinically significant postoperative pulmonary complications nor to be superior to parenteral opioids. Postoperative neuraxial analgesia is recommended after high-risk thoracic, abdominal, and major vascular surgery.

c. Mechanical Ventilation during the immediate postoperative period may be necessary in patients with severe COPD (FEV_1/FVC ratios less than 0.5 or with a preoperative $PaCO_2$ of more than 50 mm Hg).

IV. CHRONIC OBSTRUCTIVE PULMONARY DISEASE AND ACUTE RESPIRATORY FAILURE

Acute deterioration in lung function is most often triggered by events such as pneumonia, congestive heart failure, and increased metabolic production of carbon dioxide as produced by febrile states.

A. Treatment

1. Supplemental Oxygen is administered to maintain the PaO_2 at more than 60 mm Hg.

2. Bronchopulmonary Drainage is achieved by encouragement to cough, administration of inhaled bronchodilators and systemic corticosteroids, and treatment of underlying infection with antibiotics.

3. Mechanical Support of Ventilation is necessary when hypercarbia is severe enough to decrease the pHa below 7.2, patients show signs of mental status deterioration or respiratory muscle fatigue, there is hemodynamic instability, or somnolence or secretions cannot be cleared.

B. Risk Factors for Postoperative Pulmonary Complications (Table 9-10)

V. LESS COMMON CAUSES OF EXPIRATORY AIRFLOW OBSTRUCTION

A. Bronchiectasis is a chronic suppurative disease of the airways that may cause expiratory airflow obstruction similar to that seen with COPD.

1. Pathophysiology. Bacterial or mycobacterial infections are presumed responsible for most cases of bronchiectasis.

2. Diagnosis. The history of a chronic cough productive of purulent sputum is highly suggestive of bronchiectasis. Digital clubbing occurs in

TABLE 9-10	Major Risk Factors Associated with Postoperative Pulmonary Complications
Patient Related	
1. Age >60 years	
2. ASA class >II	
3. Congestive heart failure	
4. Preexisting pulmonary disease (COPD)	
5. Functionally dependent	
6. Cigarette smoking	
Procedure Related	
1. Emergency surgery	
2. Abdominal, thoracic surgery, head and neck surgery, neurosurgery, vascular/aortic aneurysm surgery	
3. Prolonged duration of anesthesia (>2.5 hours)	
4. General anesthesia	
Test Predictors	
1. Albumin level <3.5 g/dL	

ASA, American Society of Anesthesiologists.
Adapted from Smetana GW, Lawrence VA, Cornell JE: Preoperative pulmonary risk stratification for noncardiothoracic surgery. A systematic review for the American College of Physicians. Ann Intern Med 2006;144:581–595.

most patients with significant bronchiectasis and is a valuable clue, especially because this change is not characteristic of COPD. Computed tomography provides excellent images of bronchiectatic airways.

3. Treatment. Bronchiectasis is treated with antibiotics and postural drainage. Massive hemoptysis (>200 mL over a 24-hour period) may require surgical resection of the involved lung or selective bronchial arterial embolization.

4. Management of Anesthesia may include use of a double-lumen endobronchial tube to prevent spillage of purulent sputum into normal areas of the lungs and avoidance of nasal intubation due to high rates of sinusitis.

B. Cystic Fibrosis (CF)

1. Pathophysiology. CF is caused by a mutation in a single gene on chromosome 7 that encodes the cystic fibrosis transmembrane conductance regulator. The result is defective chloride ion transport in epithelial cells in the lungs (bronchiectasis, COPD, sinusitis), pancreas (diabetes mellitus), liver (cirrhosis), gastrointestinal tract (meconium ileus), and reproductive organs (azoospermia).

2. Diagnosis. Sweat chloride concentration higher than 80 mEq/L plus the characteristic clinical manifestations (cough, chronic purulent sputum production, exertional dyspnea) or a family history of the disease confirm the diagnosis of CF.

3. Treatment is similar to bronchiectasis and is directed toward symptomatic relief (mobilization and clearance of lower airway secretions and treatment of pulmonary infection) and correction of organ dysfunction (pancreatic enzyme replacement).

4. Management of Anesthesia invokes the same principles as outlined for patients with COPD and bronchiectasis. Elective surgical procedures should be delayed until optimal pulmonary function can be ensured by controlling bronchial infection and facilitating removal of airway secretions. Vitamin K treatment may be necessary if hepatic function is poor or if absorption of fat-soluble vitamins is impaired. Volatile anesthetics permit the use of high inspired concentrations of oxygen, decrease airway resistance, and decrease the responsiveness of hyperreactive airways. Humidification of inspired gases, hydration, and avoidance of anticholinergic drugs is important for maintaining secretions in a less viscous state. Frequent tracheal suctioning is often necessary.

C. Primary Ciliary Dyskinesia is characterized by congenital impairment of ciliary activity in respiratory and reproductive tract ciliated cells and sperm tails (spermatozoa are alive but immobile). As a result of impaired ciliary activity in the respiratory tract, chronic sinusitis, recurrent respiratory infections, and bronchiectasis develop. Both male and female fertility is impaired. The triad of chronic sinusitis, bronchiectasis, and situs inversus is known as Kartagener's syndrome. Preoperative preparation is directed at treating active pulmonary infection and determining the presence of any significant organ involvement. In view of the high incidence of sinusitis, nasopharyngeal airways should be avoided.

D. Bronchiolitis Obliterans is a disease of childhood and is most often the result of infection with respiratory syncytial virus. It may accompany viral pneumonia, collagen vascular disease (especially rheumatoid arthritis), and inhalation of nitrogen dioxide ("silo filler's disease"), or it may be a sequela of graft-versus-host disease after bone marrow transplantation.

E. Tracheal Stenosis may develop after prolonged endotracheal intubation.

1. Diagnosis. Tracheal stenosis becomes symptomatic when the lumen of the adult trachea is decreased to <5 mm. Dyspnea is prominent even at rest. Peak expiratory flow rates are decreased. Stridor is usually audible. Flow-volume loops display flattened inspiratory and expiratory curves.

2. Management of Anesthesia. Surgical resection of the stenotic tracheal segment with primary anastomosis is often required. Translaryngeal endotracheal intubation is initially established, and after surgical exposure the distal normal trachea is opened and a sterile cuffed tube inserted and attached to the anesthetic circuit. Maintenance of anesthesia with volatile anesthetics is useful for ensuring maximum inspired concentrations of oxygen. High-frequency ventilation is useful in selected patients. Addition of helium to the inspired gases may improve gas flow through the area of tracheal narrowing.

VI. RESTRICTIVE LUNG DISEASE

Restrictive lung disease is characterized by decreases in all lung volumes, decreased lung compliance, and preservation of expiratory flow rates (**Fig. 9-4**). Causes are summarized in **Table 9-11.**

A. Acute Intrinsic Restrictive Lung Disease is usually due to leakage of intravascular fluid into the interstitium of the lungs and into the alveoli (pulmonary edema). Acute pulmonary edema can be caused by increased capillary pressure (hydrostatic or cardiogenic pulmonary edema) or by increased capillary permeability. Diffuse alveolar damage is typically present with the increased permeability pulmonary edema associated with acute respiratory distress syndrome (ARDS).

    1. Aspiration Pneumonitis. Aspirated acidic gastric fluid is rapidly distributed throughout the lung, destroying surfactant-producing cells and

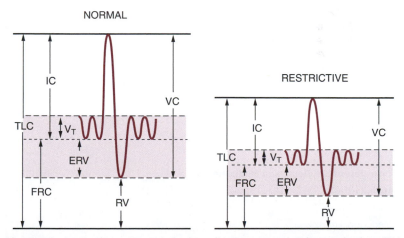

Figure 9-4 • Lung volumes in restrictive lung disease compared with normal values. ERV, expiratory reserve volume; IC, inspiratory capacity; RV, residual volume; TLC, total lung capacity; VC, vital capacity; V_T, tidal volume.

TABLE 9-11 Causes of Restrictive Lung Disease

Acute Intrinsic Restrictive Lung Disease (Pulmonary Edema)

Acute respiratory distress syndrome

Aspiration

Neurogenic problems

Opioid overdose

High altitude

Re-expansion of collapsed lung

Upper airway obstruction (negative pressure)

Congestive heart failure

Chronic Intrinsic Restrictive Lung Disease

Sarcoidosis

Hypersensitivity pneumonitis

Eosinophilic granuloma

Alveolar proteinosis

Lymphangioleiomyomatosis

Drug-induced pulmonary fibrosis

Chronic Extrinsic Restrictive Lung Disease

Obesity

Ascites

Pregnancy

Deformities of the costovertebral skeletal structures

Kyphoscoliosis

Ankylosing spondylitis

Deformities of the sternum

Flail chest

Neuromuscular disorders

Spinal cord transaction

Guillain-Barré syndrome

Myasthenia gravis

Eaton-Lambert syndrome

Muscular dystrophies

Disorders of the Pleura and Mediastinum

Pleural effusion

Pneumothorax

Mediastinal mass

Pneumomediastinum

damaging the pulmonary capillary endothelium with resulting atelectasis and leakage of intravascular fluid into the lungs. The clinical picture is similar to that of ARDS, with arterial hypoxemia, tachypnea, bronchospasm, and acute pulmonary hypertension. Chest radiographs may not demonstrate evidence of aspiration pneumonitis for 6 to 12 hours after the event.

   a. Treatment is endotracheal intubation, delivery of supplemental oxygen and positive end-expiratory pressure (PEEP), and administration of bronchodilators. There is no evidence that prophylactic antibiotics decrease the incidence of pulmonary infection or alter outcome, and corticosteroid treatment is controversial.

2. Neurogenic Pulmonary Edema develops in a small proportion of patients experiencing acute brain injury, due to massive outpouring of sympathetic impulses from the injured central nervous system that results in generalized vasoconstriction and a shift of blood volume into the pulmonary circulation.

   a. Diagnosis. The association of pulmonary edema with a recent central nervous system injury suggests neurogenic pulmonary edema. The principal entity in the differential diagnosis is aspiration pneumonitis.

   b. Treatment is directed at decreasing intracranial pressure, and support of oxygenation and ventilation.

3. Drug-Induced Pulmonary Edema can occur after administration of a number of drugs, especially heroin and cocaine. High-permeability pulmonary edema is suggested by high protein concentrations in the pulmonary edema fluid. Treatment is supportive and may include tracheal intubation for airway protection and mechanical ventilation.

4. High-Altitude Pulmonary Edema is presumed to be hypoxic pulmonary vasoconstriction, which increases pulmonary vascular pressures. Treatment includes administration of oxygen and prompt descent from the high altitude. Inhalation of nitrous oxide may improve oxygenation.

5. Re-expansion of Collapsed Lung may lead to pulmonary edema in that lung.

6. Negative-Pressure Pulmonary Edema may follow relief of acute upper airway obstruction caused by postextubation laryngospasm, epiglottitis, tumors, obesity, hiccups, or obstructive sleep apnea in spontaneously breathing patients. The time at onset after relief of airway obstruction ranges from a few minutes to as long as 2 to 3 hours. Tachypnea, cough, and failure to maintain oxygen saturation above 95% are common presenting signs and may be confused with pulmonary aspiration or pulmonary embolism.

   a. Pathogenesis is the development of high negative intrapleural pressure caused by vigorous inspiratory efforts against an obstructed upper airway. This decreases interstitial hydrostatic pressure, increases venous return, and increases left ventricular afterload. In addition, such negative pressure leads to intense sympathetic nervous system activation, hypertension, and central displacement of blood volume. Together these factors produce acute pulmonary edema by increasing the transcapillary pressure gradient.

   b. Treatment is maintenance of a patent upper airway and administration of supplemental oxygen. This form of pulmonary edema is typically transient and self-limited.

129

7. Management of Anesthesia in Patients with Acute Restrictive Lung Disease

a. Preoperative. Elective surgery should be delayed in patients with acute restrictive pulmonary disease to optimize cardiorespiratory function. Large pleural effusions may need to be drained. Persistent hypoxemia may require mechanical ventilation and PEEP.

b. Intraoperative. These patients are critically ill. It is reasonable to ventilate with low tidal volumes (e.g., 6 mL/kg) with a compensatory increase in ventilatory rate (14–18 breaths per minute) to keep the end-inspiratory plateau pressure less than 30 cm H_2O.

B. Chronic Intrinsic Restrictive Lung Disease is characterized by pulmonary fibrosis and loss of pulmonary vasculature, with pulmonary hypertension, cor pulmonale, dyspnea, and tachypnea.

1. Sarcoidosis is a systemic granulomatous disorder involving many tissues (liver, spleen, heart) but with a predilection for intrathoracic lymph nodes and the lungs. Laryngeal sarcoidosis occurs in up to 5% of patients and may interfere with tracheal intubation. Hypercalcemia is an uncommon but classic manifestation.

a. Mediastinoscopy provides lymph node tissue for the diagnosis of sarcoidosis.

b. Corticosteroids are administered to suppress the manifestation of sarcoidosis and to treat hypercalcemia.

2. Hypersensitivity Pneumonitis is characterized by diffuse interstitial granulomatous reactions in the lungs after inhalation of dust containing fungi, spores, animal, or plant material. Repeated episodes can lead to pulmonary fibrosis.

3. Eosinophilic Granuloma (Histiocytosis X) is associated with pulmonary fibrosis. No know treatment exists.

4. Pulmonary Alveolar Proteinosis is characterized by the deposition of lipid-rich proteinaceous material in the alveoli, resulting in dyspnea and hypoxemia. Treatment of severe cases requires whole-lung lavage through a double-lumen endobronchial tube.

5. Lymphangioleiomyomatosis is a proliferation of smooth muscle in airways, lymphatics, and blood vessels that occurs in females of reproductive age. Clinical presentation is progressive dyspnea, hemoptysis, recurrent pneumothorax, and pleural effusions. Most patients die within 10 years of the onset of symptoms.

6. Management of Anesthesia with Chronic Intrinsic Restrictive Lung Disease

a. Preoperative. Patients present with dyspnea and cough. Cor pulmonale may be present. A vital capacity of less than 15 mL/kg indicates severe pulmonary dysfunction. Infection should be treated, secretions cleared, and smoking stopped preoperatively.

b. Intraoperative. Patients tolerate apneic periods poorly due to their small FRC. Uptake of inhaled anesthetics is faster in these patients because of the small FRC. Peak airway pressures should be kept as low as possible to minimize the risk of barotrauma.

C. Chronic Extrinsic Restrictive Lung Disease is usually due to disorders of the thoracic cage (chest wall) that interfere with lung expansion, compress the lungs, and reduce lung volumes.

1. Obesity restricts the thoracic cage directly by the weight added to the rib cage and indirectly by the large abdominal panniculus, which impedes movement of the diaphragm in the supine position. FRC is decreased and the likelihood of ventilation-to-perfusion mismatching and hypoxemia is increased.

2. Deformities of the Costovertebral Skeletal Structures include scoliosis (lateral curvature with rotation of the vertebral column) and kyphosis (anterior flexion of the vertebral column). Severe deformities (scoliotic angle >100 degrees) may lead to chronic alveolar hypoventilation, hypoxemia, secondary erythrocytosis, pulmonary hypertension, and cor pulmonale. Patients with severe kyphoscoliosis are at increased risk for pneumonia and hypoventilation due to central nervous system depressant drugs.

3. Deformities of the Sternum and Costochondral Articulations include pectus excavatum (inward concavity of the lower sternum) and pectus carinatum (outward protuberance of the upper, middle, or lower sternum). Surgical correction is indicated when the sternal deformity is accompanied by evidence of pulmonary restriction or cardiovascular dysfunction.

4. Flail Chest. Multiple rib fractures, especially when they occur in a parallel vertical orientation, can produce a flail chest, with paradoxical inward movement of the unstable portion of the thoracic cage during inspiration, as the remainder of the thoracic cage moves outward. The result is progressive hypoxemia and alveolar hypoventilation. Treatment is positive-pressure ventilation until definitive stabilization procedures can be accomplished or rib fractures stabilize.

5. Neuromuscular Disorders that interfere with the transfer of central nervous system input to respiratory muscles can result in restrictive lung disease. Vital capacity is an important indicator of the total impact of a neuromuscular disorder on ventilation.

a. Diaphragmatic Paralysis. In the absence of respiratory disease, most adult patients with unilateral diaphragmatic paralysis are asymptomatic. Transient diaphragmatic dysfunction may occur after abdominal surgery. Atelectasis and arterial hypoxemia may occur. Incentive spirometry may alleviate these abnormalities.

b. Spinal Cord Transection. Breathing is maintained solely or predominantly by the diaphragm in quadriplegic patients (transection must be at or below C4 or the diaphragm is paralyzed). Because the diaphragm is active only during inspiration, cough, which requires activity by expiratory muscles, including those of the abdominal wall, is almost totally absent. Respiratory failure almost never occurs in quadriplegic patients in the absence of complications such as pneumonia.

c. Guillain-Barré Syndrome may result in respiratory insufficiency that requires mechanical ventilation in 20% to 25% of patients.

d. Disorders of Neuromuscular Transmission. Myasthenia gravis is the most common of the disorders affecting neuromuscular transmission that may result in respiratory failure. The myasthenic syndrome (Eaton-Lambert syndrome) may be confused with myasthenia gravis. Prolonged skeletal

131

muscle paralysis or weakness may occur following administration of nondepolarizing neuromuscular blocking drugs.

e. Muscular Dystrophy predisposes patients to pulmonary complications and respiratory failure. Chronic alveolar hypoventilation caused by inspiratory muscle weakness may develop. Expiratory muscle weakness impairs cough and accompanying weakness of the swallowing muscles may lead to pulmonary aspiration.

6. Disorders of the Pleura and Mediastinum may contribute to mechanical changes that interfere with optimal lung expansion (**Table 9-12**).

7. Management of Anesthesia

a. Preoperative Evaluation. In the presence of mediastinal tumors, severity of preoperative pulmonary symptoms bears no relationship to the degree of respiratory compromise that can be encountered during anesthesia. CT scan and/or flexible fiberoptic bronchoscopy under topical anesthesia may be useful for evaluating airway obstruction. Preoperative radiation therapy should be considered whenever possible. Under anesthesia, tumor compression of the airway, vena cava, pulmonary artery, or atria can cause life-threatening hypoxemia, hypotension, or even cardiac arrest.

b. Intraoperative. Restrictive lung disease does not influence the choice of drugs used for induction or maintenance of anesthesia. The method of induction of anesthesia and tracheal intubation in the presence of mediastinal tumors depends on the preoperative assessment of the airway. Symptomatic patients may need to be induced while sitting. Superior vena cava syndrome can cause upper airway edema. Invasive blood pressure monitoring should be considered. Spontaneous ventilation throughout surgery is recommended whenever possible. Surgical bleeding is often increased due to increased central venous pressure.

c. Postoperative tumor swelling as a result of partial resection or biopsy may increase airway obstruction and require reintubation of the trachea.

VII. DIAGNOSTIC PROCEDURES IN PATIENTS WITH LUNG DISEASE

A. **Fiberoptic Bronchoscopy** has generally replaced rigid bronchoscopy for visualizing the airways and obtaining tissue samples from the lung. The principal contraindication to pleural biopsy is a coagulopathy.

B. **Mediastinoscopy** is performed under general anesthesia through a small transverse incision just above the suprasternal notch. Complications include pneumothorax, mediastinal hemorrhage, venous air embolism, and injury to the recurrent laryngeal nerve leading to hoarseness and vocal cord paralysis. The mediastinoscope can also press against the right innominate artery, causing loss of pulses in the right arm and compromise of right carotid artery blood flow.

VIII. ACUTE RESPIRATORY FAILURE

Respiratory failure is the inability to provide adequate arterial oxygenation and/or elimination of carbon dioxide. Diagnostic criteria are summarized in **Table 9-13**.

TABLE 9-12	Disorders of the Pleura and Mediastinum that Cause Restrictive Pattern of Pulmonary Dysfunction

Pleural fibrosis (following hemothorax, empyema, surgical pleurodesis)

Pleural effusion

Pneumothorax (treatment indicated in larger (>15%) pneumothoraces or if symptomatic)

Tension pneumothorax

Mediastinal tumors

Pneumomediastinum

Mediastinitis

Bronchogenic cysts

IX. ACUTE/ADULT RESPIRATORY DISTRESS SYNDROME (ARDS)

Adult ARDS is characterized by acute inflammatory lung injury (aspiration, sepsis, trauma, multiple blood transfusions) and arterial hypoxemia. There is an influx of protein-rich edema fluid into the alveoli as a result of increased alveolar capillary membrane permeability and evidence of neutrophil-mediated lung injury.

A. Signs and Symptoms. Arterial hypoxemia resistant to treatment with supplemental oxygen is often the first sign. Radiographic signs are indistinguishable from cardiogenic pulmonary edema. Pulmonary hypertension can cause right-sided heart failure.

B. Diagnosis of ARDS is dependent on the presentation of acute, refractory hypoxemia, diffuse infiltrates on chest radiography consistent with pulmonary edema, and a pulmonary capillary wedge pressure less than 18 mm Hg. The PaO_2/FiO_2 ratio is typically less than 200 mm Hg.

C. Treatment of acute respiratory failure is directed at initiating specific therapies that support oxygenation and ventilation. The three principal goals in the management of acute respiratory failure are (1) correction of hypoxemia, (2) removal of excess carbon dioxide, and (3) provision of a patent upper

TABLE 9-13	Diagnosis of Acute Respiratory Failure

PaO_2 <60 mm Hg despite supplemental oxygen and absence of right-to-left cardiac shunt

$PaCO_2$ >50 mm Hg in the absence of respiratory compensation for metabolic alkalosis

Decreased pHa (distinguishes acute from chronic respiratory failure, in which pHa is usually 7.35–7.45).

Decreased FRC and lung compliance

Increased pulmonary vascular resistance and pulmonary artery hypertension often present

airway. Additional measures include provision of adequate nutrition and prevention of gastrointestinal bleeding and thromboembolic events.

1. Tracheal Intubation and Mechanical Ventilation

a. Inspired Oxygen Concentrations are adjusted to maintain the PaO_2 between 60 and 80 mm Hg.

2. Tidal Volumes are adjusted so that increases in peak airway pressure do not exceed 35 to 40 cm H_2O. Ideal tidal volume is determined by assessing lung mechanics rather than by measuring arterial blood gases.

a. PEEP is indicated when high concentrations of inspired oxygen ($FiO_2 > 0.5$) are needed for prolonged periods, and risk of oxygen toxicity increases. PEEP helps prevent alveolar collapse at end-expiration and thereby increases lung volumes (especially FRC), improves ventilation-to-perfusion matching, and decreases the magnitude of right-to-left intrapulmonary shunting. A pulmonary artery catheter is useful for monitoring the adequacy of intravascular fluid replacement, myocardial contractility, and tissue oxygenation in patients being treated with PEEP.

b. Inverse-Ratio Ventilation is characterized by an inspiratory time that exceeds the expiratory time due to an end-inspiratory pause to maintain the alveolar pressure briefly at the plateau level. Prospective studies have not confirmed a specific benefit in most patients.

3. Fluid and Hemodynamic Management. A reasonable goal is to maintain the intravascular fluid volume at the lowest level consistent with adequate organ perfusion as assessed by metabolic acid-base balance and renal function. If organ perfusion cannot be maintained after restoration of intravascular fluid volume, as in patients with septic shock, treatment with vasopressors may be necessary to improve organ perfusion pressures and normalize tissue oxygen delivery.

4. Corticosteroids. The value of corticosteroid administration early in the course of the disease remains unproven. Corticosteroids may have value in the treatment of the later fibrosing-alveolitis phase of ARDS or as rescue therapy in patients with severe ARDS that is not resolving.

5. Removal of Secretions, including tracheal suctioning, chest physiotherapy, and postural drainage. Fiberoptic bronchoscopy may be indicated to remove thicker accumulated secretions that are contributing to atelectasis.

6. Control of Infection using specific antibiotic therapy based on sputum culture and sensitivity is important, but the use of prophylactic antibiotics is not recommended.

7. Nutritional Support is important to prevent skeletal muscle weakness.

D. Mechanical Support of Ventilation (Fig. 9-5)

1. Modes of Mechanical Ventilation

a. Volume-Cycled Ventilation. Tidal volume (TV) is fixed, and inflation pressure varies. TV is maintained despite smaller changes in peak airway pressure, in contrast to pressure-cycled ventilators.

1.) Assist-Control Ventilation (ACV). In the control mode, the patient receives a predetermined number of mechanically delivered breaths even if there are no inspiratory efforts. In the assist mode, if the patient can create a small negative airway pressure, a breath at the preset tidal volume will be delivered (assisted).

134

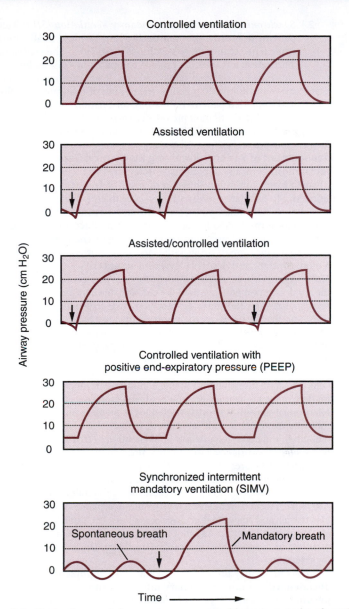

Figure 9-5 • Tidal volume and airway pressures produced by various modes of ventilation delivered through an endotracheal tube. *Arrows* indicate initiation of a spontaneous breath by the patient who triggers the ventilator to deliver a mechanically assisted breath.

    2.) *Synchronized Intermittent Mandatory Ventilation (SIMV)* allows patients to breathe spontaneously at any rate and tidal volume while a preset minute ventilation is provided by the ventilator. Theoretical advantages of SIMV compared to ACV include continued use of respiratory muscles, lower mean airway and mean intrathoracic pressure, prevention of respiratory alkalosis, and improved patient-ventilator coordination.

  b. Pressure-Cycled Ventilation provides gas flow into the lungs until a preset airway pressure is reached. TV is variable and changes with alterations in lung compliance and airway resistance.

2. Management of Patients Receiving Mechanical Support of Ventilation.
Critically ill patients who require mechanical ventilation may benefit from continuous infusion of sedative drugs to treat anxiety and agitation and to facilitate coordination with ventilator-delivered breaths.

  a. Sedation. Benzodiazepines, propofol, and narcotics are the drugs most commonly administered to decrease anxiety, produce amnesia, increase patient comfort, and provide analgesia during mechanical ventilation. Continuous infusion of drugs rather than intermittent injection provides a more constant and desirable level of drug effect.

  b. Paralysis. When sedation is inadequate or hypotension accompanies the administration of drugs used for sedation, the administration of nondepolarizing neuromuscular-blocking drugs to produce skeletal muscle relaxation may be necessary to permit optimal mechanical ventilation. A risk of prolonged drug-induced skeletal muscle paralysis is accentuation of the diffuse polyneuropathy that may accompany critical illness.

3. Complications of Mechanical Ventilation

  a. Infection. In mechanically ventilated patients with acute respiratory failure, tracheal intubation is the single most important predisposing factor for developing nosocomial pneumonia (ventilator-associated pneumonia). Nosocomial sinusitis is strongly related to the presence of a nasotracheal tube, and treatment includes antibiotics, replacement of nasal tubes with oral tubes, and decongestants and head elevation to facilitate sinus drainage.

  b. Alveolar Overdistension due to large tidal volumes (10–12 mL/kg) and high airway pressures (>50 cm H_2O) may cause alveolar rupture and hemorrhage. Tidal volumes of 5 to 8 mL/kg and airway pressures 30 cm H_2O or less may be indicated for treating acute respiratory failure and ARDS. This form of ventilation may require acceptance of some hypercarbia and respiratory acidosis as well as a PaO_2 of less than 60 mm Hg. Permissive hypercapnia is not recommended in patients with increased intracranial pressure, cardiac dysrhythmias, or pulmonary hypertension.

  c. Barotrauma may present as subcutaneous emphysema, pneumomediastinum, pulmonary interstitial emphysema, pneumoperitoneum, pneumopericardium, arterial gas embolism, or tension pneumothorax.

  d. Atelectasis is a common cause of hypoxemia that develops during mechanical ventilation that is not responsive to an increase in FiO_2.

  e. Critical Illness Myopathy. Patients who undergo mechanical ventilation are at risk of neuromuscular weakness that persists after the cause of the respiratory failure has resolved and may be exacerbated by prolonged use of muscle relaxants.

4. Monitoring of Treatment

a. Weaning from the Ventilator. Some guidelines that indicate the feasibility of discontinuing mechanical ventilation include (1) vital capacity greater than 15 mL/kg; (2) $PAO_2 - PaO_2$ less than 350 cm H_2O while breathing 100% oxygen; (3) PaO_2 more than 60 mm Hg with FiO_2 less than 0.5; (4) negative inspiratory pressure greater than -20 cm H_2O; (5) normal pHa; (6) respiratory rate less than 20 bpm; and (7) dead-space ventilation/tidal volume ratio (V_D/V_T) less than 0.6. Tachypnea and low tidal volumes usually signify an inability to tolerate extubation.

b. Tracheal Extubation should be considered when patients tolerate 2 hours of spontaneous breathing during tracheotomy tube (T-tube) weaning or when a synchronized intermittent mandatory ventilation rate of 1 to 2 breaths per minute is tolerated without deterioration of arterial blood gases, mental status, or cardiac function. The PaO_2 should remain higher than 60 mm Hg while breathing less than 50% oxygen. $PaCO_2$ should remain less than 50 mm Hg, and the pHa should remain higher than 7.30.

c. Supplemental Oxygen is often needed after tracheal extubation and is weaned while monitoring SpO_2 by pulse oximetry.

d. Oxygen Exchange and Arterial Oxygenation are reflected by the PaO_2. Calculation of $PAO_2 - PaO_2$ is useful for distinguishing among various mechanisms of arterial hypoxemia (**Table 9-14**).

e. Carbon Dioxide Elimination. The adequacy of alveolar ventilation relative to the metabolic production of carbon dioxide is reflected by the $PaCO_2$ (**Table 9-15**). The efficacy of carbon dioxide transfer across alveolar-capillary membranes is reflected by the V_D/V_T, reflecting areas in the lungs

TABLE 9-14	Mechanisms of Arterial Hypoxemia			
Mechanism	**PaO_2**	**$PaCO_2$**	**$PAO_2 - PaO_2$**	**Response to Supplemental Oxygen**
Low inspired oxygen concentration (altitude)	Decreased	Normal to decreased	Normal	Improved
Hypoventilation (drug overdose)	Decreased	Increased	Normal	Improved
Ventilation-to-perfusion mismatching (COPD, pneumonia)	Decreased	Normal to decreased	Increased	Improved
Right-to-left shunt (pulmonary edema)	Decreased	Normal to decreased	Increased	Poor to none
Diffusion impairment (pulmonary fibrosis)	Decreased	Normal to decreased	Increased	Improved

COPD, chronic obstructive pulmonary disease; $PAO_2 - PaO_2$, alveolar-arterial difference in partial pressure of oxygen.

TABLE 9-15	Mechanisms of Hypercarbia		
Mechanism	**$PaCO_2$**	**V_D/V_T**	**$PAO_2 - PaO_2$**
Drug overdose	Increased	Normal	Normal
Restrictive lung disease (kyphoscoliosis)	Increased	Normal to increased	Normal to increased
Chronic obstructive pulmonary disease	Increased	Increased	Increased
Neuromuscular disease	Increased	Normal to increased	Normal to increased

$PAO_2 - PaO_2$, alveolar-arterial difference in partial pressure of oxygen; V_D/V_T, dead space ventilation/tidal volume ratio.

that receive adequate ventilation but inadequate blood flow. Acute increases in $PaCO_2$ are associated with increased cerebral blood flow and increased intracranial pressure. Extreme increases in the $PaCO_2$ to more than 80 mm Hg may result in central nervous system depression and seizures.

f. Mixed Venous Partial Pressure of Oxygen (PvO₂) and the arterial-to-venous oxygen difference ($CaO_2 - CVO_2$) reflect the overall adequacy of the oxygen transport system (cardiac output) relative to tissue oxygen extraction. A PvO_2 less than 35 mm Hg or a $CaO_2 - CvO_2$ greater than 6 mL/dL indicates the need to increase the cardiac output to facilitate tissue oxygenation.

g. Arterial pH Measurements detect acidemia or alkalemia. Metabolic acidosis predictably accompanies arterial hypoxemia and inadequate delivery of oxygen to tissues. Acidemia due to respiratory or metabolic derangements is associated with dysrhythmias and pulmonary hypertension.

h. Intrapulmonary Shunt. Right-to-left intrapulmonary shunting occurs when there is perfusion of alveoli that are not ventilated. The net effect is a decrease in PaO_2, reflecting dilution of oxygen in blood exposed to ventilated alveoli with blood containing less oxygen coming from unventilated alveoli. Physiologic shunt normally comprises 2% to 5% of the cardiac output.

X. PULMONARY EMBOLISM (PE)

A. Diagnosis. The differential diagnosis of PE is extensive (**Table 9-16**), and clinical signs are often nonspecific (**Table 9-17**).

1. Transthoracic Echocardiography can help identify right ventricular pressure overload as well as myocardial infarction, dissection of the aorta, and pericardial tamponade, which may mimic pulmonary embolism. Echocardiography may show acute dilation of the right atrium and right ventricle, pulmonary arterial hypertension, and occasionally even thrombus in the main pulmonary arteries.

2. Laboratory Tests. A positive D-dimer test means that a PE is possible. A negative D-dimer test strongly suggests that thromboembolism is absent (negative predictive value >99%). Troponin levels may also be elevated and

TABLE 9-16 Differential Diagnosis of Pulmonary Embolism

Myocardial infarction

Pericarditis

Congestive heart failure

Chronic obstructive pulmonary disease

Pneumonia

Pneumothorax

Pleuritis

Thoracic herpes zoster

Anxiety/hyperventilation syndrome

Thoracic aorta dissection

Rib fractures

may represent right ventricular myocyte damage due to acute right ventricular strain.

3. Imaging. Spiral computed tomography scanning with contrast can diagnose both acute and chronic PE and has replaced ventilation-perfusion scanning in many centers. Pulmonary arteriography, the gold standard for the diagnosis of PE, is used when other preliminary testing is inconclusive. Ventilation-perfusion lung scanning and ultrasonography of leg veins are other noninvasive tests that can aid in the diagnosis of deep vein thrombosis and/or PE.

B. Treatment of Acute PE

1. Anticoagulation. An intravenous bolus of unfractionated heparin (5000–10,000 units) followed by a continuous intravenous infusion should be administered immediately to any patient considered to have a high

TABLE 9-17 Signs and Symptoms of Pulmonary Embolism

Sign/Symptom	Incidence (%)
Acute dyspnea	75
Tachypnea (>20 breaths per minute)	70
Pleuritic chest pain	65
Rales	50
Nonproductive cough	40
Tachycardia (>100 bpm)	30
Accentuation of pulmonic component of second heart sound	25
Hemoptysis	15
Fever (38°–39°C)	10
Homans' sign	5

clinical likelihood of PE. An alternative is low-molecular-weight heparin given subcutaneously. Extended anticoagulation is usually accomplished with warfarin to maintain an international normalized ratio of 2.0 to 3.0.

2. Thrombolytic Therapy may be considered if there is hemodynamic instability or severe hypoxemia. Inotropic support, pulmonary vasodilators, tracheal intubation and mechanical ventilation, and analgesics may also be warranted.

3. Inferior Vena Caval Filter Placement can be considered for patients who cannot be anticoagulated, have significant bleeding while being anticoagulated, or have recurrent PE despite being anticoagulated.

4. Surgical Embolectomy is reserved for patients with a massive PE who are unresponsive to medical therapy and cannot receive thrombolytic therapy.

C. **Management of Anesthesia** for the surgical treatment of life-threatening PE is designed to support vital organ function and to minimize myocardial depression. Monitoring of intra-arterial pressure and cardiac filling pressures is necessary. Cardiac inotropic support may be needed. The phosphodiesterase inhibitors amrinone and milrinone increase myocardial contractility and are also excellent pulmonary artery vasodilators. Induction and maintenance of anesthesia must avoid any accentuation of arterial hypoxemia, systemic hypotension, and pulmonary hypertension. Removal of embolic fragments from the distal pulmonary artery may be facilitated by the application of positive pressure while the surgeon applies suction through the arteriotomy in the main pulmonary artery.

XI. FAT EMBOLISM

The syndrome of fat embolism typically appears 12 to 72 hours (lucid interval) after long-bone fractures, especially of the femur or tibia. The triad of hypoxemia, mental confusion, and petechiae, especially over the neck, shoulders, and chest, in patients with tibia or femur fractures should arouse suspicion of fat embolism. Treatment includes management of acute respiratory distress syndrome and immobilization of long-bone fractures. Prophylactic administration of corticosteroids for patients at risk may be useful, but the efficacy of corticosteroids has not been proven.

XII. LUNG TRANSPLANTATION

A. Indications (**Table 9-18**)
B. Management of Anesthesia

1. Preoperative Evaluation. Smokers should have quit smoking at least 6 to 12 months before transplantation. The ability of the right ventricle to maintain an adequate stroke volume in the presence of the acute increase in pulmonary vascular resistance produced by clamping the pulmonary artery before pneumonectomy must be evaluated. Evaluation of oxygen dependence, steroid use, hematologic and biochemical analyses, and tests of lung and other major organ system function are also required.

2. Intraoperative and Postoperative Management (Table 9-19)
3. Physiologic Effects of Lung Transplantation (Table 9-20)
4. Complications of Lung Transplantation (Table 9-21)

TABLE 9-18 Indications for Lung Transplantation

1. Chronic obstructive pulmonary disease
2. Cystic fibrosis
3. Idiopathic pulmonary fibrosis
4. Primary pulmonary hypertension
5. Bronchiectasis
6. Eisenmenger's syndrome
7. Retransplantation

Adapted from Singh H, Bossard RF: Perioperative anaesthetic considerations for patients undergoing lung transplantation. Can J Anaesth 1997;44:284–299.

TABLE 9-19 Management of Anesthesia and Postoperative Period for Lung Transplantation

Practice strict aseptic technique.

Insert pulmonary artery catheter.

Avoid drugs causing histamine release.

Insert double-lumen endobronchial tube.

Arterial hypoxemia may accompany one-lung ventilation (trial of PEEP if it occurs).

Pulmonary artery hypertension may occur with clamping of the pulmonary artery (prostacyclin infusion, cardiopulmonary bypass).

Bronchospasm may occur.

Maintain postoperative ventilatory support—loss of cough reflex predisposes to pneumonia.

Principal causes of mortality are bronchial dehiscence or respiratory failure secondary to infection or rejection.

TABLE 9-20 Physiologic Effects of Lung Transplantation

Peak improvement in lung function in 3–6 months

Normalization of arterial oxygenation

Normalization of pulmonary vascular resistance and pulmonary vascular pressures

Increased cardiac output

Improved exercise tolerance

Lung denervation
  • Loss of cough reflex
  • Inhaled β-agonists cause bronchodilation
  • Mucociliary clearance is impaired
  • Blunted ventilatory response to carbon dioxide

TABLE 9-21	Complications of Lung Transplantation
Pulmonary edema	
Dehiscence of the bronchial anastomosis	
Anastomotic stenosis	
Infection	
Acute rejection (most likely in the first 100 days)	
Chronic rejection (bronchiolitis obliterans)	

5. Anesthetic Considerations in Lung Transplant Recipients should focus on (1) the function of the transplanted lung, (2) the possibility of rejection or infection in the transplanted lung, (3) the effect of immunosuppressive therapy on other organ systems and the effect of other organ system dysfunction on the transplanted lung, (4) the disease in the native lung, and (5) the planned surgical procedure and its likely effects on the lungs.

   a. Preoperative Evaluation. If rejection or infection is suspected, elective surgery should be postponed. The side effects of immunosuppressive drugs should be noted. Hypertension and renal dysfunction related to cyclosporine are present in many patients.

      1.) Chronic Rejection. The FEV_1, vital capacity, and total lung capacity decrease and arterial blood gases show an increased alveolar-to-arterial oxygen gradient, but carbon dioxide retention is rare.

      2.) Premedication is acceptable if pulmonary function is adequate. Hypercarbia is common during the early posttransplantation period, and increased sensitivity to opioids. Supplemental corticosteroids may be needed. Prophylactic antibiotics are indicated, and strict aseptic technique is required for placement of intravascular catheters. Bronchial hyperreactivity and bronchoconstriction are common. Response to carbon dioxide rebreathing is normal.

   b. Intraoperative Evaluation. Because of the diminished cough reflex, the potential for bronchoconstriction, and the increased risk of pulmonary infection, it is recommended that regional anesthesia be selected whenever possible. The importance of sterile technique in this high-risk population cannot be overemphasized. Fluid preloading before regional block may be risky in patients with a transplanted lung because disruption of the lymphatic drainage in the transplanted lung causes interstitial fluid accumulation.

      1.) Transesophageal Echocardiography is useful for monitoring volume status and cardiac function.

      2.) Anesthetic Management. An important goal is prompt recovery of adequate respiratory function and early extubation. Volatile anesthetics are well tolerated. Immunosuppressive drugs may interact with neuromuscular-blocking drugs, and the impaired renal function caused by immunosuppressive drugs may prolong the effects of certain muscle relaxants. The effects of nondepolarizing neuromuscular blockers are routinely antagonized pharmacologically because even minimal residual weakness can compromise ventilation in these patients.

3.) *When Positioning an Endotracheal Tube,* it is best to place the cuff just beyond the vocal cords to minimize the risk of traumatizing the tracheal anastomosis. If the surgical procedure requires a double-lumen endobronchial tube, it is preferable to place the endobronchial portion of the tube in the native bronchus, thus avoiding contact with the tracheal anastomosis.

CHAPTER 10

Diseases of the Nervous System

Part I: Diseases Affecting the Brain

Coexisting nervous system diseases often have important implications when selecting anesthetic drugs, techniques, and monitors. Concepts of cerebral protection and resuscitation may assume unique importance in these patients.

CEREBRAL BLOOD FLOW, BLOOD VOLUME, AND METABOLISM

I. CEREBRAL BLOOD FLOW

Cerebral blood flow (CBF) is governed by cerebral metabolic rate (CMR), cerebral perfusion pressure (CPP) (i.e., cerebral mean arterial pressure [CMAP] minus intracranial pressure [ICP]), arterial blood carbon dioxide ($PaCO_2$) and oxygen (PaO_2) tensions, the influence of various drugs, and intracranial pathology. CBF is normally constant over a given range of CPPs (autoregulation). CBF is normally 50 mL/100 g brain tissue per minute over a CPP range of 50 to 150 mm Hg.

  A. Cerebral Metabolic Rate (the rate of oxygen consumption [$CMRO_2$]) is 3.0 to 3.8 mL O_2/100 g brain tissue per minute. CMR decreases with decreased temperature and some anesthetic agents, and increases with temperature and seizures.

  B. Cerebral Blood Volume (CBV). Intracranial volume and pressure are influenced by CBV but not directly by CBF. Vasodilatory anesthetics and hypercapnia may produce parallel increases in CBF and CBV. Moderate systemic hypotension may reduce CBF but, because of vessel dilation, increase CBV. Partial cerebral arterial occlusion may reduce regional CBF but increase CBV distal to the occlusion due to compensatory vasodilation.

C. Arterial Carbon Dioxide Partial Pressure. Variations in $PaCO_2$ produce corresponding changes in CBF (**Fig. 10-1**) via vasodilation and constriction. CBF increases 1 mL/100 g per minute for every 1 mm Hg increase in the $PaCO_2$. CBF is decreased approximately 50% when the $PaCO_2$ is acutely lowered to 20 mm Hg. Vasoconstricting anesthetics attenuate the effects of $PaCO_2$ on CBV.

D. Arterial Oxygen Partial Pressure. Decreased PaO_2 does not affect CBF until a threshold value of approximately 50 mm Hg is reached (**Fig. 10-1**). Below this value, there is abrupt cerebral vasodilation and increased CBF. Arterial hypoxemia plus hypercarbia exerts a synergistic effect (increases in CBF exceed the increase that would be produced by either factor alone).

E. Cerebral Perfusion Pressure and Cerebral Autoregulation. The ability of the brain to maintain constant CBF despite changes in CPP is known as autoregulation (**Fig. 10-1**). This is an active vascular response (arterial constriction with increased blood pressure and arterial dilation during decreased blood pressure). In normotensive patients, the lower limit of CPP associated with autoregulation is about 50 mm Hg. Below that pressure, cerebral blood vessels are maximally vasodilated and as the pressure drops further, CBF decreases (flow becomes pressure dependent). The upper limit of autoregulation in normotensive patients is believed to be approximately 150 mm Hg. Above this blood pressure, the cerebral blood vessels are maximally constricted and CBF increases with increased pressure (pressure dependent flow). Autoregulation of CBF is shifted to the right (i.e., pressure dependence occurs at higher blood pressure at both upper and lower limits

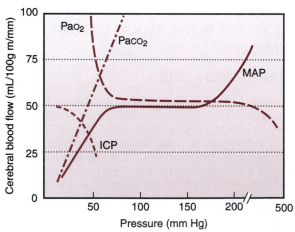

Figure 10-1 • Impact of intracranial pressure (ICP), PaO_2, $PaCO_2$, and mean arterial pressure (MAP) on cerebral blood flow.

of autoregulation) in chronic, but not acute, hypertension. Decreases in systemic blood pressure are not as well tolerated in patients with chronic hypertension (i.e., stroke, cerebral ischemia can occur at higher pressures than in normal subjects). Autoregulation improves with antihypertensive therapy. Other conditions that may cause loss or impairment of autoregulation include intracranial tumors, head trauma, and volatile anesthetic agent administration.

F. Venous Blood Pressure has little effect on CPP or CBF but may profoundly affect CBV. In order for blood to continue to flow out of the cranial vault, ICP must be greater than central venous pressure (CVP). Increases in CVP at a steady ICP lead to increases in CBV. Other causes of increased intracranial venous pressure include venous sinus thrombosis, jugular compression (extreme neck flexion or rotation), and superior vena cava syndrome.

G. Anesthetic Drugs

1. Anesthetic Gases. Changes in $CMRO_2$ usually cause parallel changes in CBF (CBF/$CMRO_2$ coupling). But volatile anesthetics administered in concentrations greater than 0.6 to 1.0 minimum alveolar concentration (MAC) are potent cerebral vasodilators that produce dose-dependent increases in CBF despite concomitant *decreases* in $CMRO_2$. This can cause increases in CBF, CBV, and ICP. With all volatile anesthetics, arterial hypocapnia or supplemental vasoconstricting agents (thiopental, propofol) minimize increases in CBV. Nitrous oxide has less effect on CBF and does not interfere with CBF autoregulation. The initiation of nitrous oxide after closure of the dura may cause a tension pneumocephalus (diffusion into and expansion of the gas bubble left in the intracranial vault), which may present as a delayed emergence from anesthesia after craniotomy.

2. Intravenous Anesthetic Agents. Ketamine is probably a cerebral vasodilator. Barbiturates, etomidate, propofol, and opioids are cerebral vasoconstrictors in the absence of hypercapnia and predictably decrease CBV and ICP. Nondepolarizing neuromuscular blocking drugs do not meaningfully alter ICP but may prevent acute increases in ICP due to movement or coughing. Succinylcholine may further raise ICP in the setting of elevated ICP through increases in muscle afferent activity and cerebral arousal, independent of visible muscle fasciculations.

II. INCREASED INTRACRANIAL PRESSURE

The pressure within the dura and cranium is referred to as the ICP. Normal combined volume intracranial contents is approximately 1200 to 1500 mL, and normal ICP is usually 5 to 15 mm Hg. An increase in one component of intracranial volume (brain tissue, CSF, blood) must be offset by a decrease in another to prevent an increase in ICP. Normally, these changes are well compensated, but at some point even a small change in intracranial contents results in a large change in ICP (**Fig. 10-2**). Homeostatic mechanisms increase MAP to overcome an increase in ICP; when this mechanism eventually fails, CPP falls and cerebral ischemia results.

A. Cerebrospinal Fluid (CSF) is produced by ultrafiltration and secretion by the cells of the choroid plexus and via the passage of water, electrolytes, and other substances across the blood-brain barrier at a constant rate of 500 to 600 mL/day in adults. CSF is absorbed by cells within the dura mater bordering venous

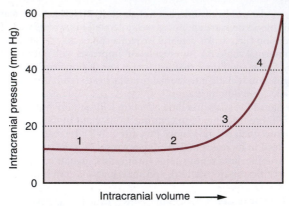

Figure 10-2 • The intracranial elastance curve depicts the impact of increasing intracranial volume on intracranial pressure (ICP). As intracranial volume increases from point 1 to 2, ICP does not increase because cerebrospinal fluid is shifted from the cranium into the spinal subarachnoid space. Patients on the rising portion of the curve (point 3) can no longer compensate for increases in intracranial volume; the ICP begins to increase and is likely to be associated with clinical symptoms. Additional increases in intracranial volume at this point (point 3), as produced by anesthetic drug-induced increases in cerebral blood volume, can precipitate abrupt increases in ICP (point 4).

sinusoids and by sinuses. The intracranial vault is compartmentalized by meningeal barriers, and increases in the contents of one region of brain may cause regional increases in ICP and potential herniation of the contents of that compartment into a different compartment. Such herniations may lead to evidence of compromise of regional brain function.

B. Signs and Symptoms of Increased ICP include headache, nausea, vomiting, and papilledema; decreased levels of consciousness and coma can be observed. Acute increases in ICP are not tolerated as well as chronically elevated ICP.

C. Diagnosis of Increased ICP is based on the symptoms and radiographic evidence (mass, hematoma, midline shift) and by directly measuring ICP.

D. Monitoring ICP. Pressure transducers can be placed into the subdural space (known as a subdural bolt), brain parenchyma, or ventricle (ventriculostomy). Ventriculostomy also allows the withdrawal of CSF in order to analyze CSF and regulate ICP. A lumbar CSF drain will also allow this, but there is a risk of tonsillar herniation in certain clinical settings (i.e., tumor) with lumbar CSF drainage.

E. Methods to Decrease ICP (Table 10-1)

F. Specific Causes of Increased Intracranial Pressure (Table 10-2)

III. INTRACRANIAL TUMORS

Intracranial tumors may be classified as primary (those arising from the brain and its coverings) or metastatic. Supratentorial tumors are more common in adults and often present with headache, seizures, or new neurologic deficits. Infratentorial tumors are more common in children and often present with obstructive hydrocephalus and ataxia.

148

TABLE 10-1	Measures to Lower ICP
Head position	• Elevate 30 degrees above the heart • Avoid extreme flexion or rotation • Avoid head-down position
Hyperventilation	• Goal is $PaCO_2$ 30–35 mm Hg • Effect wanes after 6–12 hours
CSF drainage	• Ventriculostomy ("bolt"—permits ICP monitoring) • Lumbar drain (risk of cerebral herniation) • Ventriculoperitoneal, ventriculoatrial, and ventriculopleural shunts
Administration of hyperosmolar drugs	• Mannitol (0.25–0.5 g/kg over 15–30 minutes, maximum effect 1–2 hours and duration 6 hours); osmotic diuresis. Risk of cerebral edema if blood-brain barrier broken
Loop diuretics	• Furosemide; useful in patients with increased vascular volume, such as congestive heart failure
Corticosteroids	• Not effective in closed head injury, may increase blood glucose concentration, which is detrimental in cerebral ischemia
Barbiturates and propofol	• Very useful in acute head injury

TABLE 10-2	Causes of Increased ICP
Intracranial tumors	• Mass effect, related to size • Associated edema • Obstruction of CSF flow (third ventricle tumors)
Intracranial hematomas	• Similar to mass lesions • Blood interferes with CSF reabsorption
Infection (meningitis, encephalitis)	• Edema • Obstruction of CSF reabsorption
Aqueductal stenosis (connects third and fourth ventricles)	• Common cause of obstructive hydrocephalus • Treated with ventricular shunting
Benign intracranial hypertension (pseudotumor cerebri)	• No identifiable cause; ICP >20 mm Hg, normal CSF composition, normal sensorium. Symptoms are headaches and bilateral visual disturbances • Treatment is removal of 20–40 mL of CSF, administration of acetazolamide to decrease CSF formation and (rarely) surgical shunt
Normal pressure hydrocephalus	• Triad of dementia, gait changes, and urinary incontinence • Impaired CSF reabsorption • Lumbar puncture shows normal or low CSF pressure while CT or MRI shows large ventricles • Treatment is drainage of CSF via shunt

A. Tumor types

1. Astrocytoma

a. Well-Differentiated (Low-Grade) Gliomas often present in young adults with new-onset seizures. Surgical or radiation treatment of low-grade gliomas usually results in symptom-free long-term survival.

b. Pilocytic Astrocytomas affect children and young adults. They arise in the cerebellum, cerebral hemispheres, hypothalamus, or optic pathways (optic glioma) and appear as a contrast-enhancing, well-demarcated lesion with minimal to no surrounding edema. If the local permits surgical resection, prognosis is very good.

c. Anaplastic Astrocytomas are poorly differentiated, contrast-enhancing lesions on imaging (due to disruption of the blood-brain barrier) that usually evolve into glioblastoma multiforme. Treatment is resection, radiation, or chemotherapy. Prognosis is intermediate between low-grade gliomas and glioblastoma multiforme.

d. Gliobastoma Multiforme (Grade IV Glioma) often appear as ring-enhancing lesions due to central necrosis and surrounding edema. Treatment typically involves surgical debulking combined with radiation and chemotherapy and is aimed at palliation, not cure. Life expectancy is usually on the order of weeks.

2. Oligodendrogliomas
arise from myelin-producing cells in the central nervous system. Seizures predate the appearance of tumor often by many years. Initial treatment involves resection.

3. Ependymomas
arise from cells lining the ventricles and central canal of the spinal cord. Symptoms include obstructive hydrocephalus, headache, nausea, vomiting, and ataxia. Treatment is resection and radiation.

4. Primitive Neuroectodermal Tumor
represents a diverse class of tumors including retinoblastoma, medulloblastoma, pineoblastoma, and neuroblastoma. Presentation of medulloblastoma (the most common pediatric primary malignant brain tumor) is similar to ependymoma. Treatment is a combination of resection and radiation. Prognosis is very good in children if there is disappearance of both tumor on magnetic resonance imaging (MRI) and tumor cells within the CSF.

5. Meningiomas
are usually slow-growing, well-circumscribed, benign tumors arising from arachnoid cap cells, not the dura mater. Surgical resection is the mainstay of treatment. Prognosis is usually excellent. Malignant meningiomas are rare.

6. Pituitary Tumors
usually arise from cells of the anterior pituitary gland and may occur with tumors of the parathyroids and pancreatic islet cells as part of multiple endocrine neoplasia (MEN) type 1. Panhypopituitarism can be caused by either functional or nonfunctional tumors. Tumors can invade the cavernous sinus or internal carotid artery or compress various cranial nerves, causing an array of symptoms.

a. Functional Tumors (i.e., hormone secreting) usually present as a result of an endocrinologic disturbance related to the hormone secreted by the tumor and are usually smaller (<1 cm in diameter) at the time of diagnosis (microadenomas).

b. Nonfunctional Tumors are usually less than 1 cm in diameter when diagnosed (macroadenomas) and present with symptoms related to their mass (headache, visual changes due to compression of the optic chiasm).

c. Pituitary Apoplexy is a symptom complex (abrupt onset of headache, visual changes, ophthalmoplegia, altered mental status) secondary to hemorrhage, necrosis, or infarction within the tumor.

d. Treatment depends on tumor type. Prolactinomas are often initially treated medically with bromocriptine. Surgical resection via the transsphenoidal or open craniotomy approach is often curative.

7. Acoustic Neuroma is usually a benign schwannoma involving the vestibular component of cranial nerve VIII within the internal auditory canal. Bilateral tumors may occur as part of neurofibromatosis type 2.

a. Symptoms include hearing loss, tinnitus, and disequilibrium. Larger tumors may cause symptoms related to compression of cranial nerves, most commonly the facial nerve (cranial nerve VII), as well as the brainstem.

b. Treatment is surgical resection with or without radiation therapy. Surgery usually involves intraoperative cranial nerve monitoring with electromyography or brainstem auditory evoked potentials.

c. Prognosis is usually very good; however, recurrence of tumor is not uncommon.

8. Central Nervous System Lymphoma is a rare tumor that can arise as a primary brain tumor, also known as a microglioma, or via metastatic spread from a systemic lymphoma. It may be associated with systemic lupus erythematosus, Sjögren's syndrome, rheumatoid arthritis, immunosuppressed states, and infection with Epstein-Barr virus.

a. Symptoms depend on the location of the tumor.

b. Diagnosis is via imaging and biopsy. Steroid treatment should be withheld until pathologic findings are obtained, because steroid-associated tumor lysis prior to biopsy may result in inadequate sample size for diagnosis.

c. Treatment is chemotherapy (including intraventricularly delivered drugs) and whole-brain radiation.

d. Prognosis is poor.

9. Metastatic Brain Tumors originate most often from the lungs or breasts. Malignant melanoma, hypernephroma, and carcinoma of the colon may also spread to the brain. Metastatic brain tumor is likely if more than one intracranial lesion is present.

B. Management of Anesthesia for Tumor Resection (Table 10-3). Goals are maintenance of adequate perfusion and oxygenation of normal brain, optimization of operative conditions to facilitate resection, assurance of a rapid emergence from anesthesia to facilitate neurologic assessment, and accommodation of intraoperative electrophysiologic monitoring.

1. Sitting Position and Venous Air Embolism. The sitting position is often used for exploration of the posterior cranial fossa because of excellent surgical exposure and enhanced cerebral venous and CSF drainage. These advantages are offset by the decreases in systemic blood pressure, decreased cardiac output, and the potential hazard of venous air embolism. The cut edge of cranial bone is a common site for the entry of air into veins. Death

TABLE 10-3	Anesthetic Considerations for Brain Tumor Resection
Preoperative	• Identify the presence or absence of increased ICP (nausea, vomiting, altered consciousness, mydriasis, decreased pupil reactivity, papilledema, bradycardia, systemic hypertension, breathing disturbances, midline shifts on CT or MRI) • Sedation may mask neurologic deficits or cause hypoventilation, hypercarbia, and further elevate ICP
Induction	• Thiopental, etomidate propofol (rapid unconsciousness without increases in ICP) • Nondepolarizing muscle relaxants (succinylcholine may transiently increase ICP) • Mechanical hyperventilation (avoid hypercapnia)
Laryngoscopy, placement of skull pinions, skin incision	• Adequate anesthesia depth for laryngoscopy (avoid increased CBF, CBV, ICP) • Intravenous lidocaine (1.5 mg/kg), potent short-acting opioids to blunt response
Maintenance anesthesia	• Maintain $PaCO_2$ around 35 mm Hg • Use PEEP with caution • Use of nitrous oxide is controversial; may enlarge air embolism, cause tension pneumocephalus after closure • Vasodilators can increase CBV, ICP—best used after dura is open
Fluid therapy	• Avoid hypo-osmolar solutions • Aim for euvolemia • Correct blood loss with red packed cells or colloid • Use glucose-containing solutions with caution (hyperglycemia exacerbates neuronal injury)
Monitoring	• Arterial catheter for blood pressure monitoring, blood gas, pH, and repeated blood sampling • Capnography to monitor $PaCO_2$, air embolism • Continuous ICP monitoring not routine but can be useful • Urinary catheter • Central venous catheter for sitting craniotomy (aspiration of air) • Transesophageal echocardiography may help detect air embolism • PA catheter for cardiac indications • Peripheral nerve stimulator may falsely indicate inadequate paralysis
Postoperative	• Limit reaction to endotracheal tube (narcotics, lidocaine 0.5–1.5 mg/kg IV) • Delayed wakeup can be due to anesthetic drugs, hypothermia, residual neuromuscular block, cerebral ischemia, hematoma, or tension pneumocephalus

is usually secondary to a vapor lock causing right-sided cardiac output to plummet, acute cor pulmonale, or arterial hypoxemia from combined cardiac and pulmonary insults. Paradoxical air embolism (embolism into the systemic circulation through a patent foramen ovale or other cardiopulmonary shunt) can occur. For that reason, known right-to-left cardiopulmonary shunts are relative contraindications to use of the sitting position. When the likelihood of venous air embolism is increased, it is useful, but not mandatory, to place a right atrial catheter (for air aspiration) before beginning surgery.

a. Detection of Air Embolism (Table 10-4)
b. Treatment of Air Embolism (Table 10-5)

TABLE 10-4   Detection of Venous Air Embolism

Doppler transducer over right heart structures	Very sensitive May detect clinically unimportant emboli Does not quantify emboli
Transesophageal echocardiography	Detects and quantifies air emboli Evaluates cardiac function
$PaCO_2$	Sudden decrease can mean increase in alveolar dead space or cardiac impairment due to air emboli
Decreased end-expired nitrogen concentration	Precede changes in $PaCO_2$ or increased PA pressures
Clinical findings	Hypotension, tachycardia, cardiac arrhythmias, cyanosis (late signs) Gasp reflex (early sign) Millwheel murmur

TABLE 10-5   Treatment of Air Embolism

Surgeon should flood the operative site with fluid, apply occluding material to bone edges, and identify other sources of air entry

Anesthesiologist:

1. Aspirate right atrial catheter to evacuate air (multi-orifice catheters are better than single-orifice catheters).

2. Discontinue nitrous oxide, ventilate with 100% oxygen.

3. PEEP or jugular venous compression may be helpful (increases venous back pressure at the surgical site).

4. Provide hemodynamic support (sympathomimetic drugs).

5. Left lateral decubitus position is rarely possible and should not be pursued first.

6. Hyperbaric therapy may be useful for severe venous air embolism or paradoxical air embolism (must be done within 8 hours to be meaningful).

IV. DISORDERS RELATED TO VEGETATIVE BRAIN FUNCTION

A. Coma is a state of profound unconsciousness produced by drugs, disease, or injury affecting the central nervous system. The causes of coma include structural lesions (tumor, stroke, abscess, intracranial bleeding) or diffuse disorders (hypothermia, hypoglycemia, hepatic or uremic encephalopathy, postictal state following seizures, encephalitis, drug effects). The most common means used to assess the overall severity of coma is by using the Glasgow Coma Scale (**Table 10-6**).

   1. Initial Management is establishment of a patent airway and ensuring the adequacy of oxygenation, ventilation, and circulation.

   2. Determining Cause of Coma

   a. Vital signs may suggest a cause such as hypothermia.

   b. Respiratory Patterns can also aid in diagnosis. Irregular breathing patterns may reflect an abnormality at a specific site in the central nervous system (**Table 10-7**).

   c. Neurologic Examination

   1.) Pupillary Responses. Compression of the diencephalon or thalamic structures leads to small (2 mm) but reactive pupils, unresponsive midsize pupils (5 mm) may indicate midbrain compression, and a fixed and dilated pupil (>7 mm) usually indicates oculomotor nerve compression (herniation,

TABLE 10-6	Glasgow Coma Scale	
Response	**Score**	
Eye Opening		
Spontaneous	4	
To speech	3	
To pain	2	
Nil	1	
Best Motor Response		
Obeys	6	
Localizes	5	
Withdraws (flexion)	4	
Abnormal flexion	3	
Extensor response	2	
Nil	1	
Verbal Responses		
Oriented	5	
Confused conversation	4	
Inappropriate words	3	
Incomprehensible sounds	2	
Nil	1	

TABLE 10-7	Abnormal Patterns of Breathing	
Ataxic (Biot's breathing)	Unpredictable sequence of breaths varying in rate and tidal volume	Medulla
Apneustic breathing	Repetitive gasps and prolonged pauses at full inspiration	Pons
Cheyne-Stokes breathing	Cyclic crescendo-decrescendo tidal volume pattern interrupted by apnea	Cerebral hemispheres Congestive heart failure
Central neurogenic hypoventilation	Hypocarbia	Cerebral thrombosis or embolism
Posthyperventilation apnea	Awake apnea following moderate decreases in $PaCO_2$	Frontal lobes

anticholinergic or sympathomimetic drug intoxication). Pinpoint pupils (1 mm) may indicate opioid or organophosphate intoxication, focal pontine lesions, or neurosyphilis.

2.) *Extraocular Muscles Function* tests brainstem function via assessment of the function of the oculomotor, trochlear, and abducens nerves (cranial nerves III, IV, and VI).

   a.) **Passive Head Rotation** (oculocephalic reflex or doll's head maneuver) in comatose patients with normal brainstem function will show full conjugate horizontal eye movements.

   b.) **Cold Water Irrigation** of the tympanic membrane (oculovestibular reflex or cold caloric testing) with intact brainstem function will result in tonic conjugate eye movement toward the side of cold water irrigation. Unilateral oculomotor nerve or midbrain lesions result in failed adduction but intact contralateral abduction. Complete absence of responses can indicate pontine lesions or diffuse disorders.

3.) *Evaluation of Motor Responses to Painful Stimuli* may help localize the cause of coma. Those with mild to moderate diffuse brain dysfunction above the level of the diencephalon will react with purposeful or semipurposeful movements toward the painful stimulus. Unilateral reactions may indicate unilateral lesions such as stroke or tumor.

   a.) **Decorticate Responses** (flexion of the elbow, adduction of the shoulder, extension of the knee and ankle) are usually indicative of diencephalic dysfunction.

   b.) **Decerebrate Responses** (extension of the elbow, internal rotation of the forearm, leg extension) usually imply more severe brain dysfunction. Patients with pontine or medullary lesions often exhibit no response to painful stimuli.

4.) *Laboratory Evaluation and Other Tests.* Laboratory evaluation should include blood electrolytes and glucose to assess for disorders of sodium and glucose. Liver and renal function tests help evaluate

155

hepatic or uremic encephalopathy. Drug and toxicology screens may help to identify exogenous intoxicants. A complete blood cell count and coagulation studies may suggest intracranial bleeding (i.e., thrombocytopenia or coagulopathy). Computed tomography (CT) or MRI may suggest a structural cause such as tumor or stroke. A lumbar puncture can be performed if meningitis or subarachnoid hemorrhage is suspected.

5.) *Management of Anesthesia.* Comatose patients may present to the operating suite either for treatment of the cause of their coma (e.g., burr hole drainage of an intracranial hematoma) or for treatment of injuries that are associated with their comatose state. Goals are establishment of an airway, provision of adequate cerebral perfusion and oxygenation, and optimization of operating conditions. Monitoring of ICP and arterial catheterization for blood pressure monitoring and blood sampling may be indicated. Anesthetic agents that increase ICP (halothane, ketamine) should be avoided, but other potent volatile agents used at low doses (<1 MAC), and intravenous cerebral vasoconstrictive anesthetics, are acceptable. Succinylcholine is best avoided because it may transiently increase ICP.

B. Brain Death
1. Criteria (Table 10-8)
2. Management of Anesthesia for Organ Donation (Table 10-9)

V. CEREBROVASCULAR DISEASE

Stroke is characterized by sudden neurologic deficits due to ischemia (88%) or hemorrhage (12%) (Table 10-10). Ischemic stroke is described by the area of the brain affected and the etiologic mechanisms. Hemorrhagic strokes are classified as intracerebral (15%) or subarachnoid (85%).

TABLE 10-8 Criteria for Brain Death
All reversible causes of coma ruled out
Lack of spontaneous movement (spinal cord reflexes may be intact)
Lack of cranial nerve reflexes and function
• Failure of heart rate to increase more than 5 beats per minute in response to intravenous atropine 0.04 mg/kg (loss of vagal nuclear function)
• Apnea test indicating lack of respiratory control. Test is initiated at $PaCO_2$ 40 ± 5 mm Hg, arterial pH 7.35–7.4, and patient is ventilated with 100% oxygen for >10 minutes. Ventilation is discontinued for 10 minutes, with continued tracheal insufflation with 100% oxygen. Arterial blood gases are checked at 5 and 10 minutes (to ensure $PaCO_2$ >60 mm Hg). If no respirations, test is considered confirmatory
• Isoelectric EEG
• Demonstration of absence of cerebral blood flow

TABLE 10-9	**Anesthetic Management of the Brain Dead Organ Donor**
Hypotension (may be due to drugs, third space losses, diabetes insipidus)	Provide aggressive fluid resuscitation. Avoid hypervolemia (pulmonary edema, cardiac failure, hepatic congestion). Avoid vasoconstrictors if possible. Inotropic agents (dobutamine, dopamine) are first-line pharmacologic therapy.
ECG changes	Moniter for electrolyte abnormalities. Monitor for increased ICP. Assess for cardiac contusion (if death is due to trauma). Consider antiarrhythmic drugs and pacing if needed.
Hypoxemia	Aim for normoxia and normocarbia. Avoid excessive PEEP. Treat anemia and coagulopathy.
Diabetes insipidus	Common in brain death. Provide volume replacement with hypotonic solutions. Administer vasopressin (0.4–0.1U/hr IV) or desmopressin (0.3 mcg/kg IV).
Temperature regulation	Poikilothermia is common.
Rule of 100s	Systolic BP >100, urine output >100 mL/hr, PaO_2 >100 mm Hg, hemoglobin >100 g/L.

ECG, electrocardiogram.

A. Cerebrovascular Anatomy. Blood supply to the brain is via the internal carotid arteries and the vertebral arteries (**Fig. 10-3**), which join to form the circle of Willis. The vessels arising from the carotid arteries comprise the anterior circulation and supply the frontal, parietal, and lateral temporal lobes, the basal ganglia, and most of the internal capsule. Vessels that receive their blood supply from the vertebral-basilar system comprise the posterior circulation and typically supply the brainstem, occipital lobes, cerebellum, medial portions of the temporal lobes, and most of the thalamus. Occlusion of specific arteries distal to the circle of Willis results in predictable clinical neurologic deficits (**Table 10-11**).

B. Acute Stroke

    1. Transient Ischemic Attack (TIA) is a sudden vascular-related focal neurologic deficit that resolves promptly (<24 hours) and represents an impending ischemic stroke. Stroke is a medical emergency. Prognosis depends on minimizing time from the onset of symptoms to thrombolytic intervention if thrombosis is the cause.

TABLE 10-10	Characteristics of Stroke Subtypes				
Parameter	Systemic Hypoperfusion	Embolism	Thrombosis	Subarachnoid Hemorrhage	Intracerebral Hemorrhage
Risk factors	Hypotension Hemorrhage Cardiac arrest	Smoking Ischemic heart disease Peripheral vascular disease Diabetes mellitus White men	Smoking Ischemic heart disease Peripheral vascular disease Diabetes mellitus White men	Often absent Hypertension Coagulopathy Drugs Trauma	Hypertension Coagulopathy Drugs Trauma
Onset	Parallels risk factors	Sudden	Often preceded by a TIA	Sudden, often during exertion	Gradually progressive
Signs and symptoms	Pallor Diaphoresis Hypotension	Headache	Headache	Headache Vomiting Transient loss of consciousness	Headache Vomiting Decreased level of consciousness Seizures
Imaging	CT (black) MRI	CT (black) MRI	CT (black) MRI	CT (white) MRI	CT (white) MRI

TIA, transient ischemic attack.
Adapted from Caplan LR: Diagnosis and treatment of ischemic stroke. JAMA 1991;266:2413–2418.

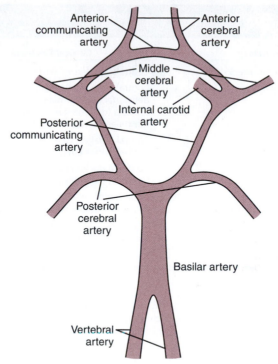

Figure 10-3 • Cerebral circulation and circle of Willis. The cerebral blood supply is from the vertebral arteries (arising from the subclavian arteries) and the internal carotid arteries (arising from the common carotid arteries).

2. Risk Factors include systemic hypertension, cigarette smoking, hyperlipidemia, diabetes mellitus, excessive alcohol consumption, and increased serum homocysteine concentrations.

3. Diagnosis. Imaging with noncontrast CT reliably distinguishes acute intracerebral hemorrhage from ischemia, which have very different treatments. Conventional angiography is useful in demonstrating arterial occlusion. Other tests include magnetic resonance angiography and transcranial Doppler sonography.

  a. Acute Ischemic Strokes are due to embolism occurring from a cardiac source, large-vessel atherothromboembolism (often from the carotid bifurcation in the neck), and small-vessel occlusive disease (lacunar infarction). Echocardiography is useful for evaluating the patient's cardiac status and looking for sources of embolism.

   1.) Management of Acute Ischemic Stroke includes aspirin. Intravenous recombinant tissue plasminogen activator (tPA) is used in patients who meet specific eligibility requirements if treatment can be initiated within 3 hours of the onset, or infusion of thrombolytic

TABLE 10-11   Clinical Features of Cerebrovascular Occlusive Syndromes

Occluded Artery	Clinical Features
Anterior cerebral artery	Contralateral leg weakness
Middle cerebral artery	Contralateral hemiparesis and hemisensory deficit (face and arm more than leg) Aphasia (dominant hemisphere) Contralateral visual field defect
Posterior cerebral artery	Contralateral visual field defect Contralateral hemiparesis
Penetrating arteries	Contralateral hemiparesis Contralateral hemisensory
Basilar artery	Oculomotor deficits and/or ataxia with "crossed" sensory and motor deficits
Vertebral artery	Lower cranial nerve deficits and/or ataxia with crossed sensory deficits

Adapted from Morgenstern LB, Kasner SE: Cerebrovascular disorders. Sci Am Med 2000:1–15.

drugs (prourokinase or tPA) into occluded blood vessels. Supportive therapy includes airway management, oxygenation, ventilation, and control of systemic blood pressure, blood glucose concentrations, and body temperature.

a.) **Blood Pressure Control.** Systemic hypertension is common. Rapid lowering of systemic blood pressure can impair CBF and worsen ischemic injury. Antihypertensive drug therapy (small intravenous doses of labetalol) may be used when necessary to maintain the systemic blood pressure at less than 185/110 mm Hg to lessen myocardial work and irritability. Hypervolemic hemodilution may be considered in attempts to increase CBF while decreasing blood viscosity without significant decreases in oxygen delivery.

b.) **Hyperglycemia.** Normalization of blood glucose concentrations is recommended, using insulin when appropriate, and the administration of parenteral glucose should be minimized.

c.) **Temperature Control.** Benefits of hypothermia are not proven in humans. Fever should be avoided.

b. *Acute Hemorrhagic Stroke* results from either intracerebral or subarachnoid hemorrhage.

1.) *Intracerebral Hemorrhage* is four times more likely than ischemic stroke to cause death and cannot be reliably distinguished from ischemic stroke by clinical criteria. A noncontrast CT evaluation is needed. Intravenous administration of recombinant activated factor VIIA within 4 hours of onset has been shown to decrease hematoma volume and improve clinical outcome. Intraventricular hemorrhage may occlude CSF drainage. Prompt ventricular drainage is performed for any signs of hydrocephalus. An ICP monitor is often recommended for patients who are obtunded. Systemic blood pressure management is controversial, as there is concern about decreasing CPP in those with increased ICP. In patients with coexisting essential hypertension, a goal may be to keep the MAP at less than 130 mm Hg.

2.) *Subarachnoid Hemorrhage (SAH).* Spontaneous subarachnoid hemorrhage most commonly results from rupture of intracranial aneurysms. Risk factors for aneurysm rupture are aneurysm size (>25 mm), systemic hypertension, cigarette smoking, cocaine abuse, female sex, and use of oral contraceptives.

   a.) **Diagnosis of SAH** is based on clinical symptoms (e.g., "worst headache of my life") and CT demonstration of subarachnoid blood. Rapid onset of photophobia, stiff neck, decreased level of consciousness, and focal neurologic changes also suggest SAH. Establishing the diagnosis promptly followed by treatment of the aneurysm can decrease morbidity and mortality. Two common methods used to grade the severity of subarachnoid hemorrhage are the Hunt and Hess classification and the World Federation of Neurologic Surgeons grading system (**Table 10-12**). These systems help predict severity and outcome and help to evaluate the efficacy of various therapies.

   b.) **Treatment** involves localizing the aneurysm with conventional or magnetic resonance angiography and excluding the aneurysmal sac from the intracranial circulation while preserving the parent artery, either by surgical or endovascular techniques. Supportive treatment includes anticonvulsants, control of systemic blood pressure, and ventricular drainage.

   c.) **Vasospasm.** The incidence and severity of vasospasm correlate with the amount of subarachnoid blood seen on CT. Vasospasm typically occurs 3 to 15 days after SAH. Triple H therapy (hypertension, hypervolemia, passive hemodilution) is initiated if vasospasm occurs. Nimodipine, a calcium channel blocker, has been shown to improve outcome when initiated on the first day and continued for 21 days after SAH.

   d.) **Management of Anesthesia.** The goals of anesthesia are to limit the risks of aneurysm rupture, prevent cerebral ischemia, and facilitate surgical exposure (**Table 10-13**).

VI. VASCULAR MALFORMATIONS

A. Arteriovenous Malformations (AVMs) are abnormal blood vessels with multiple direct arterial-to-venous connections without intervening capillaries. Rupture is not clinically associated with acute or chronic hypertensive episodes. Although often congenital, they commonly present in adulthood as either hemorrhage or new-onset seizures (stealing of blood away from normal brain toward the low-resistance AVM, gliosis due to previous hemorrhage).

TABLE 10-12	Common Grading Systems for Subarachnoid Hemorrhage	
Hunt & Hess Classification		
Score	**Neurologic Finding**	**Mortality**
0	Unruptured aneurysm	0%–2%
1	Ruptured aneurysm with minimal headache and no neurologic deficits	2%–5%
2	Moderate to severe headache, no deficit other than cranial nerve palsy	5%–10%
3	Drowsiness, confusion, or mild focal motor deficit	5%–10%
4	Stupor, significant hemiparesis, early decerebration	25%–30%
5	Deep coma, decerebrate rigidity	40%–50%
World Federation of Neurologic Surgeons Grading System		
Score	**GCS**	**Presence of Major Focal Deficit**
0		Intact, unruptured aneurysm
1	15	No
2	13–14	No
3	13–14	Yes
4	7–12	Yes or no
5	3–6	Yes or no

GCS, Glasgow Coma Scale.
Adapted from Lam AM: Cerebral aneurysms: Anesthetic considerations. In Cottrell JE, Smith DS (eds): Anesthesia and Neurosurgery, 4th ed. St. Louis, Mosby, 2001.

1. Diagnosis is made by either MRI or angiography.

2. Treatment can involve surgical resection, highly focused (gamma knife) radiation, angiographically guided embolization, or a combination of these.

3. Prognosis can be estimated using the Spetzler-Martin AVM grading system (**Table 10-14**).

B. **Venous Angiomas** are of tufts of veins that may present as hemorrhage or new-onset seizures.

C. **Cavernous Angioma** are benign lesions that consist of vascular channels without large feeding arteries or large veins that may present as new-onset seizures or occasionally as hemorrhage. Treatment usually involves surgical resection for symptomatic lesions.

D. **Capillary Telangiectasias** represent low-flow, enlarged capillaries and are probably one of the least understood vascular lesions of the central nervous system. The risk of hemorrhage is low, except for lesions occurring in the brainstem. These lesions are usually not treatable.

162

TABLE 10-13	**Anesthesia Considerations for Cerebral Aneurysm Surgery**
Induction	Avoid increases in systemic blood pressure. Avoid excessive decreases in ICP prior to dural opening (increases transmural pressure). Avoid hyperventilation. Avoid decreases in systemic blood pressure if patient has high ICP or vasospasm (decreased CPP).
Monitoring	Use arterial catheter for blood pressure monitoring and frequent blood sampling. Check CVP for monitoring central volume. Use PA catheter and/or transesophageal echocardiogram in patients with cardiac indications. EEG, somatosensory or motor evoked potentials are of limited use.
Induction	Administer IV thiopental, propofol, or etomidate. Administer nondepolarizing muscle relaxants.
Intubation	IV short-acting beta-blockers, lidocaine, propofol, barbiturates or short-acting opioids may blunt response.
Intravenous access	Prepare for possible large volume fluid and blood resuscitation in case of aneurysm rupture.
Management in case of rupture	Perform aggressive volume resuscitation. Create controlled hypotension (e.g., nitroprusside) until clipped, then return blood pressure to normal or slightly elevated.
Maintenance	Volatile anesthetic agents with narcotic supplementation. Muscle paralysis during clipping. For elevated ICP: monitor hyperventilation, CSF drainage, diuretics, patient positioning to maximize exposure. Avoid glucose-containing intravenous solutions (hyperglycemia exacerbates cerebral neural injury) Barbiturates may be protective if the parent vessel must be clamped for >10 minutes.
Emergence	Administer labetolol or esmolol to control BP. Use lidocaine during airway manipulation. Extubate early if possible. Delayed emergence may indicate vasospasm, surgical complication.

BP, blood pressure, EEG, electroencephalogram; ICP, intracranial pressure; IV, intravenous.

E. Arteriovenous Fistulas (AVFs) are direct communications between an artery and a vein that may arise spontaneously, as the result of trauma, or in association with a previous rupture of an intracavernous carotid artery. They commonly present with tinnitus. Treatment is angiographic embolization, or surgical ligation. Diagnosis is made by magnetic resonance or conventional angiography.
F. Management of Anesthesia. Surgical resection of low-flow vascular malformations (i.e., venous angiomas and cavernous angiomas) is generally

TABLE 10-14	Spetzler-Martin Arteriovenous Malformation Grading System

Graded Feature	Points Assigned
Nidus size	
Small (<3 cm)	1
Medium (3–6 cm)	2
Large (>6 cm)	3
Eloquence of adjacent brain*	
Noneloquent	0
Eloquent	1
Pattern of venous drainage	
Superficial only	0
Deep only or deep andsuperficial	1

Surgical Outcome Based On Spetzler-Martin AVM Grading System	
Grade	Percent of Patients With No Postoperative Neurologic Deficit
1	100
2	95
3	84
4	73
5	69

*Eloquent brain refers to sensory, motor, language, or visual areas as well as hypothalamus, thalamus, internal capsule, brainstem cerebellar peduncles, and deep nuclei.
AVM, arteriovenous malformations.
Adapted from Spetzler RF, Martin NA: A proposed grading system for arteriovenous malformations. J Neurosurg 65:476;1986.

not associated with the degree of both intraoperative and postoperative complications as associated with the resection of high-flow vascular lesions (i.e., AVMs and AV fistulas). Considerations include management of high ICP and meticulous blood pressure control (hypotension may result in ischemia in hypoperfused areas, and hypertension may increase the risk of rupture). A smooth, hemodynamically stable induction of general anesthesia is paramount. Muscle relaxation should be accomplished with nondepolarizing neuromuscular blocking. Techniques to blunt the hemodynamic responses to stimulating events such as laryngoscopy, pinion placement, and incision should be used. Hypotonic and glucose-containing solutions should be avoided; mild hyperventilation ($PaCO_2$ of 30–35 mm Hg) will help facilitate surgical exposure. Lumbar CSF drainage may also help to decrease intracranial volume and improve exposure. Diuretics such as mannitol and furosemide, or, in extreme cases, high-dose barbiturate or propofol anesthesia, may be used to treat cerebral edema.

VII. MOYAMOYA DISEASE

Progressive stenosis of intracranial vessels with the secondary development of an anastomotic capillary network is the hallmark of moyamoya disease. It may be seen following head trauma or in association with other disorders such as neurofibromatosis, tuberous sclerosis, and fibromuscular dysplasia. Intracranial aneurysms occur with increased frequency. Symptoms can be ischemic or hemorrhagic in nature.

A. Diagnosis is typically made by conventional or magnetic resonance angiography.

B. Medical Treatment usually consists of a combination of vasodilators and anticoagulants.

C. Surgical Treatment includes direct anastomosis of the superficial temporal artery to the middle cerebral artery (also known as an extracranial-intracranial bypass).

D. Prognosis is not good; only 58% of patients ever attain normal neurologic function.

E. Management of Anesthesia. Preoperative assessment should document preexisting neurologic deficits. Anticoagulants or antiplatelet drug should be discontinued, if possible, to avoid bleeding complications intraoperatively.

The goals of induction and maintenance of anesthesia include hemodynamic stability (hypotension could lead to ischemia in the distribution of the abnormal vessels, and hypertension may cause hemorrhagic complications); avoidance of factors that lead to cerebral or peripheral vasoconstriction (hypocapnia and phenylephrine), which can compromise blood flow in the feeding or recipient vessels; and provision of a rapid emergence from anesthesia so that neurologic function can be assessed. Excessive hyperventilation should be avoided due to its cerebral vasoconstrictive effect. Hypovolemia should be treated with colloid or nonhypotonic crystalloid. Dopamine and ephedrine are reasonable options for the pharmacologic treatment of hypotension. Anemia should be treated to prevent ischemia in already compromised brain regions. Postoperative complications include stroke, seizure, and hemorrhage.

VIII. TRAUMATIC BRAIN INJURY

Traumatic brain injury is the leading cause of disability and death in young adults in the United States.

A. Diagnosis is usually by CT scan. The Glasgow Coma Scale score provides a reproducible method for assessing the seriousness of brain injury (scores of <8 points indicate severe injury) and for following the patient's neurologic status (**Table 10-6**). Head injury patients with scores less than 8 are by definition in coma, and approximately 50% of these patients die or remain in vegetative states.

B. Perioperative Management of patients with acute head trauma must consider the risks of secondary injury due to cerebral ischemia as well as injuries affecting organ systems other than the brain. CBF is usually initially decreased and then gradually increases with time. Factors contributing to poor outcome in head injury patients are increased ICP and systolic blood pressures less than 70 mm Hg. Hyperventilation, although effective in controlling ICP, may contribute to cerebral ischemia in head injury patients and it is a common recommendation to avoid hyperventilation. Barbiturate coma may be useful in some patients as a means to control intracranial hypertension. Associated lung injuries may impair oxygenation and ventilation in these patients and necessitate mechanical ventilation. Neurogenic pulmonary edema may also contribute to acute pulmonary dysfunction. Disseminated intravascular coagulation can occur following severe head injury, possibly due to the release of brain thromboplastin into the systemic circulation.

C. Management of Anesthesia includes efforts to optimize CPP, minimize the occurrence of cerebral ischemia, and avoid drugs and techniques that could increase ICP. CPP is maintained above 70 mm Hg if possible, and hyperventilation is not used unless it is needed as a temporizing measure to control ICP. Glucose-containing solutions should be avoided unless specifically indicated. In moribund patients, the establishment of a safe and effective airway takes priority over concerns for anesthetic selection, as drugs may not be needed. One should also be aware of the possible presence of hidden extracranial injuries (i.e., bone fractures, pneumothorax) as they may lead to problems such as excessive blood loss and perturbations in ventilation and circulation. Nitrous oxide should be avoided because of the risk of pneumocephalus and concern for non-neurologic injuries such as pneumothorax. If acute brain swelling develops, correctable causes such as hypercapnia, arterial hypoxemia, systemic hypertension, and venous obstruction must be considered and corrected if present. Intra-arterial monitoring of systemic blood pressure is helpful, whereas time constraints may limit the use of CVP or pulmonary artery catheter monitoring. During the postoperative period, it is common to maintain skeletal muscle paralysis to facilitate mechanical ventilation.

D. Hematomas. Four major types of intracranial hematoma are described based on their location: epidural, subarachnoid, subdural, and intraparenchymal.

   1. Epidural Hematoma results from arterial bleeding into the space between the skull and dura. The cause is usually a tear in a meningeal artery (may be associated with skull fracture). Often, patients experience loss of consciousness in association with the injury, followed by return of consciousness. Hemiparesis, mydriasis, and bradycardia then suddenly develop a few hours after the head injury, reflecting uncal herniation and brainstem compression. Treatment is prompt drainage.

   2. Traumatic Subarachnoid Hematoma, like subarachnoid hemorrhage associated with aneurysmal rupture, is also associated with the development of cerebral vasospasm.

   3. Subdural Hematoma results from lacerated or torn bridging veins that bleed into the space between the dura and arachnoid. Examination of the CSF reveals clear fluid as subdural blood does not typically have access to the subarachnoid CSF. Diagnosis of a subdural hematoma is confirmed by CT. Head trauma is the most common cause. Patients may view the causative head trauma as trivial, and it may have been forgotten by the patient.

   a. Signs and Symptoms evolve gradually over several days (in contrast to epidural hematomas). Headache is a universal complaint. Drowsiness and obtundation are characteristic findings. Lateralizing neurologic signs eventually occur, manifesting as hemiparesis, hemianopsia, and language disturbances. Elderly patients may have unexplained progressive dementia.

166

b. Treatment. Conservative medical management of subdural hematomas may be acceptable for patients whose condition stabilizes. The most likely treatment is surgical evacuation of the clot, as the prognosis is poor if coma develops. Because venous bleeding in usually the cause of a subdural hematoma, following evacuation of the hematoma, normocapnia is usually the goal to allow for a larger brain volume in an attempt to tamponade any sites of venous bleeding.

4. Intraparenchymal Hematoma is an abnormal collection of blood within the brain tissue proper. Treatment is usually conservative.

IX. CONGENITAL ANOMALIES OF THE BRAIN

A. Chiari Malformations are a group of disorders consisting of congenital displacement of the cerebellum. A Chiari I malformation is downward displacement of the cerebellar tonsils over the cervical spinal cord; Chiari II malformations consist of downward displacement of the cerebellar vermis and are often associated with a meningomyelocele. Chiari III malformations are extremely rare and represent displacement of the cerebellum into an occipital encephalocele.

1. Signs and Symptoms of Chiari I malformation are an occipital headache made worse by coughing or moving the head, often extending into the shoulders and arms, with corresponding cutaneous dysasthesia. Visual disturbances, intermittent vertigo, ataxia, and signs of syringomyelia can occur. Chiari II malformations usually present in infancy with obstructive hydrocephalus plus lower brainstem and cranial nerve dysfunction.

2. Treatment consists of surgical decompression by freeing adhesions and enlarging the foramen magnum. Management of anesthesia must consider the possibility of associated increases in ICP as well as significant intraoperative blood loss, especially in the case of Chiari II malformations.

B. Tuberous Sclerosis (Bourneville's disease) is characterized by mental retardation, seizures, and facial angiofibromas. Pathologically, tuberous sclerosis can be viewed as a condition in which a constellation of benign hamartomatous proliferative lesions and malformations occur in virtually every organ of the body (cortical brain tubors, giant cell astrocytomas, cardiac rhabdomyomas, angiomyolipomas, renal cysts, oral lesions [nodular tumors, fibromas, papillomas]). Prognosis depends on the organ systems involved, ranging from no symptoms to life-threatening complications.

1. Anesthesia Management considers the likely presence of mental retardation and treatment of seizures with antiepileptic drugs. Upper airway abnormalities are determined preoperatively. Cardiac involvement may be associated with intraoperative cardiac arrhythmias. Impaired renal function may have implications when selecting drugs that depend on renal clearance mechanisms.

C. Von Hippel–Lindau Disease is characterized by retinal angiomas, hemangioblastomas, and central nervous system (typically cerebellar) and visceral tumors. Management of anesthesia in patients with von Hippel–Lindau disease must consider the increased risk of pheochromocytomas. The possibility of spinal cord hemangioblastomas may limit the use of spinal anesthesia, although epidural anesthesia has been described for cesarean section. Exaggerated systemic hypertension during direct laryngoscopy or with surgical stimulation may require intervention with esmolol, labetalol, or sodium nitroprusside.

D. Neurofibromatosis is caused by an autosomal dominant mutation that is not limited to racial or ethnic origin and has a diversity of clinical features (**Table 10-15**). One feature common to all patients is progression of the disease with time.

    1. Treatment consists of symptomatic drug therapy, such as antiepileptic drugs, and appropriately timed surgery. Surgical removal of cutaneous neurofibromas is reserved for those that are particularly disfiguring or functionally compromising. Progressive kyphoscoliosis is best treated with surgical stabilization.

    2. Management of Anesthesia. Although rare, the possible presence of pheochromocytomas should be considered during the preoperative evaluation. Signs of increased ICP may reflect expanding intracranial tumors. Airway patency may be jeopardized by expanding laryngeal neurofibromas. Selection of regional anesthesia must recognize the possible future development of neurofibromas involving the spinal cord. Nevertheless, epidural analgesia is an effective method for producing analgesia during labor and delivery.

X. DEGENERATIVE DISEASES OF THE BRAIN

A. Alzheimer's Disease is a chronic neurodegenerative disorder and the most common cause of dementia in patients more than 65 years of age. Diffuse amyloid-rich senile plaques and neurofibrillary tangles are the hallmark pathologic findings. Early-onset Alzheimer's disease usually presents before age 60 and has an autosomal dominant mode of transmission. Late-onset

TABLE 10-15 Manifestations of Neurofibromatosis
Café au lait spots (present at birth, vary from 1 mm to >15 mm in size)
Neurofibromas (cutaneous, neural, vascular)
Intracranial tumor (presence of bilateral acoustic neuromas and café au lait spots establishes diagnosis)
Spinal cord tumor
Pseudarthrosis
Kyphoscoliosis
Short stature
Cancer (neurofibrosarcoma, malignant schwannoma, Wilms' tumor, rhabdomyosarcoma, leukemia)
Endocrine abnormalities (rare pheochromocytomas)
Learning disability
Seizures
Congenital heart disease (pulmonic stenosis)

Alzheimer's disease usually develops after age 60, and genetic transmission plays a relatively minor role. With both forms of the disease, patients develop progressive cognitive impairment (problems with memory, apraxia, aphasia, agnosia). Premortem diagnosis is one of exclusion. Treatment focuses on control of symptoms. Pharmacologic options include cholinesterase inhibitors, such as tacrine, donepezil, rivastigmine, and galantamine. Prognosis is poor.

1. Anesthesia Management. Shorter-acting sedative/hypnotic drugs, anesthetic agents, and narcotics are preferred because they may allow a more rapid return to baseline mental status. Prolongation of the effect of succinylcholine and relative resistance to nondepolarizing muscle relaxants may occur due to the use of cholinesterase inhibitors.

B. Parkinson's Disease is a neurodegenerative disorder of unknown cause marked by a characteristic loss of dopaminergic fibers in the basal ganglia; regional dopamine concentrations are also depleted. Depletion of dopamine results in diminished inhibition of neurons controlling the extrapyramidal motor system and unopposed stimulation by acetylcholine.

1. Signs and Symptoms. The classic triad of major signs of Parkinson's disease consists of skeletal muscle tremor, rigidity, and akinesia. The earliest manifestations may be loss of associated arm swings when walking and absence of head rotation when turning the body. Facial immobility and tremors occur. Dementia and depression are often present.

2. Medical Treatment is to increase dopamine in the basal ganglia or decrease the neuronal effects of acetylcholine.

a. Levodopa combined with a decarboxylase inhibitor (prevents peripheral conversion of levodopa to dopamine and optimizes the amount of levodopa available to the central nervous system) is the standard medical treatment. Side effects of levodopa include dyskinesias (the most serious side effect, developing in 80% of patients after 1 year of treatment) and psychiatric disturbances (including agitation, hallucinations, mania, and paranoia). Orthostatic hypotension may be prominent in treated patients.

b. Amantadine, an antiviral agent, is reported to help control the symptoms of Parkinson's disease.

c. Selegiline (type B monoamine oxidase inhibitor) can help control the symptoms of Parkinson's disease by inhibiting the catabolism of dopamine in the central nervous system. Selegiline is not associated with tyramine-associated hypertensive crisis.

3. Surgical Treatment is reserved for disabling and medically refractory symptoms. Stimulation of the subthalamic nuclei via an implanted deep brain stimulator device may relieve or help to control tremor. Pallidotomy is associated with significant improvement in levodopa-induced dyskinesias.

4. Management of Anesthesia. Levodopa therapy, including the usual morning dose on the day of surgery, should be continued during the perioperative period. Oral levodopa can be administered approximately 20 minutes before inducing anesthesia and may be repeated intraoperatively and postoperatively via an orogastric or nasogastric tube to minimize the likelihood of exacerbations (muscle rigidity interfering with ventilation).

Butyrophenones (e.g., droperidol, haloperidol) antagonize the effects of dopamine in the basal ganglia. An acute dystonic reaction following administration of alfentanil has been speculated to reflect opioid-induced decreases in central dopaminergic transmission. Use of ketamine is questionable because of the possible provocation of exaggerated sympathetic nervous system responses.

C. Hallervorden-Spatz Disease is a rare progressive disorder of the basal ganglia starting in childhood and leading to death in approximately 10 years. Dementia and dystonia with torticollis, as well as scoliosis, are commonly present. Skeletal muscle contractures and bony changes may lead to immobility of the temporomandibular joint and cervical spine, even in the presence of deep general anesthesia or drug-induced skeletal muscle paralysis. Noxious stimulation, as produced by attempted awake tracheal intubation, can intensify dystonia. Administration of succinylcholine is questionable. Emergence from anesthesia is predictably accompanied by return of dystonic posturing.

D. Huntington's Disease is a premature degenerative disease of the central nervous system characterized by marked atrophy of the caudate nucleus and, to a lesser degree, the putamen and globus pallidus. Manifestations include progressive dementia combined with choreoathetosis. Involvement of the pharyngeal muscles makes these patients susceptible to pulmonary aspiration. The duration of Huntington's disease, from clinical onset to death, averages 17 years and is often the result of suicide.

> **1. Treatment** is symptomatic. Haloperidol and other butyrophenones may be administered to control the chorea and emotional lability associated with the disease.

> **2. Anesthesia Management** considers the risk of pulmonary aspiration. Preoperative sedation using butyrophenones such as droperidol or haloperidol may be helpful in controlling choreiform movements. Decreased plasma cholinesterase activity, with prolonged responses to succinylcholine, has been observed.

E. Torticollis presents as spasmodic contraction of nuchal muscles, which may progress to involvement of limb and girdle muscles. Hypertrophy of the sternocleidomastoid muscles may be present. There are no known problems relative to the selection of anesthetic drugs, but spasm of nuchal muscles can interfere with maintenance of a patent upper airway before institution of skeletal muscle paralysis. Sudden appearance of torticollis after administration of anesthetic drugs has been reported, which responds dramatically to administration of diphenhydramine, 25 to 50 mg intravenously (IV).

F. Transmissible Spongiform Encephalopathies (Creutzfeldt-Jakob disease, kuru, Gerstmann-Straussler-Scheinker syndrome) are noninflammatory diseases of the central nervous system caused by transmissible slow infectious protein pathogens known as prions. Prions differ from viruses in that they lack RNA and DNA and fail to produce a detectable immune reaction. Transmissible spongiform encephalopathies are diagnosed on the basis of clinical and neuropathologic findings (diffuse or focally clustered small, round vacuoles that may become confluent). Bovine spongiform encephalopathy (mad cow disease) is a transmissible spongiform encephalopathy that occurs in animals.

> **1. Creutzfeldt-Jakob Disease (CJD)** is the most common transmissible spongiform encephalopathy. The time interval between infection and development of symptoms is months to years. The disease develops by accumulation of an abnormal protein thought to act as a neurotransmitter in the central nervous system. Rapidly progressive dementia with ataxia and

myoclonus suggests the diagnosis, although confirmation may require a brain biopsy. No vaccines or treatments are effective.

   a. Universal Infection Precautions are recommended when caring for patients with CJD, but other precautions are not necessary. Handling CSF calls for special precautions (double gloves, protective glasses, specimen labeled "infectious"), as this has been the only body fluid shown to result in transmission to primates. Surgical instruments should be disposable or should be decontaminated by soaking in sodium hypochlorite or autoclaving. Human-to-human transmission has occurred inadvertently in association with surgical procedures (corneal transplantation, stereotactic procedures with previously used electrodes, contaminated neurosurgical instruments, and human cadaveric dura mater transplantation).

   b. Management of Anesthesia includes the use of universal infection precautions, disposable equipment, and sterilization of any reusable equipment (laryngoscope blades) using sodium hypochlorite. Personnel participating in anesthesia are kept to a minimum, and they should wear protective gowns, gloves, and face masks with transparent protective visors to protect the eyes.

G. Multiple Sclerosis is an autoimmune disease affecting the central nervous system that seems to occur in genetically susceptible persons. It is characterized by diverse combinations of inflammation, demyelination, and axonal damage in the central nervous system. The loss of myelin covering the axons is followed by formation of demyelinative plaques. Peripheral nerves are not affected.

   1. Clinical Manifestations reflect sites of demyelination in the central nervous system and spinal cord and include gait disturbances, limb paresthesias and weakness, urinary incontinence, sexual impotence, optic neuritis (diminished visual acuity, defective pupillary reaction to light), ascending spastic paresis of the skeletal muscles, and Lhermitte's sign (an electrical sensation that runs down the back into the legs in response to flexion of the neck). Increases in body temperature can cause exacerbation of symptoms due to further alterations in nerve conduction in regions of demyelination. There is an increased incidence of seizure disorders. The course of multiple sclerosis is characterized by exacerbations and remissions of symptoms at unpredictable intervals over a period of several years.

   2. Diagnosis is based on clinical features alone or clinical features in combination with oligoclonal abnormalities of immunoglobulins in the CSF, prolonged latency of evoked potentials reflecting slowing of nerve conduction due to demyelination, and signal changes in white matter seen on cranial MRI.

   3. Treatment is directed at both symptom control and methods to slow the progression of disease, and includes corticosteroids, interferon-β, glatiramer acetate (a mixture of random synthetic polypeptides synthesized to mimic myelin basic protein), mitoxantrone (an immunosuppressive agent), azathioprine, and low-dose methotrexate.

   4. Management of Anesthesia considers the impact of surgical stress on the natural progression of the disease (symptoms of multiple sclerosis will likely be exacerbated postoperatively). Any increase in body temperature (e.g., as little as 1°C) that follows surgery may be more likely than drugs to be responsible for exacerbations of multiple sclerosis. Spinal anesthesia has been implicated in postoperative exacerbations of multiple sclerosis, but exacerbations of the disease after epidural anesthesia or peripheral nerve blocks have not been described. Exaggerated release of muscle potassium and hyperkalemia can follow administration of succinylcholine. Corticosteroid supplementation during the perioperative period may be indicated in patients undergoing long-term treatment with these drugs.

H. Postpolio Sequelae include fatigue, skeletal muscle weakness, joint pain, cold intolerance, dysphagia, and sleep and breathing problems (i.e., obstructive sleep apnea) that presumably reflect neurologic damage from the original poliovirus infection. Anesthesia considerations include exquisite sensitivity to sedative effects of anesthetics and delayed awakening from anesthesia, sensitivity to nondepolarizing muscle relaxants, exaggerated postoperative shivering, and increased postoperative pain. Outpatient surgery may not be appropriate for many postpolio patients because they are at increased risk of complications secondary to respiratory muscle weakness and dysphagia.

XI. SEIZURE DISORDERS

Seizures are caused by transient, paroxysmal, and synchronous discharge of groups of neurons in the brain. Epilepsy is defined as recurrent seizures resulting from congenital or acquired (e.g., cerebral scarring) factors. Simple seizures involve no loss of consciousness, whereas altered levels of consciousness are seen in complex seizures. Partial seizures appear to originate from a limited population of neurons in a single hemisphere, whereas generalized seizures appear to initially involve diffuse activation of neurons in both cerebral hemispheres. A partial seizure that is initially evident in one region of the body (e.g., the right arm) may subsequently become generalized, involving both hemispheres, a process known as the jacksonian march.

A. Pharmacologic Treatment. Seizures are treated initially with antiepileptic drugs, starting with a single drug and achieving seizure control by increasing the dose as necessary. Drugs effective for the treatment of partial seizures include carbamazepine, phenytoin, and valproate. Generalized seizure disorders can be managed with carbamazepine, phenytoin, valproate, barbiturates, gabapentin, or lamotrigine. Except for gabapentin, all the useful antiepileptic drugs are metabolized in the liver before undergoing renal excretion. Gabapentin is excreted unchanged by the kidneys. Carbamazepine, phenytoin, and barbiturates cause enzyme induction, and long-term treatment with these drugs can alter the rate of their own metabolism and that of other drugs.

B. Surgical Treatment is considered in patients who do not respond to antiepileptic drugs, including resection of a single pathologic region of the brain, corpus callosotoy, and hemispherectomy. A more conservative surgical approach to medically intractable seizures involves the implantation of a left vagal nerve stimulator. The left side is chosen because the right vagal nerve usually has significant cardiac innervation, which could lead to severe bradyarrhythmias. The mechanism by which vagal nerve stimulation produces its effects is unclear.

C. Status Epilepticus is a life-threatening condition that manifests as continuous seizure activity or two or more seizures occurring in sequence without recovery of consciousness between them.

The goal of treatment of status epilepticus is prompt establishment of venous access and subsequent pharmacologic suppression of seizure activity combined with support of the patient's airway, ventilation, and circulation and correction of hypoglycemia if present.

D. Management of Anesthesia in patients with seizure disorders includes considering the impact of antiepileptic drugs on organ function, the effect of anesthetic drugs on seizures, and alterations in pharmacokinetics of drugs due to antiepileptic drug-induced enzyme induction. Methohexital, alfentanil, ketamine, Enflurane, isoflurane, and sevoflurane may stimulate epileptiform brainwave activity. Various antiepileptic drugs (phenytoin, carbamazepine) shorten the duration of action of nondepolarizing muscle relaxants. Topiramate may cause unexplained metabolic acidosis. Most inhaled anesthetics, including nitrous oxide, have been reported to produce seizure activity. Thiobarbiturates, opioids, and benzodiazepines are preferred drugs. It is important to maintain treatment with the existing antiepileptic drugs throughout the perioperative period.

XII. NEURO-OCULAR DISORDERS

A. Leber's Optic Atrophy is characterized by degeneration of the retina and atrophy of the optic nerves, culminating in blindness. This rare disorder exhibits mitochondrial inheritance and usually presents as loss of central vision in adolescence or early adulthood, often associated with other neuropathologic conditions, including multiple sclerosis and dystonia.

B. Retinitis Pigmentosa is a genetically and clinically heterogeneous group of inherited retinopathies characterized by degeneration of the retina.

C. Kearns-Sayre Syndrome is characterized by retinitis pigmentosa associated with progressive external ophthalmoplegia, typically manifesting before 20 years of age. Cardiac conduction abnormalities (from bundle branch block to complete atrioventricular heart block) are common. Management of anesthesia requires a high index of suspicion for, and previous preparation to treat, new-onset third-degree atrioventricular heart block.

D. Ischemic Optic Neuropathy should be suspected in patients who complain of visual loss during the first week following surgery of any form. If ischemic optic neuropathy is suspected, urgent ophthalmologic consultation should be obtained. Ischemic injury to the optic nerve can result in loss of both central and peripheral vision. The optic nerve can be functionally divided into an anterior and a posterior segment based on difference in blood supply.

1. Anterior Ischemic Optic Neuropathy. The visual loss associated with anterior ischemic optic neuropathy is due to infarction within the watershed perfusion zones between the small branches of the short posterior ciliary arteries. The usual presentation involves sudden, painless, monocular visual deficits varying in severity from slight decreases in visual acuity to blindness. Prognosis is poor for recovery of visual function. Nonarteritic anterior ischemic optic neuropathy is usually attributed to decreased oxygen delivery to the optic disk in association with hypotension and/or anemia. Arteritic anterior ischemic optic neuropathy, which is less common, is associated with inflammation and thrombosis of the short posterior ciliary arteries and may respond to high-dose corticosteroid therapy.

2. Posterior Ischemic Optic Neuropathy is more common than anterior ischemic optic neuropathy as a cause of visual loss in the perioperative period. It presents as acute loss of vision and visual field defects similar to anterior ischemic optic neuropathy. The etiology of postoperative ischemic optic neuropathy appears to be multifactorial (hypotension, anemia, congenital absence of the central retinal artery, altered optic disk anatomy, air embolism, venous obstruction, infection). It has been described following prolonged spine surgery performed in the prone position, cardiac surgery, radical neck dissection, and hip arthroplasty. Associated nonsurgical, but potentially contributory, factors include cardiac arrest, acute treatment of malignant hypertension, blunt trauma, and severe anemia.

E. Cortical Blindness may follow profound hypotension or circulatory arrest as a result of hypoperfusion and infarction of watershed areas in the parietal or occipital lobes and may also result from air or particulate emboli during cardiopulmonary bypass. Cortical blindness is characterized by loss of vision but retention of pupillary reactions to light and normal funduscopic examinations. CT or MRI abnormalities in the parietal or occipital lobes confirm the diagnosis.

F. Retinal Artery Occlusion presents as painless monocular blindness and occlusion of a branch of the retinal artery that results in limited visual field defects or blurred vision. Visual field defects are often severe initially but improve with time. Central retinal artery occlusion is often caused by emboli from an ulcerated atherosclerotic plaque of the ipsilateral carotid artery.

G. Ophthalmic Venous Obstruction may occur intraoperatively when patient positioning results in external pressure on the orbits. The prone position and use of headrests during neurosurgical procedures require careful attention to ensure that the patient's orbits are free from external compression.

Part II: Spinal Cord Disorders

I. ACUTE TRAUMATIC SPINAL CORD INJURY

A. Spinal Cord Transection. Acute spinal cord transection initially produces flaccid paralysis, with total absence of sensation below the level of the spinal cord injury. The cord is not usually anatomically transected, but complete or nearly complete neuronal dysfunction occurs below a sentinel dermatomal level. The physiologic effects depend on the level of injury. Severe physiologic derangements occur with injury to the cervical cord, and lesser perturbations occur with more caudal cord injuries. The effects of spinal cord injury collectively known as spinal shock include loss of temperature regulation below the level of the injury, hypotension, and bradycardia. Spinal shock typically last 1 to 3 weeks.

1. Acute Cervical Spinal Cord Injury

   a. Diagnosis. Cervical spine radiographs are obtained in a large fraction of patients who present with various forms of trauma for fear of missing occult cervical spine injuries. The probability of cervical spine injury is minimal in patients who meet the following criteria: (1) no midline cervical spine tenderness, (2) no focal neurologic deficits, (3) normal sensorium, (4) no intoxication, and (5) no painful distracting injury. Routine imaging studies are not needed in these patients. The sensitivity of plain radiographs is less than 100%, and therefore the likelihood of cervical spine injury must be interpreted in conjunction with other clinical symptoms and risk factors.

b. Treatment is immediate immobilization to limit neck flexion and extension (halo-thoracic devices are most effective). Manual in-line immobilization is recommended to help minimize cervical spine flexion and extension during direct laryngoscopy for tracheal intubation.

c. Management of Anesthesia

1.) *Direct Laryngoscopy and Tracheal Intubation.* Cervical spine movement during direct laryngoscopy is likely to be concentrated at the occipitoatlantoaxial area.

a.) The key principle when performing direct laryngoscopy is to minimize neck movements during the procedure. Extensive clinical experience supports the use of direct laryngoscopy for orotracheal intubation, provided that (1) maneuvers are taken to stabilize the head during the procedure (avoiding hyperextension of the patient's neck) and (2) evaluation of the patient's airway did not suggest the likelihood of any associated technical difficulty.

b.) There is perhaps an even greater risk of compromise of the blood supply to the spinal cord produced by neck motion that elongates the cord, with resultant narrowing of the longitudinal blood vessels. Maintenance of perfusion pressure may be more important than positioning for preventing spinal cord injury in the presence of cervical spine injury.

c.) Topical anesthesia and awake fiberoptic laryngoscopy are alternatives to direct laryngoscopy if patients are cooperative and airway trauma—with ensuing blood, secretions, and anatomic deformities—does not preclude visualization with the fiberscope.

d.) Awake tracheostomy is reserved for the most challenging airway conditions, in which neck injury, combined with facial fractures or other severe anomalies of airway anatomy, make safely securing the airway by nonsurgical means difficult or unsafe.

2.) *Pathophysiology of Acute Spinal Cord Injury.* Patients with cervical or high thoracic spinal cord injury are vulnerable to dramatic decreases in systemic blood pressure following acute changes in body posture, blood loss, or positive airway pressure. Goals of anesthetic management are optimization of intravascular volume (fluids, blood) to minimize blood pressure changes, ventilatory support, and maintenance of body temperature. Succinylcholine is unlikely to provoke excessive release of potassium during the first few hours after spinal cord transection.

II. CHRONIC SPINAL CORD INJURY

A. Pathophysiology. Early and late sequelae of spinal cord injury are summarized in **Table 10-16**. Several weeks after acute spinal cord transection, the spinal cord reflexes gradually return. The chronic stage is characterized by overactivity of the sympathetic nervous system and involuntary skeletal muscle spasms.

   1. Treatment. Baclofen is useful for treating spasticity. Alternative therapies include diazepam and other benzodiazepines, surgical treatment via dorsal rhizotomy or myelotomy, or implantation of a spinal cord stimulator or subarachnoid baclofen pump.

   2. Management of Anesthesia focuses on preventing autonomic hyperreflexia. Nondepolarizing muscle relaxants are used because succinylcholine is likely to provoke hyperkalemia, particularly during the initial 6 months following spinal cord transection.

TABLE 10-16	Early and Late Complications in Patients with Spinal Cord Injury	
Complication		**Incidence (%)**
2 Years after Injury		
Urinary tract infection		59
Skeletal muscle spasticity		38
Chills and fever		19
Decubitus ulcer		16
Autonomic hyperreflexia		8
Skeletal muscle contractures		6
Heterotopic ossification		3
Pneumonia		3
Renal dysfunction		2
Postoperative wound infection		2
30 Years after Injury		
Decubitus ulcers		17
Skeletal muscle or joint pain		16
Gastrointestinal dysfunction		14
Cardiovascular dysfunction		14
Urinary tract infection		14
Infectious disease or cancer		11
Visual or hearing disorders		10
Urinary retention		8
Male genitourinary dysfunction		7
Renal calculi		6

B. Autonomic Hyperreflexia appears following spinal shock and is triggered by cutaneous stimulation (surgical incision) or visceral stimulation (bladder distension) below the level of spinal cord transection. It is unlikely to occur in injuries below T10.

1. Mechanism. Stimulation below the level of spinal cord transection initiates afferent impulses that enter the spinal cord (**Fig. 10-4**).

2. Signs and Symptoms include systemic hypertension and reflex bradycardia, with cutaneous vasodilation above the level of the spinal cord transection. Patients may complain of headache, blurred vision, and nasal stuffiness. Cerebral, retinal, or subarachnoid hemorrhages can occur, as well as increased operative blood loss. Other effects may be loss of consciousness, seizures, cardiac arrhythmias, and pulmonary edema due to acute left ventricular failure.

3. Anesthetic Management focuses on prevention of autonomic hyperreflexia. Although epidural or spinal anesthesia may reduce the risk, epidural anesthesia may be less effective than spinal anesthesia because of its relative sparing of the sacral segments. Regardless of the technique selected for anesthesia, vasodilator drugs with short half-life (e.g., sodium nitroprusside) should be readily available to treat sudden-onset systemic hypertension. Autonomic hyperreflexia may first manifest postoperatively when the effects of the anesthetic drugs begin to wane.

III. SPINAL CORD TUMORS

Spinal cord tumors can be intramedullary (gliomas, ependymomas), extramedullary intradural (neurofibromas, meningiomas), or extramedullary extradural in location (metastatic lung, breast or prostate tumors). Other mass lesions of the spinal cord,

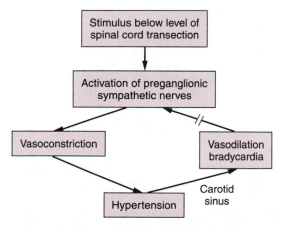

Figure 10-4 • Sequence of events associated with clinical manifestations of autonomic hyperreflexia. Because the afferent impulses that produce vasodilation cannot reach the neurologically isolated portion of the spinal cord, vasoconstriction develops below the level of the spinal cord transection, resulting in systemic hypertension.

including abscesses and hematomas, share many of the clinical signs and symptoms seen with tumors.

A. Symptoms include pain (often aggravated by coughing or straining), motor symptoms, sphincter dysfunction, and spinal tenderness.

B. Diagnosis involves spinal cord imaging (MRI, CT).

C. Management of Anesthesia involves ensuring adequate spinal cord oxygenation and perfusion (avoiding hypotension, anemia, and hypoxemia). Tumors involving the cervical spinal cord may influence the approach used to secure the airway. Airway management is similar to that discussed in the management of acute spinal cord injury. Safe resection of a tumor may require the use of intraoperative electrophysiologic monitoring of neurologic function (electromyography, somatosensory evoked potentials, motor evoked potentials). Succinylcholine should be used with caution in patients with spinal cord tumors given the risk of associated hyperkalemia.

IV. INTERVERTEBRAL DISC DISEASE

Among chronic conditions, low back pain is the most common cause for limitation of activity in patients younger than 45 years of age. Disc disease is the result of trauma or degenerative changes in the intervertebral disc, with nerve root or spinal cord compression from a protruding nucleus pulposus. Pain associated with nerve root compression is usually in a single dermatomal distribution. Spinal cord compression can lead to complex sensory, motor, and autonomic symptoms at and below the level of the insult. CT or MRI confirms the diagnosis and the location.

A. Cervical Disc Disease usually occurs at the C5–C6 or C6–C7 intervertebral spaces. Initial treatment is usually conservative involving rest, pain control, and possible epidural steroids. Surgical decompression is necessary if symptoms do not abate with conservative treatment.

B. Lumbar Disc Disease. The most common site is the L4–L5 and L5–S1 intervertebral spaces. Both sites produce low back pain, which radiates down the posterior and lateral aspects of the thighs and calves (sciatica) and is aggravated by coughing or stretching the sciatic nerve (straight-leg raising).

1. Treatment. Continuing ordinary activities within the limits permitted by the pain leads to more rapid recovery than bed rest or back-mobilizing exercises. When neurologic symptoms persist despite conservative management, surgical laminectomy or microdiscectomy can be considered. An alternative therapy is epidural steroid injection (e.g., triamcinolone, methylprednisolone), although this treatment offers no significant functional benefit, nor does it decrease the need for surgery.

V. CONGENITAL ANOMALIES AND DEGENERATIVE DISEASES OF THE VERTEBRAL COLUMN

A. Spina Bifida Occulta (incomplete formation of a single lamina in the lumbosacral spine without other abnormalities) is a congenital defect that is present in an estimated 20% of individuals. It is often an incidental finding during evaluation of another disease process. A variant of spina bifida occulta known as occult spinal dysraphism is with a tethered spinal cord (cord ending below the

L2–L3 interspace). Up to 50% of individuals with a tethered spinal cord have cutaneous manifestations overlying the anomaly (tufts of hair, hyperpigmented areas, cutaneous lipomas, skin dimples). Performance of spinal anesthesia in patients with a tethered spinal cord may increase the risk of cord injury.

B. Spondylosis is a noncongenital disorder with osteophyte formation and degenerative disc disease. Narrowing of the spinal canal (spinal stenosis) and compression of the spinal cord by transverse osteophytes or nerve root compression by bony spurs in the intervertebral foramina are seen.

1. Symptoms with cervical spondylosis include neck pain and radicular pain in the arms and shoulders that are accompanied by sensory loss and skeletal muscle wasting. Lumbar spondylosis leads to radicular pain and wasting in the lower extremities. Sphincter disturbances are uncommon regardless of the location of spondylosis.

C. Spondylolisthesis is anterior subluxation of one vertebral body on another, most commonly at the lumbosacral junction. Radicular symptoms usually involve the nerve root inferior to the pedicle of the anteriorly subluxed vertebra. Treatment is initially analgesics, anti-inflammatory medications, and physical therapy if the low back pain is the only symptom. Surgery is usually reserved for patients who present with myelopathy, radiculopathy, or neurogenic claudication.

VI. CONGENITAL ANOMALIES AND DEGENERATIVE DISEASES OF THE SPINAL CORD

A. Syringomyelia, also known as syrinx, is a disorder in which there is cystic cavitation of the spinal cord. The condition may be congenital, secondary to spinal cord trauma, or occurring in association with various neoplastic conditions (e.g., gliomas). Rostral extension into the brainstem is called syringobulbia. Cysts may have connections to cerebrospinal fluid spaces (communicating) or be isolated from the cerebrospinal fluid spaces (noncommunicating).

1. Signs and Symptoms include sensory impairment of pain and temperature in the upper extremities. Progressive cavitation of the spinal cord leads to destruction of lower motor neurons. Syringobulbia is characterized by paralysis of the palate, tongue, and vocal cords and loss of sensation over the face. MRI is the preferred diagnostic procedure. No known treatment is effective.

2. Management of Anesthesia. Lower motor neuron disease with skeletal muscle wasting raises the possibility that hyperkalemia could develop after administration of succinylcholine. Thermal regulation may be impaired. With syringobulbia, any decreased or absent protective airway reflexes may influence the timing of tracheal tube removal postoperatively.

B. Amyotrophic Lateral Sclerosis (ALS) is a degenerative disease involving (1) the lower motor neurons in the anterior horn gray matter of the spinal cord and (2) the corticospinal tracts (i.e., the primary descending upper motor neurons.

1. Signs and Symptoms initially are skeletal muscle atrophy, weakness, and fasciculations, often beginning in the intrinsic muscles of the hands.

Progressive signs eventually include atrophy and weakness of most of the patient's skeletal muscles, including the tongue, pharynx, larynx, and chest. Other problems include autonomic nervous system dysfunction (orthostatic hypotension, resting tachycardia). ALS has no known treatment, and death is likely within 6 years after the onset of clinical symptoms, usually due to respiratory failure.

2. Anesthesia Considerations include the possibility of exaggerated ventilatory depression, risk of hyperkalemia after succinylcholine, prolonged responses to nondepolarizing muscle relaxants, and predisposition to pulmonary aspiration due to bulbar palsy.

C. Friedreich's Ataxia is an autosomal recessive inherited condition characterized by degeneration of the spinocerebellar and pyramidal tracts. Other manifestations are cardiomyopathy, kyphoscoliosis with impaired pulmonary function, ataxia, dysarthria, nystagmus, skeletal muscle weakness and spasticity, and diabetes mellitus. Friedreich's ataxia is usually fatal by early adulthood, often due to cardiac failure.

1. Management of Anesthesia is similar to that described for ALS. Response to muscle relaxants seems normal.

Part III: Diseases of the Autonomic and Peripheral Nervous Systems

I. AUTONOMIC DISORDERS

A. Shy-Drager Syndrome belongs to a group of three heterogeneous disorders known as multiple-system atrophy (striatonigral degeneration, olivopontocerebellar atrophy, Shy-Drager syndrome).

1. Signs and Symptoms are related to autonomic nervous system dysfunction (orthostatic hypotension, syncope, urinary retention, bowel dysfunction, sexual impotence, failure of baroreceptor reflexes to produce increases in heart rate or vasoconstriction in response to hypotension).

2. Treatment is symptomatic and includes elastic stockings, a high-sodium diet to expand the intravascular fluid volume, and administration of α-adrenergic agonists (midodrine or yohimbine).

3. Management of Anesthesia. Most patients tolerate general and regional anesthesia without undue risk. Principles of management are prompt correction of hypovolemia and hypotension, the use of direct-acting vasopressor when needed (patients have exaggerated responses to indirect-acting agents), atropine or glycopyrrolate for bradycardia, and adjustment of doses of anesthetic agents to accommodate the patient's diminished compensatory responses.

B. Orthostatic Intolerance Syndrome is a chronic idiopathic disorder of primary autonomic system failure characterized by episodic or postural tachycardia occurring independent of alterations in systemic blood pressure. Symptoms often include palpitations, tremulousness, light-headedness, fatigue, and syncope. Management includes maintenance of circulating volume, and possibly long-term administration of α_1-adrenergic agonists, such as midodrine.

C. Glomus Tumors of the Head and Neck are paragangliomas that arise embryologically from neural crest cells and lie along the carotid artery, aorta, glossopharyngeal nerve, and middle ear. Symptoms such as unilateral pulsatile tinnitus, conductive hearing loss, aural fullness, and a bluish red mass behind the tympanic membrane are characteristic of middle ear involvement, and facial paralysis, dysphonia, hearing loss, and pain are indications of cranial nerve invasion.

    1. Glomus Jugulare Tumors can secrete a variety of hormonal substances such as norepinephrine, cholecystokinin, serotonin, kallikrein, histamine, or bradykinin, thus mimicking pheochromocytoma or carcinoid syndrome.

    2. Treatment is most often radiation. Surgery is recommended if bony destruction is present.

    3. Anesthetic Management. Preoperative determination of serum norepinephrine and catecholamine metabolite (i.e., metanephrine, vanillylmandelic acid) concentrations may detect patients likely to respond as if a pheochromocytoma were present. Administration of phenoxybenzamine or prazosin may be used preoperatively to lower blood pressure and facilitate volume expansion in patients with increased serum norepinephrine concentrations. Invasive hemodynamic monitoring may be warranted. Patients with increased serum 5-hydroxyindoleacetic acid concentration, especially those with symptoms similar to those of carcinoid syndrome, should receive preoperative octreotide, often administered subcutaneously.

D. Carotid Sinus Syndrome is an exaggeration of normal activity of the carotid baroreceptors in response to mechanical stimulation (profound bradycardia and/or hypotension). Treatment includes drugs, a demand-type artificial cardiac pacemaker, ablation of the carotid sinus, or ablation of the glossopharyngeal nerve with ethanol injection.

    1. Management of Anesthesia is complicated by hypotension, bradycardia, and cardiac arrhythmias. Infiltration of a local anesthetic-containing solution around the carotid sinus before dissection usually improves hemodynamic stability but may also interfere with determining the completeness of the ablation. Drugs such as atropine, isoproterenol, and epinephrine or electrical cardiac pacing may be more effective options.

II. DISEASES OF THE PERIPHERAL NERVOUS SYSTEM

A. Idiopathic Facial Paralysis (Bell's Palsy) is characterized by the rapid onset of motor weakness or paralysis of all the muscles innervated by the facial nerve. A viral inflammatory mechanism (perhaps herpes simplex virus) may be the cause. Spontaneous recovery usually occurs over approximately 12 weeks.

    1. Treatment. Prednisone (1 mg/kg orally each day for 5–10 days) dramatically relieves pain and decreases the number of patients experiencing complete denervation of the facial nerve. If blinking is not possible, the patient's affected eye should be covered to protect the cornea from dehydration. Surgical decompression of the facial nerve may be needed for persistent or severe cases of idiopathic facial paralysis or for facial paralysis secondary to trauma.

B. Trigeminal Neuralgia (Tic Douloureux) is characterized by the sudden onset of brief but intense unilateral facial pain triggered by local sensory stimuli to the affected side of the face. It is diagnosed based on purely clinical signs and symptoms.

1. Treatment. Antiepileptic drugs are useful. The anticonvulsant carbamazepine is the drug treatment of choice, but baclofen and lamotrigine are also effective. Surgical therapy (selective radiofrequency destruction of trigeminal nerve fibers, transection of the sensory root of the trigeminal nerve, microsurgical decompression of the trigeminal nerve root) is recommended for individuals who develop pain refractory to drug therapy.

C. Glossopharyngeal Neuralgia is characterized by intense pain in the throat, neck, tongue, and ear triggered by swallowing, chewing, coughing, or talking. Cardiac symptoms (profound bradycardia, hypotension) associated with glossopharyngeal neuralgia may be confused with sick sinus syndrome or carotid sinus syndrome.

1. Treatment of cardiovascular symptoms includes atropine, isoproterenol, an artificial external cardiac pacemaker, or a combination of these modalities). Pain associated with this syndrome is managed by chronic administration of anticonvulsant drugs such as carbamazepine and phenytoin. Permanent pain relief is possible after repeated glossopharyngeal nerve blocks, but this neuralgia is sufficiently life threatening to justify intracranial transection of the nerve in patients not responsive to medical therapy.

2. Management of Anesthesia is directed at maximizing volume status preoperatively and preparation for intraoperative cardiac pacing if necessary. Topical anesthesia of the oropharynx with lidocaine may prevent bradycardia and hypotension that can occur in response to stimulation from direct laryngoscopy. Anticholinergic drugs should be promptly available to treat vagus nerve–mediated responses. Systemic hypertension, tachycardia, and ventricular premature beats may occur after surgical transection of the glossopharyngeal nerve and the upper two roots of the vagus nerve.

D. Charcot-Marie-Tooth Disease is the most common inherited cause of chronic motor and sensory peripheral neuropathy, characterized by distal skeletal muscle weakness, wasting, and loss of tendon reflexes. Classically, this neuropathy is described as being restricted to the lower one third of the legs, producing foot deformities (high pedal arches and talipes) and peroneal muscle atrophy ("stork-leg" appearance).

1. Treatment is limited to supportive measures, including splints, tendon transfers, and various arthrodeses.

2. Management of Anesthesia is influenced by concerns about the responses to neuromuscular blocking drugs and the possibility of postoperative respiratory failure due to weakness of the muscles responsible for respiration. It appears reasonable to avoid succinylcholine based on theoretical concerns about exaggerated potassium release following administration of this drug to individuals with neuromuscular diseases.

E. Brachial Plexus Neuropathy (idiopathic brachial neuritis, Parsonage-Turner syndrome, shoulder-girdle syndrome) is characterized by the acute onset of severe pain in the upper arm and patchy paresis or paralysis of the skeletal muscles innervated by branches of the brachial plexus. Skeletal muscle wasting, particularly involving the shoulder girdle and arm, is common. Diagnosis of brachial plexus neuropathy best accomplished by electrodiagnostic studies. Recovery, though prolonged, is nearly always complete.

F. Guillain-Barré Syndrome (acute idiopathic polyneuritis) is characterized by sudden onset of skeletal muscle weakness or paralysis that typically manifests initially in the legs and spreads cephalad over the ensuing days to involve skeletal muscles of the arms, trunk, and face. Difficulty swallowing due to pharyngeal muscle weakness and impaired ventilation due to intercostal muscle paralysis are the most serious symptoms of this process. Autonomic nervous system dysfunction is seen as wide fluctuations in systemic blood pressure, sudden profuse diaphoresis, peripheral vasoconstriction, resting tachycardia, and cardiac conduction abnormalities. Complete spontaneous recovery can occur within a few weeks or may take months with some permanent paralysis remaining.

    1. Diagnosis (Table 10-17)

    2. Treatment is mainly symptomatic and supportive. Corticosteroids are not considered useful therapy for this syndrome. Plasma exchange or infusion of γ-globulin may benefit some patients.

    3. Management of Anesthesia. Compensatory cardiovascular responses may be absent, resulting in profound hypotension in response to changes in posture, blood loss, or positive airway pressure. Noxious stimulation (direct laryngoscopy) could manifest as exaggerated increases in systemic blood pressure. Patients may exhibit exaggerated responses to indirect-acting vasopressors. Succinylcholine should be avoided. Continued ventilatory support may be needed in the postoperative period.

TABLE 10-17	Diagnostic Criteria for Guillain-Barré Syndrome
Features Required for Diagnosis	
Progressive bilateral weakness in legs and arms	
Areflexia	
Features Strongly Supporting the Diagnosis	
Progression of symptoms over 2–4 weeks	
Symmetry of symptoms	
Mild sensory symptoms or signs (definitive sensory level makes diagnosis doubtful)	
Cranial nerve involvement (especially bilateral facial weakness)	
Spontaneous recovery beginning 2–4 weeks after progression ceases	
Autonomic nervous system dysfunction	
Absence of fever at onset	
Increased concentrations of protein in the cerebrospinal fluid	

G. Neuropathies. Entrapment neuropathies occur at anatomic sites where peripheral nerves pass through narrow passages (median nerve and carpal tunnel at the wrist, ulnar nerve and cubital tunnel at the elbow), making compression a possibility. Focal demyelination of nerve fibers causes slowing or blocking of nerve impulse conduction through the damaged area. Electromyography studies are adjuncts to nerve conduction studies, showing the presence of denervation impulses and ultimately reinnervation of muscle fibers by surviving axons.

1. Carpal Tunnel Syndrome is the most common entrapment neuropathy, resulting from compression of the median nerve between the transverse carpal ligament forming the roof of the carpal tunnel and the carpal bones at the wrist.

   a. Treatment is immobilizing the wrist with a splint initially. Injection of corticosteroids into the carpal tunnel may relieve symptoms but is seldom curative. Definitive treatment is decompression of the median nerve by surgical division of the transverse carpal ligament.

2. Cubital Tunnel Entrapment Syndrome results from compression of the ulnar nerve after it passes through the condylar groove and enters the cubital tunnel. Surgical treatment of cubital tunnel entrapment syndrome (by tunnel decompression and transposition of the nerve) may be helpful for relieving symptoms but may also make symptoms worse, perhaps by interfering with the nerve's blood supply.

3. Diseases Associated with Peripheral Neuropathies

   a. Diabetes Mellitus. Up to 7.5% of patients with non–insulin-dependent diabetes mellitus have clinical neuropathy at the time of diagnosis. The principal manifestations are unpleasant tingling, numbness, burning, and aching in the lower extremities; skeletal muscle weakness; and distal sensory loss. The peripheral nerves of patients with diabetes mellitus are more vulnerable to ischemia due to compression or stretch injury (such as may occur during intraoperative and postoperative positioning), despite accepted padding and positioning during these periods.

   b. Alcohol Abuse. Polyneuropathy of chronic alcoholism is nearly always associated with nutritional and vitamin deficiencies. Symptoms characteristically begin in the lower extremities, with pain and numbness in the feet. Restoration of a proper diet, abstinence from alcohol, and multivitamin therapy promote slow but predictable resolution of the neuropathy.

   c. Vitamin B_{12} Deficiency neuropathy resembles the neuropathy typically seen in patients who abuse alcohol. Nitrous oxide is known to inactivate certain vitamin B_{12}-dependent enzymes, which could lead to symptoms of altered nerve function.

   d. Uremia. Distal polyneuropathy with sensory and motor components often occurs in the extremities of patients with chronic renal failure. Symptoms tend to be more prominent in the legs than in the arms. Improved nerve conduction velocity often occurs within a few days after renal transplantation. Hemodialysis does not appear to be equally effective for reversing the polyneuropathy.

e. Cancer. Peripheral sensory and motor neuropathies occur in patients with a variety of malignancies, especially those involving the lung, ovary, and breast. Myasthenic (Eaton-Lambert) syndrome may be observed in patients with carcinoma of the lung. Invasion of the lower trunks of the brachial plexus by tumors in the apex of the lungs (Pancoast syndrome) produces arm pain, paresthesias, and weakness of the hands and arms.

f. Collagen Vascular Diseases (systemic lupus erythematosus, polyarteritis nodosa, rheumatoid arthritis, scleroderma) are commonly associated with peripheral neuropathies.

g. Sarcoidosis is a disorder of unknown etiology whereby noncaseating granulomas occur in multiple organ systems, most commonly the lung, lymphatics, bone, liver, and nervous system. Polyneuropathy, due to the presence of granulomatous lesions in peripheral nerves, is a common finding in patients with sarcoidosis.

h. Refsum's Disease is a multi-system disorder that manifests as polyneuropathies, ichthyosis, deafness, retinitis pigmentosa, cardiomyopathy, and cerebellar ataxia. Metabolic defects responsible for this disease reflect a failure to oxidize phytic acid, a fatty acid that subsequently accumulates in excessive concentrations.

CHAPTER 11

Diseases of the Liver and Biliary Tract

Diseases of the liver and biliary tract can be categorized as parenchymal liver disease (hepatitis and cirrhosis) and cholestasis with or without obstruction of the extrahepatic biliary pathway.

I. ACUTE HEPATITIS

Acute hepatitis is most often caused by a virus but can also be caused by drugs and toxins. Acute viral hepatitis is typically caused by one of five viruses: hepatitis A virus (HAV), hepatitis B virus (HBV), hepatitis C virus (HCV), hepatitis D virus (HDV), or hepatitis E virus (HEV).

A. **Viral Hepatitis.** All types of viral hepatitis are similar and cannot be distinguished reliably by clinical features or routine laboratory tests.

    1. Classification (Table 11-1)

    2. Diagnosis of viral hepatitis is dependent on clinical signs and symptoms, laboratory findings, serologic assays, and occasionally liver biopsy (**Table 11-2**).

        a. Signs and Symptoms (Table 11-2). The onset of viral hepatitis may be gradual or sudden and most often manifests as dark urine, fatigue, anorexia, and nausea. Other signs may include low-grade fever, upper quadrant pain or generalized abdominal pain, and myalgias or arthralgias. Many of the initial symptoms abate when jaundice develops. Hepatomegaly and splenomegaly may be present. If viral hepatitis is severe, there may be evidence of acute liver failure including confusion, asterixis, peripheral edema, and ascites.

        b. Laboratory Tests

            1.) General. Serum aminotransferase concentrations (aspartate aminotransferase [AST], alanine aminotransferase [ALT]) increase 7 to 14 days before the appearance of jaundice and begin to decrease shortly after jaundice develops. The degree of aminotransferase increase does not necessarily parallel the

TABLE 11-1 Characteristic Features of Viral Hepatitis

Parameter	Type A	Type B	Type C	Type D
Mode of transmission	Fecal-oral Sewage-contaminated shellfish	Percutaneous Sexual	Percutaneous	Percutaneous
Incubation period	20–37 days	60–110 days	35–70 days	60–110 days
Results of serum antigen and antibody tests	IgM early and IgG appears during convalescence	HBsAg and anti-HBc early and persists in carriers	Anti-HCV in 6 weeks to 9 months	Anti-HDV late and may be short-lived
Immunity	Antibodies in 45%	Antibodies in 5%–15%	Unknown	Protected if immune to type B
Course	Does not progress to chronic liver disease	Chronic liver disease develops in 1%–5% of adults and 80%–90% of children	Chronic liver disease develops up to 75%	Co-infection with type B
Prevention after exposure	Pooled γ-globulin Hepatitis A vaccine	Hepatitis B immunoglobulin Hepatitis B vaccine	? Interferon	Unknown
Mortality	<0.2%	0.3%–1.5%	Unknown	Acute icteric hepatitis: 2%–20%

HBc, hepatitis B core antigen; HBsAg, hepatitis B surface antigen.
Adapted from Keefe EB: Acute hepatitis. Sci Am Med 1999;1–9.

TABLE 11-2	Incidence of Signs and Symptoms in Acute Viral Hepatitis	
Symptom/Sign	**Incidence (%)**	
Dark urine	94	
Fatigue	91	
Anorexia	90	
Nausea	87	
Fever	76	
Emesis	71	
Headache	70	
Abdominal discomfort	65	
Light-colored stools	52	
Pruritus	42	

Adapted from Keefe EB: Acute hepatitis. Sci Am Med 1999;1–9.

severity of the hepatitis. Anemia and lymphocytosis are typically present. Serum bilirubin concentration rarely exceeds 20 mg/dL. Alkaline phosphatase is not increased unless cholestasis is present. Severe acute hepatitis may result in hypoalbuminemia and/or a prolonged prothrombin time.

2.) *Serologic Markers (Table 11-3)*

3.) *Liver Biopsy* typically shows spotty necrosis of hepatocytes and widespread parenchymal inflammation.

3. Clinical Course. Hepatitis typically produces symptoms for 7 to 14 days before the appearance of dark urine and jaundice. Serum bilirubin concentration increases for 10 to 14 days and then decreases during the next 14 to 28 days. Aminotransferase concentrations usually begin to decrease just before peak jaundice occurs, and then they decrease rapidly. Chronic hepatitis does not occur after hepatitis A or E but develops in 2% to 7% of patients infected with HBV and in 60% to 75% of patients infected with HCV. Cirrhosis and primary hepatocellular carcinoma are risks of chronic hepatitis B or C.

4. Treatment of acute viral hepatitis is symptomatic, with restriction of physical activity and sensible nutrition and intravenous fluids if needed. Abstinence from alcohol is recommended. Liver transplantation is a consideration for fulminant hepatic failure.

5. Prevention of viral hepatitis includes avoidance of exposure to the virus, passive immunization with γ-globulin, and active immunization with a specific vaccine. Pooled γ-globulin administered intramuscularly as soon as possible after known exposure dramatically decreases the incidence of hepatitis A. Individuals exposed to HBV by percutaneous or mucous membrane routes should receive hepatitis B immunoglobulin and hepatitis B vaccine within 24 hours.

TABLE 11-3 Serologic Markers of Hepatitis

Type of Hepatitis	Serum Marker	Comments
Hepatitis A	IgM anti-HAV	Appears early, persists for approximately 120 days
	IgG anti-HAV	Replaces IgM at about 120 days
Hepatitis B	HbsAg	Appears at 7–14 days, persists several months
	HbsAb	Appears 60–240 days, HbsAg disappears
	HbcAb	Appears early, persists 6–12 months
Hepatitis C	Anti-HCV	Present in acute and chronic infection
	HCV RNA	Indicates ongoing viremia
Hepatitis D (co-infection with type B)	Anti-HDV, HBsAg and IgM anti-HBcAg	
Hepatitis E	anti-HEV antibody	

HBcAg, hepatitis B core antibody; HBsAb, hepatitis B surface antibody; HBsAg, hepatitis B surface antigen.

a. Hepatitis A Vaccine provides protection for 10 years or longer. Travelers to endemic regions, neonatal intensive care unit staff, food handlers, children in day care centers, and military personnel should receive this vaccine.

b. Hepatitis B Vaccine is recommended for individuals at increased risk of HBV infection, including health care workers with frequent exposure to blood products, homosexual men, intravenous drug users, recipients of certain blood products, and infants born to hepatitis B surface antigen (HBsAg)-positive mothers.

B. Additional Viruses that Cause Hepatitis

1. Cytomegalovirus, a herpesvirus, is ubiquitous. It can cause a disease similar to infectious mononucleosis but without adenopathy or tonsillopharyngeal involvement.

2. Epstein-Barr Virus usually produces mild hepatitis associated with nausea and vomiting that is usually part of the typical clinical syndrome of infectious mononucleosis.

C. Drug-Induced Hepatitis.

Many drugs (analgesics, volatile anesthetics, antibiotics, antihypertensives, anticonvulsants, tranquilizers) can cause hepatitis indistinguishable histologically from acute viral hepatitis. Most of these drug reactions are idiosyncratic, rare, unpredictable, and not dose dependent.

1. Acetaminophen Overdose produces profound hepatocellular necrosis in most persons. Oral N-acetylcysteine given within 8 hours of an acetaminophen overdose can dramatically decrease the risk of hepatotoxicity.

2. Volatile Anesthetics may produce mild, self-limiting postoperative liver dysfunction that likely reflects anesthetic-induced alterations in hepatic oxygen supply relative to demand. Any anesthetic that decreases hepatic blood flow could interfere with adequate hepatocyte oxygenation. Indeed, α-glutathione-S-transferase concentration (a sensitive marker of hepatocellular damage) increases transiently after administration of isoflurane, desflurane, and sevoflurane.

> **a. Immune-Mediated Hepatotoxicity.** A rare but life-threatening form of hepatic dysfunction following administration of volatile anesthetics (most often halothane) likely involves an immune-mediated hepatotoxicity in genetically susceptible individuals. IgG antibodies are directed against microsomal proteins on the surface of hepatocytes that have been covalently modified by the reactive oxidative trifluoroacetyl halide metabolite of halothane to form neoantigens.
>
> **b. Enflurane, Isoflurane, and Desflurane** may form trifluoroacetyl metabolites, resulting in cross-sensitivity with halothane, but the incidence of hepatitis after these anesthetics is much lower than after halothane because the degree of anesthetic metabolism is substantially less.
>
> **c. Sevoflurane** does not undergo metabolism to trifluoroacetylated metabolites and would not be expected to produce immune-mediated hepatotoxicity.
>
> **d. Differential Diagnosis of Postoperative Hepatic Dysfunction.** When postoperative hepatic dysfunction (jaundice) occurs, an analysis of historical data, clinical signs and symptoms, serial liver function tests, and a search for extrahepatic causes of hepatic dysfunction facilitate development of a differential diagnosis. The causes of hepatic dysfunction can be categorized as prehepatic, intrahepatic (hepatocellular), or posthepatic (cholestatic) based on measurement of serum bilirubin, aminotransferases, and alkaline phosphatase (**Table 11-4**). Postoperative hepatic dysfunction is often multifactorial.
>
> *1.)* Review all drugs administered.
>
> *2.)* Check for sources of sepsis.
>
> *3.)* Evaluate the possibility of an increased exogenous bilirubin load.
>
> *4.)* Rule out occult hematomas.
>
> *5.)* Rule out hemolysis.
>
> *6.)* Review perioperative records for evidence of hypotension, arterial hypoxemia, hypoventilation, and hypovolemia.
>
> *7.)* Consider extrahepatic abnormalities (congestive heart failure, respiratory failure, pulmonary embolism, renal insufficiency).
>
> *8.)* Consider the possibility of benign postoperative intrahepatic cholestasis.
>
> *9.)* Consider the possibility of immune-mediated hepatotoxicity.

II. CHRONIC HEPATITIS

Chronic hepatitis encompasses a diverse group of diseases characterized by long-term (>6 months) elevation of liver chemistries and evidence of inflammation on liver biopsy.

TABLE 11-4	Causes of Hepatic Dysfunction Based on Liver Function Tests			
Hepatic Dysfunction	Bilirubin	Aminotransferase Enzymes	Alkaline Phosphatase	Causes
Prehepatic	Increased unconjugated fraction	Normal	Normal	Hemolysis Hematoma resorption Bilirubin overload from blood transfusion
Intrahepatic (hepatocellular)	Increased conjugated fraction	Markedly increased	Normal to slightly increased	Virus Drugs Sepsis Hypoxemia Cirrhosis
Posthepatic (cholestatic)	Increased conjugated fraction	Normal to slightly increased	Markedly increased	Biliary tract stones Sepsis

A. Signs and Symptoms of chronic hepatitis vary and range from asymptomatic disease to fulminant hepatic failure. The most common symptoms of chronic hepatitis are fatigue, malaise, and abdominal pain.

B. Laboratory Tests. Aminotransferase concentrations are increased, and serum bilirubin concentrations are typically normal. Serum γ-globulin concentrations are increased. Serum albumin concentrations are decreased, and prothrombin time is prolonged.

C. Autoimmune Hepatitis is characterized by hypergammaglobulinemia, increased serum aminotransferase concentrations, and the presence of antinuclear antibodies.

D. Chronic Hepatitis B is present in 5% of the world's population, and an estimated 0.5% of the U.S. population are carriers of HBsAg. The goal of treatment of chronic hepatitis B is to eradicate HBV infection and prevent the development of cirrhosis or hepatocellular cancer. Currently available therapies, such as lamivudine and adefovir, can suppress HBV replication and lead to improvement in the clinical, biochemical, and histologic features of chronic hepatitis B. Liver transplantation can be performed for liver failure, but HBV will infect the allograft in nearly all recipients. Posttransplantation prophylaxis with lamivudine and hepatitis B immunoglobulin reduces the reinfection rate to approximately 10%.

E. Chronic Hepatitis C infection follows acute HCV infection in up to 75% of patients, and an estimated 1.8% of the U.S. population are carriers of HCV.

    1. Diagnosis is based on persistently or intermittently increased serum aminotransferase concentrations in association with the presence of anti-HCV antibody. The natural history of chronic hepatitis C may span several decades, progressing insidiously with the ultimate development of cirrhosis or hepatocellular cancer after 10 to 20 years.

    2. Treatment. Interferon reduces or normalizes serum ALT concentration and decreases inflammation as indicated by liver biopsy in approximately 40% of patients with chronic hepatitis C, but a sustained response to interferon therapy is uncommon. Chronic hepatitis C with liver failure is one of the most common indications for liver transplantation.

F. Less Common Causes of Chronic Hepatitis (Table 11-5)

III. CIRRHOSIS

Cirrhosis can result from a variety of chronic, progressive liver diseases that are most often the result of excessive chronic alcohol ingestion or chronic viral hepatitis caused by HBV or HCV infection.

TABLE 11-5   Less Common Causes of Chronic Hepatitis
Drug-induced chronic hepatitis (e.g., methyldopa, trazodone, isoniazid)
Wilson's disease (diagnosed by liver biopsy and hepatic copper content)
α_1-AT deficiency
Primary biliary cirrhosis
Primary sclerosing cholangitis

A. Diagnosis. Percutaneous liver biopsy establishes the diagnosis of cirrhosis. Computed tomography, magnetic resonance imaging, and hepatic ultrasonography with Doppler flow studies may reveal findings consistent with cirrhosis (splenomegaly, ascites, irregular liver surface). Upper gastrointestinal endoscopy can establish the presence of esophagogastric varices.

B. Signs and Symptoms (Table 11-6)

C. Specific Forms of Cirrhosis

1. **Alcoholic Cirrhosis** is directly attributable to chronic ingestion of large quantities of alcohol. The diagnosis of alcoholic hepatitis is supported by an AST/ALT ratio of at least 2:1.

2. **Postnecrotic Cirrhosis** is characterized by a shrunken liver containing regenerating nodules. The most common causes of this condition are chronic viral hepatitis, autoimmune hepatitis, and cryptogenic (cause unknown) hepatitis.

3. **Primary Biliary Cirrhosis** occurs most often in women 30 to 50 years of age, and the presence of antimitochondrial antibodies suggests an immune mechanism in the pathogenesis of this disorder. It is commonly associated with autoimmune diseases such as rheumatoid arthritis, CREST syndrome, thyroiditis, pernicious anemia, Sjögren's syndrome, and renal tubular acidosis.

4. **Hemochromatosis** is an autosomal recessive disorder associated with iron deposition in various body tissues, including the liver. Hepatomegaly is found in 75% of patients even if they are asymptomatic. Signs of portal hypertension eventually develop in most patients. Primary hepatocellular cancer occurs in 15% to 20% of patients with hemochromatosis.

5. **Wilson's Disease** (hepatolenticular degeneration) is an autosomal recessive disorder due to a defect in the gene that codes for copper binding. The subsequent excretion of copper into bile is defective, leading to total body copper accumulation. Neurologic dysfunction (tremors, gait disturbances, slurring of speech) and hepatic dysfunction (fatigue, jaundice, ascites, splenomegaly, gastroesophageal varices) develop. Associated hemolytic anemia is another clue to the diagnosis as is the Kayser-Fleischer ring, a thin brown crescent of pigmentation at the periphery of the cornea.

6. α_1-**Antitrypsin Deficiency** is associated with a rare syndrome of progressive cirrhosis and, in adult patients, pulmonary emphysema. The

TABLE 11-6 Signs and Symptoms of Cirrhosis of the Liver
Fatigue and malaise
Nondiagnostic physical findings: palmar erythema, spider nevi, gynecomastia, testicular atrophy, splenomegaly, ascites
Decreased hepatic blood flow
Hepatomegaly
Decreased serum albumin concentration
Prolonged prothrombin time
Increased serum aminotransferases and alkaline phosphatase

liver disease is not due to $\alpha_1 AT$ deficiency but rather to accumulation of abnormal $\alpha_1 AT$ in the liver.

7. Nonalcoholic Steatohepatitis (fatty liver) is fat accumulation in the liver leading to cirrhosis. It is more common in women and is associated with obesity, hyperlipidemia, and diabetes mellitus.

D. Complications of Cirrhosis (Table 11-7)

E. Management of Anesthesia. It is estimated that 5% to 10% of patients with cirrhosis require surgery in the last 2 years of life. In those patients who abuse alcohol, the presence of ascites, sepsis, and chronic obstructive pulmonary disease preoperatively is associated with increased postoperative morbidity and mortality.

   1. Preoperative Preparation. Certain preoperative criteria correlate with surgical risk and postoperative outcome in patients with cirrhosis who are undergoing major surgery (**Table 11-8**). Identifying co-existing problems that can be optimized preoperatively (cardiorespiratory function, coagulation status, renal function, intravascular fluid volume, electrolyte balance, nutrition) may decrease morbidity and mortality associated with elective surgery in patients with severe liver disease.

TABLE 11-7	Complications of Cirrhosis
Portal hypertension	Hepatomegaly with or without ascites
Esophagogastric varices	Treatment is usually endoscopic therapy with banding, ligation, or sclerotherapy
Ascites	Treatment is diuresis with an aldosterone antagonist and/or paracentesis
Hyperdynamic circulation	Due to vasodilating substances such as glucagons, increased intravascular volume, decreased blood viscosity due to anemia, arteriovenous shunting especially in the lungs
Cardiomyopathy	Congestive heart failure
Anemia	Antagonism of folate by alcohol
Coagulopathy	Decreased coagulation factor synthesis
Hepatorenal syndrome	95% mortality
Malnutrition	
Spontaneous bacterial peritonitis	Fever, leukocytosis, abdominal pain, decreased bowel sounds
Arterial hypoxemia	Impaired diaphragm movement due to ascites, right-to-left intrapulmonary shunting in the presence of portal vein hypertension, chronic obstructive pulmonary disease, pneumonia
Hypoglycemia	
Impaired immune defense	Alcohol ingestion suppresses immune mechanisms
Hepatic encephalopathy	Mental obtundation, asterixis, fetor hepaticus; treatment is dietary protein restriction, lactulose, liver transplantation

TABLE 11-8	Prediction of Perioperative Risk in the Patient with Liver Disease		
Parameter	**Low Risk**	**Moderate Risk**	**High Risk**
Bilirubin (mg/dL)	<2	2–3	>3
Albumin (g/dL)	>3.5	3.0–3.5	<3
Prothrombin time (seconds prolonged)	1–4	4–6	>6
Encephalopathy	None	Moderate	Severe
Nutrition	Excellent	Good	Poor
Ascites	None	Moderate	Marked

Adapted from Strunin I: Preoperative assessment of the patient with liver dysfunction. Br J Anaesth 1978;50:25–34.

> *a. Parenteral Vitamin K* is administered if the prothrombin time is prolonged.
> *b. Thrombocytopenia* may require treatment.
> *c. Administration of a Glucose Solution* is a consideration perioperatively.
> *d. Proper Hydration and Urine Output* should be maintained prior to surgery.
> *e. Intoxicated Patients* require less anesthetic, may be more vulnerable to aspiration, and may experience increased bleeding due to alcohol-induced platelet dysfunction.

2. Intraoperative Management. Optimal anesthetic drug choices or techniques in the presence of liver disease are unknown. A constant feature of chronic liver disease is decreased hepatic blood flow due to portal hypertension (hepatic blood flow and hepatocyte oxygenation are more dependent on hepatic artery blood flow). It is prudent to limit the dose of volatile anesthetic to minimize the likelihood of a persistent decrease in mean arterial pressure. Regional anesthesia can be useful in patients with advanced liver disease if the coagulation status is acceptable.

> *a. Muscle Relaxants.* Hepatic clearance of muscle relaxant drugs may be altered. Succinylcholine or mivacurium are acceptable choices, although severe liver disease may decrease plasma cholinesterase activity and prolong their action. The increased volume of distribution that accompanies cirrhosis will result in the need for a larger initial dose to produce the required plasma concentration. Hepatic dysfunction does not alter the elimination half-time of atracurium or cisatracurium.
> *b. Monitoring* of arterial blood gases and urine output is often necessary. Fluid administration must be carefully titrated (consider monitoring central venous pressure or pulmonary artery occlusion pressure). Intraoperative maintenance of an acceptable urine output may help decrease the risk of postoperative acute renal failure.

3. Postoperative Management. Regardless of the drugs selected for anesthesia, postoperative liver dysfunction/jaundice is likely in patients with

196

chronic liver disease. Cholestasis and sepsis can also be causes of postoperative jaundice. Manifestations of alcohol withdrawal usually appear 24 to 72 hours after cessation of drinking and can constitute a medical emergency in the postoperative period.

IV. HYPERBILIRUBINEMIA (Table 11-9)

Unconjugated hyperbilirubinemia will occur with an increase in bilirubin production, decreased hepatic uptake of bilirubin, or decreased conjugation of bilirubin. *Conjugated hyperbilirubinemia* occurs with decreased canalicular transport of bilirubin, acute or chronic hepatocellular dysfunction, or obstruction of the bile ducts.

V. ACUTE LIVER FAILURE

Acute hepatic failure is characterized by jaundice, hypoalbuminemia, coagulopathy, malnutrition, susceptibility to infection, and renal dysfunction in the clinical setting of acute hepatic disease. Fulminant hepatic failure refers to acute liver failure with superimposed hepatic encephalopathy that develops within 2 to 8 weeks of the onset of illness in a patient without preexisting liver disease (**Table 11-10**).

A. Signs and Symptoms. Typically, nonspecific symptoms such as malaise or nausea develop in a previously healthy individual and are followed by jaundice, altered mental status, and even coma. The progression of symptoms is rapid. Altered mentation and a prolonged prothrombin time are hallmarks of acute liver failure.

   1. Acute Fatty Liver of Pregnancy is characterized by accumulation of fat in hepatocytes. Approximately one half of patients have evidence of pregnancy-induced hypertension and/or laboratory evidence of HELLP syndrome (hemolysis, elevated liver enzymes, and low platelet count occurring in association with preeclampsia).

TABLE 11-9	Unusual Causes of Hyperbilirubinemia
Gilbert Syndrome	Hereditary (present in 7%–12% of the population). Unconjugated hyperbilirubinemia. Bilirubin concentrations seldom exceed 5 mg/dL, but can increase two- to threefold during fasting or illness.
Crigler-Najjar Syndrome	Decreased or absent glucuronyl transferase. Unconjugated hyperbilirubinemia. Causes perinatal jaundice.
Dubin-Johnson Syndrome	Conjugated hyperbilirubinemia with benign prognosis.
Benign Postoperative Intrahepatic Cholestasis	Conjugated hyperbilirubinemia. Occurs after prolonged surgery, especially if complicated by hypotension, hypoxemia, transfusion.
Progressive Familial Intrahepatic Cholestasis	Hereditary cholestatic jaundice of uncertain etiology. Presents in infancy; may be associated with severe pruritus. Liver transplantation is the only curative treatment.

TABLE 11-10 Some Causes of Acute Liver Failure
Viral hepatitis
Drug-induced hepatitis, such as with acetaminophen overdose
Toxin-induced hepatitis, such as from carbon tetrachloride
Hepatic ischemia
Acute fatty liver of pregnancy
Reye's syndrome

B. Treatment. No specific treatments exist for managing acute liver failure. Antidotes must be administered early for acetaminophen or mushroom poisoning. Glucose administration may be indicated. Cerebral edema requires aggressive intervention in the hope of preventing brain herniation. When survival seems unlikely, the only curative treatment is liver transplantation.

C. Management of Anesthesia (Table 11-11)

D. Liver Transplantation is the only curative therapy for patients with severe acute liver failure or end-stage liver disease with cirrhosis. At present, the typical 1-year survival rate for liver transplant recipients is approximately 85% and the 5-year survival rate is approximately 70%.

1. Management of Anesthesia. Candidates for liver transplantation may present with severe multiorgan dysfunction. Many of the physiologic derangements are not correctable until after successful liver transplantation. The likely presence of HBV or HBC in the transplant recipient must be considered by the health care providers.

a. Induction of Anesthesia can be affected by the presence of ascites compromising lung volumes and delaying gastric emptying. Anesthesia can be maintained with opioids and/or inhaled anesthetics combined with

TABLE 11-11 Anesthetic Considerations for Patients with Acute Liver Failure
Only life-saving surgery should be undertaken.
Coagulopathy should be corrected preoperatively.
Low doses of volatile agents, or nitrous oxide alone, may be sufficient for anesthesia.
Consider metabolism and clearance when selecting muscle relaxants.
Glucose may be indicated for hypoglycemia.
Transfuse blood slowly to avoid citrate intoxication.
Judicious fluid management may be needed to maintain urine output (mannitol if necessary).
Invasive monitoring as needed based on cardiovascular status.
Practice strict aseptic techniques.
Initiate lactulose therapy to prevent hepatic encephalopathy.

muscle relaxants that are not dependent on hepatic clearance mechanisms (atracurium, cisatracurium). Nitrous oxide is usually avoided because of concerns regarding bowel distension that can compromise surgical exposure.

b. Fluid Warming Devices and Rapid Infusion Systems designed to deliver warmed fluids or blood products at rates exceeding 1 L per minute are routinely employed.

c. Invasive Monitoring of systemic blood pressure and cardiac filling pressures and placement of several large-bore intravenous catheters to optimize fluid replacement are important parts of anesthetic management.

d. Surgical Stages during Liver Transplantation

   1.) Prehepatic or Dissection Phase involves mobilizing the vascular structures around the liver (hepatic artery, portal vein, supra- and infrahepatic vena cava), isolating the common bile duct, and removing the native liver. Cardiovascular instability due to hemorrhage, venous pooling, and impaired venous return is common.

   2.) Anhepatic Phase begins when the blood supply to the native liver is interrupted by clamping of the hepatic artery and portal vein. To support cardiac output and aid venous return to the heart, a venovenous bypass system is often used. Metabolic acidosis, decreased drug metabolism, and citrate intoxication are likely.

   3.) Reperfusion or Neohepatic Phase begins after reanastomosis of the major vascular structures. Unclamping can cause significant hemodynamic instability, dysrhythmias, severe bradycardia, hypotension, and hyperkalemic cardiac arrest. Once the allograft begins to function, hemodynamic and metabolic stability are gradually restored and urine output increases.

E. Anesthetic Considerations in the Patient after Liver Transplantation. Potential adverse effects (systemic hypertension, anemia, thrombocytopenia) and drug interactions related to chronic immunosuppressive therapy are important considerations. There is no evidence of an increased risk of developing hepatitis after administration of volatile anesthetics to liver transplant recipients.

VI. DISEASES OF THE BILIARY TRACT

Cholelithiasis and inflammatory biliary tract disease constitute major health problems in the United States, affecting more than 30 million Americans.

A. Cholelithiasis and Cholecystitis. Patients who have gallbladder or biliary tract stones can exhibit no symptoms (silent disease), display acute symptomatic disease, or have chronic intermittently symptomatic disease.

   1. Acute Cholecystitis. Obstruction of the cystic duct, which is nearly always due to a gallstone, produces acute inflammation of the gallbladder. Cholelithiasis is present in 95% of patients with acute cholecystitis.

   a. Signs and Symptoms of acute cholecystitis include nausea, vomiting, fever, abdominal pain, and right upper quadrant tenderness. Patients may notice dark urine and scleral icterus.

   b. Diagnosis. Ultrasonography is the principal diagnostic procedure used in patients with suspected gallstones and acute cholecystitis.

c. Differential Diagnosis (Table 11-12)

d. Treatment. Patients with a clinical diagnosis of acute cholecystitis are treated with intravenous fluids and opioids. Febrile patients with leukocytosis are given antibiotics. Laparoscopic cholecystectomy has almost completely replaced open cholecystectomy due to less postoperative pain, fewer pulmonary complications, and more rapid convalescence. Common duct stones can be removed concurrently or subsequently by endoscopic retrograde cholangiopancreatography (ERCP). Operative common bile duct exploration and stone removal may occasionally be needed.

e. Complications. Localized perforation and abscess formation are likely if symptoms persist for several days. Gallstone ileus results from obstruction of the small bowel, often at the ileocecal valve, by a large gallstone.

f. Management of Anesthesia. Anesthetic considerations for laparoscopic cholecystectomy are similar to those for other laparoscopic procedures. Insufflation of the abdominal cavity (pneumoperitoneum) may impede ventilation and venous return. The reverse Trendelenburg position favors movement of abdominal contents away from the operative site and may improve ventilation. Mechanical ventilation is recommended to prevent atelectasis, ensure adequate ventilation in the presence of increased intra-abdominal pressure, and offset the effects of systemic absorption of carbon dioxide. Endotracheal intubation with a cuffed tube minimizes the risk of pulmonary aspiration. Intraoperative decompression of the stomach with a nasogastric or orogastric tube may decrease the risk of visceral puncture during needle insertion to produce the pneumoperitoneum. Capnography is important for recognizing carbon dioxide embolism. There is no evidence that nitrous oxide significantly expands bowel gas or interferes with surgical working conditions during laparoscopic cholecystectomy. The use of opioids during anesthesia for this operation is controversial because these drugs can cause spasm of the sphincter of Oddi.

2. Chronic Cholecystitis is usually accompanied by evidence of chronic cholecystitis. Ultrasonography is a mainstay of diagnosis. Treatment is usually elective cholecystectomy.

a. Alternative Therapies include oral dissolution therapy with ursodeoxycholic acid and extracorporeal shockwave lithotripsy.

TABLE 11-12 Differential Diagnosis of Acute Cholecystitis
Pancreatitis
Penetrating duodenal ulcer
Appendicitis
Acute viral hepatitis
Alcoholic hepatitis
Pyelonephritis
Right lower lobe pneumonia
Acute myocardial infarction

3. Choledocholithiasis occurs when gallstones are present in the common bile duct. Stones typically lodge at the point of insertion of the duct into the ampulla of Vater.

   a. Signs and Symptoms may include signs of cholangitis (fever, shaking chills, jaundice, right upper quadrant pain) or jaundice alone and a history of pain suggestive of cholecystitis.

   b. Diagnosis. Ultrasonography may reveal a dilated common bile duct.

   c. Differential Diagnosis. Acute obstruction of the common bile duct by a stone may mimic ureterolithiasis, pancreatitis, acute myocardial infarction or viral hepatitis.

   d. Treatment. Endoscopic sphincterotomy is the initial treatment for the patient with choledocholithiasis. ERCP can be used to identify the cause of common bile duct obstruction and to remove a stone or place a stent.

CHAPTER 12

Diseases of the Gastrointestinal System

I. ESOPHAGEAL DISEASES

Dysphagia is the classic symptom of all disorders of the esophagus (evaluate by barium contrast study and upper gastrointestinal [GI] endoscopy).

A. **Diffuse Esophageal Spasm** occurs most often in elderly patient, may mimic angina pectoris, and may respond to treatment with nitroglycerin. Nifedipine and isosorbide, which decrease lower esophageal sphincter (LES) pressure, may also relieve pain produced by esophageal spasm.

B. **Gastroesophageal Reflux Disease**

1. **Physiology and Pathophysiology.** The underlying pathology of esophageal reflux is a decrease in the resting tone of the LES (average 13 mm Hg vs. 29 mm Hg in normal patients). Reflux occurs only when the gradient of pressure between the LES and the stomach is lost. Reflux can result in chronic cough, bronchoconstriction, pharyngitis, laryngitis, morning hoarseness, bronchitis, or pneumonia. Persistent dysphagia suggests development of a peptic stricture.

2. **Drug Effects on LES (Table 12-1)**

3. **Incidence of Reflux.** More than one third of healthy adults experience symptoms of heartburn at least once every 30 days. The incidence of aspiration during anesthesia is between 0.7 and 4.7 per 10,000 general anesthetics.

4. **Anesthesia Considerations (Table 12-2)**

C. **Hiatal Hernia** is a herniation of part of the stomach into the thoracic cavity through the esophageal hiatus in the diaphragm. A sliding hernia is found in approximately 30% of patients undergoing upper GI radiographic examination. Most patients with hiatal hernia do not have symptoms of reflux esophagitis, emphasizing the importance of the integrity of the LES.

TABLE 12-1	Effect of Agents on Lower Esophageal Sphincter Tone	
Increase	**Decrease**	**No Change**
Metoclopramide	Atropine	Propranolol
Domperidone	Glycopyrrolate	Oxprenolol
Prochlorperazine	Dopamine	Cimetidine
Cyclizine	Sodium nitroprusside	Ranitidine
Edrophonium	Ganglion blockers	Atracurium
Neostigmine	Thiopental	Nitrous oxide
Succinylcholine	Tricyclic antidepressants	
Pancuronium	β-adrenergic stimulants	
Metoprolol	Halothane	
α–adrenergic stimulants	Enflurane	
Antacids	? Nitrous oxide	
	Propofol	
	Opioids	

D. Esophageal Diverticula are outpouchings of the wall of the esophagus. Zenker's diverticulum appears in the posterior hypopharyngeal wall (Killian's triangle). Regurgitation of previously ingested food from a Zenker's diverticulum can predispose a patient to pulmonary aspiration, even without recent food intake. A mid-esophageal diverticulum can result from traction from old adhesions or by propulsion associated with esophageal motor abnormalities. An epiphrenic diverticulum may be associated with achalasia.

TABLE 12-2	Some Anesthesia Considerations in Patients with Esophageal Reflux
Anticholinergic medications	Can decreased LES tone and may increase the risk of silent aspiration
Succinylcholine	Increases LES pressure, but trans-LES pressure is unchanged.
Prophylactic premedications—histamine blockers	Cimetidine, ranitidine, famotidine, nizatidine all decrease gastric acid secretion and increase gastric pH
Preoperative protein pump inhibitors	Omeprazole (given the night before surgery), rabeprazole, and lansoprazole (both given the morning of surgery).
Sodium citrate	Oral nonparticulate antacid
Metoclopramide	Gastrokinetic agent to facilitate gastric emptying
Cricoid pressure	Should be applied during induction to prevent aspiration
Tracheal intubation	To protect the airway from aspiration in the anesthetized patient

E. Mucosal Tear (Mallory-Weiss Syndrome) This tear is usually caused by vomiting, retching, or vigorous coughing. Patients present with upper GI bleeding, which usually resolves spontaneously.

II. PEPTIC ULCER DISEASE

Burning epigastric pain exacerbated by fasting and improved with meals is a symptom complex associated with peptic ulcer disease (PUD). Benign gastric ulcers are a form of PUD, occurring with one third the frequency of benign duodenal ulceration.

A. Pathophysiology. The mucus-bicarbonate layer serves as a physicochemical barrier to multiple agents including hydrogen ions. Surface epithelial cells provide the next line of defense through several factors, including mucus production, epithelial cell ionic transporters that maintain intracellular pH and bicarbonate production, and intracellular tight junctions. Prostaglandins play a central role in gastric epithelial defense and repair.

B. Causes of Injury

1. Hydrochloric Acid and Pepsinogen are the two principal gastric secretory products capable of inducing mucosal injury.

2. *Helicobacter Pylori* is a major factor in the pathogenesis of duodenal ulcerations, although early *H. pylori* infection is associated with a decrease in gastric acid secretion. *H. pylori* might induce increased acid secretion through both direct and indirect actions of *H. pylori* and proinflammatory cytokines (interleukin [IL]-8, tumor necrosis factor, and IL-1) on G, D, and parietal cells. *H. pylori* also decreases duodenal mucosal bicarbonate production.

C. Complications of Peptic Ulcer Disease

1. Bleeding is the leading cause of death associated with PUD, and the incidence of this complication has not changed since the introduction of H_2-receptor antagonists.

2. Perforation occurs in about 10% of patients. Mortality of emergent ulcer operations is correlated with preoperative shock, co-existing medical illness, and perforation for more than 48 hours.

3. Gastric Outlet Obstruction can occur acutely or chronically in patients with duodenal ulcer disease; hence, they should be treated as full stomach when they present for surgery. Pyloric obstruction is suggested by recurrent vomiting, dehydration, and hypochloremia. Treatment usually consists of nasogastric suction, rehydration, and intravenous administration of antisecretory agents, but surgery may be necessary.

D. Stress Gastritis. Major trauma accompanied by shock, sepsis, respiratory failure, hemorrhage, transfusion requirement of more than 6 units, or multi-organ injury is often accompanied by the development of acute stress gastritis. The major complication of stress gastritis is hemorrhage.

E. Treatment of Peptic Ulcer Disease

1. Medical Treatment (Table 12-3)

2. Surgical Treatment is reserved for the treatment of the most complicated ulcer disease. Three procedures, truncal vagotomy and drainage, truncal vagotomy and antrectomy, and proximal gastric vagotomy, have been most widely used for the operative treatment of peptic ulcer disease.

TABLE 12-3	Treatment of Peptic Ulcer Disease
Antacids	For Symptomatic Relief
H_2-Receptor antagonists	Cimetidine, ranitidine, famotidine, nizatidine; bind to cytochrome P-450 and can affect metabolism of other medications and, rarely, affect bone marrow function
Proton-pump inhibitors (PPIs)	Omeprazole, esomeprazole, lansoprazole, rabeprazole, pantoprazole; rapid onset and long duration
Prostaglandin analogues	Misoprostol; enhance mucosal bicarbonate secretion, stimulate mucosal blood flow, and decrease mucosal cell turnover
Cytoprotective agents	Sucralfate provides physicochemical barrier to acid and pepsin; bismuth-containing preparations may exert positive effects through ulcer coating, prevention of further damage, stimulation of prostaglandins
Miscellaneous drugs	Anticholinergics (weak acid-inhibiting effect)
H. pylori treatment	Combination therapy with amoxicillin, metronidazole, tetracycline, clarithromycin, and bismuth compounds: typical triple therapy includes a PPI, and two antibiotics

III. ZOLLINGER-ELLISON SYNDROME

Zollinger-Ellison syndrome includes gastroduodenal and intestinal ulceration, with gastric hypersecretion and non–beta islet cell tumor of the pancreas. The incidence of Zollinger-Ellison syndrome varies from 0.1% to 1% of individuals presenting with PUD.

A. Pathophysiology. Excess gastrin stimulates acid secretion and exerts a trophic action on gastric epithelial cells. Gastric acid secretion is markedly increased through both parietal cell stimulation and increased parietal cell mass. This increased gastric acid output leads to the peptic ulcer disease, erosive esophagitis, and diarrhea.

B. Clinical Manifestations. Abdominal pain and peptic ulceration are seen in up to 90% of patients. Diarrhea and gastroesophageal reflux is seen in up to half of patients. Gastrinomas can develop in the presence of multiple endocrine neoplasia type I (MEN I) syndrome, a disorder involving primarily three organ sites: the parathyroid glands (80%–90%), pancreas (40%–80%), and pituitary gland (30%–60%). An additional distinguishing feature in Zollinger-Ellison syndrome patients with MEN I is the higher incidence of gastric carcinoid tumor development compared with patients with sporadic gastrinomas.

C. Diagnosis is established by clinical presentation and elevated fasting gastrin level. Multiple processes can lead to an elevated fasting gastrin level (**Table 12-4**).

D. Treatment is initially with proton pump inhibitors. Curative surgical resection of the gastrinoma is indicated in the absence of evidence of MEN I

TABLE 12-4	Causes of Increased Fasting Serum Gastrin	
Hypo- and achlorhydria (± pernicious anemia)	*H. pylori*
	Retained gastric antrum
	Gastric outlet obstruction
G-cell hyperplasia	Massive small bowel obstruction
Renal insufficiency	Vitiligo, diabetes mellitus
Rheumatoid arthritis	Patients on antisecretory drugs
Pheochromocytomas	Diabetes mellitus

syndrome and metastatic disease. Anesthetic considerations for gastrinoma resection include the presence of gastric hypersecretion and reflux, and depletion of intravascular fluid volume and electrolyte imbalance (hypokalemia, metabolic alkalosis) due to diarrhea. Associated endocrine abnormalities (MEN I syndrome) should be considered. A preoperative coagulation screen and liver function test may be needed, as alterations in fat absorption could influence clotting factors. Intravenous administration of ranitidine is useful for preventing gastric acid hypersecretion during surgery.

IV. POSTGASTRECTOMY SYNDROMES

A. Dumping Symptoms (nausea, epigastric discomfort, palpitations, reactive hypoglycemia, and, in extreme cases, dizziness or syncope) occur immediately after a meal (early) or after 1 to 3 hours (late). Octreotide may be effective treatment.
B. Alkaline Reflux Gastritis is the clinical triad of postprandial epigastric pain, evidence of reflux of bile into the stomach, and an associated histologic evidence of gastritis. The only proven treatment is operative diversion of intestinal contents from contact with the gastric mucosa (Roux-en-Y gastrojejunostomy).

V. IRRITABLE BOWEL SYNDROME

Patients with irritable bowel syndrome complain of generalized bowel discomfort, usually confined to the left lower quadrant. Commonly, the frequency of stools is increased and the stool is covered with mucus. Many patients have associated symptoms of vasomotor instability, including tachycardia, hyperventilation, fatigue, diaphoresis, and headaches. There is no known specific etiologic agent or structural or biochemical defect.

VI. INFLAMMATORY BOWEL DISEASE

Inflammatory bowel diseases are the second most common chronic inflammatory disorders after rheumatoid arthritis.
A. Classification of Inflammatory Bowel Disease
   1. Ulcerative Colitis is a mucosal disease involving the rectum and all or part of the colon. Major symptoms are diarrhea, rectal bleeding, tenesmus, passage

of mucus, and crampy abdominal pain. Other symptoms in moderate to severe disease include anorexia, nausea, vomiting, fever, and weight loss.

 a. *Complications* include catastrophic illness, hemorrhage, toxic megacolon, perforation, peritonitis, and colonic obstruction.

2. Crohn's Disease (CD) usually presents as acute or chronic bowel inflammation. CD usually follows one of two patterns of disease: a penetrating-fistulous pattern or an obstructing pattern, each with different treatments and prognoses. Presentation is usually right lower quadrant pain with diarrhea but can mimic appendicitis. Obstruction, strictures, and fistulae all occur. Jejunal involvement can lead to malabsorption, steatorrhea, and nutritional deficiencies. Colitis and toxic megacolon can occur. Associated gastritis can result in nausea, vomiting, and epigastric pain. Patients with perianal CD are at higher risk of developing extraintestinal manifestations (**Table 12-5**).

B. Treatment of Inflammatory Bowel Disease
 1. Surgical Treatment (Table 12-6)
 2. Medical Treatment (Table 12-7)

VII. PSEUDOMEMBRANOUS ENTEROCOLITIS

Pseudomembranous enterocolitis is often associated with antibiotic therapy (especially clindamycin and lincomycin), bowel obstruction, uremia, congestive heart failure, and intestinal ischemia. Clinical manifestations include fever,

TABLE 12-5	Extraintestinal Manifestation of Inflammatory Bowel Disease
Dermatologic	Erythema nodosum in 10%–15% of IBD; pyoderma gangrenosum in 1%–12%
Rheumatologic	Peripheral arthritis develops in 15%–20% of IBD patients
Ocular	1%–10% of IBD; conjunctivitis, anterior uveitis/iritis, and episcleritis
Hepatobiliary	Approximately 50% of IBD; hepatomegaly; fatty liver due to chronic debilitating illness, malnutrition, and glucocorticoid therapy; cholelithiasis caused by malabsorption of bile acids; primary sclerosing cholangitis leading to biliary cirrhosis and hepatic failure
Urologic	Calculi in 10%–20%; ureteral obstruction
Others	Thromboembolic disease (pulmonary embolism, cerebrovascular accidents, and arterial emboli) due to thrombocytosis; increased levels of fibrinopeptide A, factor V, factor VIII, and fibrinogen; accelerated thromboplastin generation; antithrombin III deficiency due to increased gut losses or increased catabolism; free protein S deficiency, endocarditis, myocarditis, pleuropericarditis, and interstitial lung disease, secondary/reactive amyloidosis

IBD, inflammatory bowel disease.

TABLE 12-6	Surgical Indications: Inflammatory Bowel Disease
Ulcerative Colitis	
Massive hemorrhage, perforation, toxic megacolon obstruction, intractable and fulminant disease, cancer	
Crohn's Disease	
Stricture, obstruction, hemorrhage, abscess, fistulas, intractable and fulminant disease, cancer and unresponsive perianal disease	

watery diarrhea, dehydration, hypotension, cardiac dysrhythmias, skeletal muscle weakness, intestinal ileus, and metabolic acidosis.

VIII. CARCINOID TUMORS

A. Carcinoid Tumors can occur in almost any GI tissue, but most originate in the bronchus, jejunoileum, or colon/rectum. Carcinoid tumors secrete a variety of amine and neuropeptide hormones (**Table 12-8**), which may be released in sufficient amounts to cause significant systemic symptoms (carcinoid syndrome). Most carcinoid tumors are found incidentally during surgery for suspected appendicitis (**Table 12-9**).

B. Carcinoid Syndrome occurs in about 20% of patients. The two most common symptoms are flushing and diarrhea. Flushing may be associated with pruritus, lacrimation, diarrhea, or facial edema, and may be precipitated by stress, alcohol, exercise, certain foods such as cheese, or agents such as catecholamines, pentagastrin, and serotonin reuptake inhibitors. Cardiac manifestations are caused by fibrosis involving the endocardium, primarily on the right side. The carcinoid triad is cardiac involvement with flushing and

TABLE 12-7	Medical Treatment of Inflammatory Bowel Disease
Sulfasalazine	Antibacterial and anti-inflammatory (5-acetylsalicylic acid). Effective at inducing remission in UC and CD, and maintains remission in UC. Newer agents include Asacol and Pentasa (mesalamine).
Oral, topical, or parenteral glucocorticoids	Used in both UC and CD to induce remission. No role in maintenance therapy.
Antibiotics	Used to treat pouchitis in UC patients after colectomy (metronidazole or ciprofloxacin).
Immunomodulatory drugs	Azathioprine, 6-mercaptopurine (inhibit cell proliferation), cyclosporine (inhibits T-cell–mediated responses).

CD, Crohn's disease; UC, ulcerative colitis.

TABLE 12-8	Substances Produced by Carcinoid Tumors at Various Locations		
	Foregut	**Midgut**	**Hindgut**
Serotonin (5HTP)	Low	High	Rarely
Other substances	ACTH, 5HTP, GRF	Tachykinins (substance P, neuropeptide K, substance K); rarely 5HTP, ACTH	Rarely 5HTP, ACTH; contains numerous peptides
Carcinoid syndrome	Atypical	Typical	Rare

ACTH, corticotropin; GRF, growth hormone releasing factor; 5HTP, 5-hydroxyl-L-tryptophan.

diarrhea. Asthma-like wheezing can also occur. Carcinoid crisis, which can be fatal, is characterized by intense flushing, diarrhea, abdominal pain, and cardiovascular instability. Provocative events can include stress, biopsy, and certain drugs (**Table 12-10**).

1. Diagnosis relies on measurement of urinary or plasma serotonin or its metabolites in the urine.

2. Management of Anesthesia. Administration of octreotide, 150 to 250 µg subcutaneously (SC) every 6 to 8 hours for 24 to 48 hours prior to anesthesia and throughout the procedure, will attenuate most adverse hemodynamic responses. Use of epidural analgesia in patients who have been adequately treated with octreotide is a safe technique, although the sympathetic blockade produced by epidural or spinal anesthesia may worsen hypotension. Ondansetron, a serotonin antagonist, is a useful and logical antiemetic choice. Invasive arterial blood pressure monitoring may be necessary.

3. Medical Treatment of Carcinoid includes avoiding conditions that precipitate flushing, dietary supplementation with nicotinamide, treatment of heart failure and wheezing, and controlling the diarrhea (loperamide or

TABLE 12-9	Location and Presentation of Carcinoid Tumors
Carcinoid Location	**Presentation**
Small intestine	Abdominal pain (51%), intestinal obstruction (31%), tumor (17%), gastrointestinal bleed (11%)
Rectal	Bleeding (39%), constipation (17%), diarrhea (17%)
Bronchial	Asymptomatic (31%)
Thymic	Anterior mediastinal masses
Ovarian and testicular	Masses discovered on physical examination or ultrasonography
Metastatic	In the liver; often presents as hepatomegaly

TABLE 12-10	Pharmacologic Agents Associated with Carcinoid Crisis
Drugs that May Provoke Mediator Release	
Succinylcholine, mivacurium, atracurium, and d-tubocurarine	
Epinephrine, norepinephrine, dopamine, isoproterenol, and thiopental	
Drugs Not Known to Release Mediators	
Propofol, etomidate, vecuronium, cisatracurium, rocuronium, sufentanil, alfentanil, fentanyl, and remifentanil; all inhalation agents; desflurane may be the better choice in patients with liver metastasis because of its low rate of metabolism	

diphenoxylate). 5-HT$_3$ receptor antagonists (ondansetron, tropisetron, alosetron) may control diarrhea and nausea. A combination of histamine H$_1$- and H$_2$-receptor antagonists (diphenhydramine and cimetidine or ranitidine) may control flushing in patients with foregut carcinoids. Somatostatin analogues octreotide and lanreotide control symptoms in most patients and are effective in treating carcinoid crises.

4. Other Treatment. Hepatic artery embolization alone or with chemotherapy (chemoembolization) has been used to control the symptoms of carcinoid syndrome. Surgery is the only potentially curative therapy for nonmetastatic carcinoid tumors.

IX. ACUTE PANCREATITIS

Acute pancreatitis is characterized as an inflammatory disorder of the pancreas in which pancreatic autodigestion is the most likely cause. Normal pancreatic function is restored after the acute event resolves.

A. Etiology. Gallstones and alcohol abuse are etiologic factors in most patients with acute pancreatitis. Acute pancreatitis is common in patients with acquired immunodeficiency syndrome and those with hyperparathyroidism and associated hypercalcemia.

B. Signs and Symptoms (Table 12-11)

C. Diagnosis. The hallmark of acute pancreatitis is an increased serum amylase concentration. Contrast-enhanced computed tomography can document the morphologic changes associated with acute pancreatitis. The differential diagnosis includes a perforated duodenal ulcer, acute cholecystitis, mesenteric ischemia, and bowel obstruction.

D. Prognosis. Ranson's criteria can be used to estimate mortality (**Table 12-12**).

E. Complications include shock, arterial hypoxemia, acute respiratory distress syndrome (20%), renal failure (25%), GI hemorrhage, coagulation defects from disseminated intravascular coagulation, and pancreatic infection (>50% mortality).

F. Treatment includes aggressive intravenous fluid administration (up to 10 L of crystalloid), resting the gut by stopping oral intake, opioids to manage the severe pain, prophylactic antibiotic therapy, endoscopic removal of obstructing gallstones within the first 24 to 72 hours of the onset of symptoms to decrease

211

TABLE 12-11	Signs and Symptoms of Acute Pancreatitis
Mid-epigastric abdominal pain radiating to the back, improved by leaning forward	
Nausea and vomiting	
Abdominal distension and ileus	
Dyspnea due to pleural effusions or ascites	
Fever	
Shock	
Tetany (with development of hypocalcemia)	
Obtundation and psychosis (if withdrawing from alcohol)	

the risk of cholangitis, and parenteral nutrition if it is anticipated that patients will experience a protracted course.

X. CHRONIC PANCREATITIS

Chronic pancreatitis is characterized by chronic inflammation that leads to irreversible damage to the pancreas.

TABLE 12-12	Ranson's Criteria for Acute Pancreatitis
Criteria	
Age >55	
White blood cell count $>16 \times 10^{-9}$/L	
Blood urea nitrogen >16 mmol/L	
Aspartate transaminase >250 U/L	
Arterial PO_2 <8 kPa (60 mm Hg)	
Fluid deficit >6 L	
Blood glucose >200 mg/dL, no history of diabetes mellitus	
Lactate dehydrogenase >350 IU/L	
Corrected calcium <8 mg/dL	
Decrease in hematocrit >10	
Metabolic acidosis with base deficit >4 mmol/L	
(Note: serum amylase is NOT a criteria)	
Mortality	
0–2 criteria: <5%	
3–4 criteria: 20%	
5–6 criteria: 40%	
7–8 criteria: 100%	

A. Etiology. Chronic pancreatitis is most often caused by chronic alcohol abuse. Idiopathic chronic pancreatitis is the second most common form of this disease. Chronic pancreatitis occasionally occurs in association with cystic fibrosis or hyperparathyroidism (hypercalcemia) or as a hereditary disease transmitted by an autosomal dominant gene.

B. Signs and Symptoms. Chronic pancreatitis is often characterized by epigastric abdominal pain that radiates to the back and is often postprandial. Steatorrhea is present when at least 90% of the pancreas is destroyed. Diabetes mellitus eventually occurs.

C. Diagnosis of chronic pancreatitis is based on the history of chronic alcohol abuse and presence of pancreatic calcifications. Serum amylase concentrations are usually normal. Ultrasonography may document the presence of an enlarged pancreas or identify a fluid-filled pseudocyst. Computed tomography demonstrates dilated pancreatic ducts and changes in the size of the pancreas. Endoscopic retrograde cholangiopancreatography is the most sensitive imaging test for detecting early changes in the pancreatic ducts caused by chronic pancreatitis.

D. Treatment includes management of pain, malabsorption, and diabetes mellitus. Internal surgical drainage (pancreaticojejunostomy) or endoscopic placement of stents may be helpful in patients who are resistant to medical management of pain. Enzyme supplement (lipase) allows fat digestion.

XI. MALABSORPTION AND MALDIGESTION

Malabsorption of nutrients is reflected by impaired absorption of fat (steatorrhea), fat developing hypoalbuminemia due to a protein leak through diseased intestinal mucosa, fat-soluble vitamin deficiencies (vitamins A, D, E, K), hypocalcemia, and hypomagnesemia.

A. Gluten-Sensitive Enteropathy (previously termed celiac disease or nontropical sprue) is a disease of the small intestine resulting in malabsorption (steatorrhea), weight loss, abdominal pain, and fatigue. Treatment is removal of gluten (wheat, rye, barley) from the diet.

B. Small Bowel Resection may result in malabsorption if the small intestinal surface area that remains for absorption is decreased below critical levels. Diarrhea, steatorrhea, trace element deficiencies, and electrolyte imbalance (hyponatremia, hypokalemia) can result. Total parenteral nutrition is needed only if multiple small feedings are not effective.

XII. GASTROINTESTINAL BLEEDING (Table 12-13)

A. Upper Gastrointestinal Bleeding. Patients with acute upper GI bleeding may experience hypotension and tachycardia if blood loss exceeds approximately 25% of the total blood volume (1500 mL in adults). Most patients with evidence of acute hypovolemia (orthostatic hypotension characterized by decreases in systolic blood pressure of 10 to 20 mm Hg and corresponding increases in heart rate) have hematocrits less than 30%. The hematocrit may be normal early in the course of acute hemorrhage because of the insufficient time for equilibration of the plasma volume.

TABLE 12-13 Causes of Upper and Lower Gastrointestinal Bleeding

Causes	Incidence (%)
Upper gastrointestinal bleeding	
Peptic ulcer	
Duodenal ulcer	36
Gastric ulcer	24
Mucosal erosive disease	
Gastritis	6
Esophagitis	6
Esophageal varices	6
Mallory-Weiss tear	3
Malignancy	2
Lower gastrointestinal bleeding	
Colonic diverticulosis	42
Colorectal malignancy	9
Ischemic colitis	9
Acute colitis of unknown causes	5
Hemorrhoids	5

Adapted from Young HS: Gastrointestinal bleeding. Sci Am Med 1998;1–10.

1. **Melena** usually indicates that bleeding has occurred at a site above the cecum. The blood urea nitrogen concentration is usually higher than 40 mg/dL because of the absorbed nitrogen load in the small intestine.

2. **Treatment.** For patients with bleeding peptic ulcers, endoscopic coagulation (thermotherapy, injection with epinephrine or a sclerosant) is indicated when active bleeding is visible. Surgical treatment of nonvariceal upper GI bleeding (oversewing an ulcer, gastrectomy for diffuse hemorrhagic gastritis) is used in patients who continue to bleed despite optimal supportive therapy and in whom endoscopic coagulation is unsuccessful.

B. **Lower Gastrointestinal Bleeding** typically presents as abrupt passage of bright red blood and clots.

1. **BUN Concentration** is not likely to be significantly increased in these patients.

2. **Sigmoidoscopy** to exclude anorectal lesions is indicated as soon as patients are hemodynamically stable. If bleeding is persistent and brisk, angiography and possibly embolic therapy may be attempted. Lower GI bleeding may require surgical intervention to control it.

C. **Occult Gastrointestinal Bleeding** may present as unexplained iron deficiency anemia or as intermittent positive tests for blood in the patient's feces. Peptic ulcer disease and colonic neoplasm are the most common causes of occult GI bleeding.

XIII. DIVERTICULOSIS AND DIVERTICULITIS

Colonic diverticula, herniations of the mucosa and submucosa through the muscularis propria, occur most often in individuals who consume low-fiber diets. Diverticulitis occurs with inflammation of one or more diverticula, usually in sigmoid or descending colon.

A. Signs and Symptoms include fever, and lower abdominal pain and tenderness. Nausea, vomiting, constipation, diarrhea, dysuria, tachycardia, and an elevated white blood cell count with a left shift may be noted. Right-sided colonic diverticulitis is usually indistinguishable from appendicitis. Severe diverticulitis can present with purulent peritonitis. Abdominal computed tomography is the most useful study for early evaluation of suspected diverticulitis.

B. Treatment includes 7 to 10 days of oral broad-spectrum antimicrobial therapy, which includes anaerobic coverage. Intravenous fluids, bowel rest, broad-spectrum antibiotics, and analgesics may be needed. Surgical treatment (resection of diseased colon) may be required if the patient does not improve within 48 hours despite maximal therapy.

XIV. APPENDICITIS

Appendicitis is often associated with obstruction of the lumen of the appendix by a fecalith, followed by bacterial invasion of the appendiceal wall and arterial compromise to the appendix because of high intraluminal pressures. Peak incidence is in the second and third decades of life.

A. Clinical Manifestations include mild, poorly localized abdominal pain, often cramping in nature. As inflammation spreads, pain becomes steadier, more severe, and localized to the right lower quadrant. Anorexia is very common, and nausea and vomiting occur in 50% to 60% of cases. The temperature is usually normal or slightly elevated (high temperature suggests perforation). For differential diagnosis, see **Table 12-14**.

B. Treatment is early surgery and appendectomy.

XV. PERITONITIS

Peritonitis is an inflammation of the peritoneum caused by spontaneous bacterial hematogenous spread or secondary to an intra-abdominal process (**Table 12-15**).

A. Clinical Features are acute abdominal pain and tenderness, usually with fever, diffuse abdominal tenderness and rebound, rigidity of the abdominal

TABLE 12-14	Differential Diagnosis: Appendicitis	
Mesenteric lymphadenitis	Ureteral calculus	Pelvic inflammatory disease
Ruptured graafian follicle	Acute cholecystitis	Corpus luteum cyst
Acute pancreatitis	Acute gastroenteritis	Strangulating intestinal obstruction
Perforated ulcer	Acute diverticulitis	No organic disease

215

TABLE 12-15	Causes of Peritonitis
Bowel Perforation	
Trauma, iatrogenic, endoscopic perforation, ischemia, anastomotic leak, catheter perforation, ingested foreign body, inflammatory bowel disease, vascular embolus, strangulated hernias, volvulus, intussusception	
Other Organ Leak	
Pancreatitis, cholecystitis, salpingitis, bile leak after biopsy, urinary bladder rupture	
Peritoneal Disruption	
Peritoneal dialysis, intraperitoneal chemotherapy, postoperative foreign body, penetrating-fistulous pattern, trauma	

wall, absence of bowel sounds, and often tachycardia, hypotension, and signs of dehydration. Leukocytosis and acidosis are common laboratory findings. Ascites may show high numbers of neutrophils, and increased protein and lactate dehydrogenase levels.

B. Treatment is rehydration, correction of electrolyte abnormalities, antibiotics, and surgical correction of the underlying defect.

XVI. ACUTE COLONIC PSEUDO-OBSTRUCTION

Acute colonic pseudo-obstruction is a clinical syndrome characterized by massive dilation of the colon in the absence of mechanical obstruction. It occurs most often in hospitalized patients with medical or surgical disease. A current hypothesis is that an imbalance in neural input to the colon distal to the splenic flexure, with an excess of sympathetic stimulation and a paucity of parasympathetic input, results in a spastic contraction of the distal colon and functional obstruction. Patients who fail conservative therapy (hydration, mobilization, enemas, nasogastric suction) for more than 48 hours should be considered for active intervention consisting of decompressive colonoscopy and/or intravenous administration of the cholinesterase inhibitor neostigmine at a dose of 2.0 to 2.5 mg given over 3 to 5 minutes, which results in immediate colonic decompression in 80% to 90% of patients.

CHAPTER 13

Nutritional Diseases and Inborn Errors of Metabolism

The presence of nutritional disorders or inborn errors of metabolism will significantly influence the management of anesthesia.

I. OBESITY

Obesity (body weight ≥20% above ideal weight) is associated with increased morbidity and mortality and a wide spectrum of medical and surgical diseases (**Tables 13-1** and **13-2**). A body mass index (BMI) greater than 28 is associated with increased morbidity due to stroke, ischemic heart disease, and diabetes that is 3 to 4 times the risk in the general population.

A. **Pathogenesis.** Obesity is a complex, multifactorial disease (mechanisms of fat storage, genetic, psychological). Most simply, it occurs when net energy intake exceeds net energy expenditure over a prolonged period of time.

1. **Fat Storage.** Surplus calories are converted to triglycerides and stored in adipocytes. Central or android distribution of fat (more common in men) manifests as abdominal obesity. Abdominal fat deposits are metabolically more active than peripheral or gynecoid fat distribution (hips, buttocks, thighs) and are associated with a higher incidence of metabolic complications (dyslipidemias, glucose intolerance and diabetes mellitus, ischemic heart disease, congestive heart failure, stroke).

2. **Metabolic Effects of Weight Change.** Small decreases in body weight result in decreased energy expenditures that persist despite a caloric intake that is sufficiently decreased to maintain the lower weight. Thus, a formerly obese person requires approximately 15% fewer calories to maintain normal body weight than persons of the same body composition who have never been obese.

TABLE 13-1	Medical and Surgical Conditions Associated with Obesity
Organ System	**Side Effects**
Respiratory system	Obstructive sleep apnea Obesity hypoventilation syndrome Restrictive lung disease
Cardiovascular system	Systemic hypertension Cardiomegaly Congestive heart failure Ischemic heart disease Cerebrovascular disease Peripheral vascular disease Pulmonary hypertension Deep vein thrombosis Pulmonary embolism Hypercholesterolemia Hypertriglyceridemia Sudden death
Endocrine system	Diabetes mellitus Cushing syndrome Hypothyroidism
Gastrointestinal system	Hiatal hernia Inguinal hernia Gallstones Fatty liver infiltration
Musculoskeletal system	Osteoarthritis of weight-bearing joints Back pain
Malignancy	Breast Prostate Cervical Uterine Colorectal

Adapted from Adams JP, Murphy PG: Obesity in anaesthesia and intensive care. Br J Anaesth 2000;85:91–108.

TABLE 13-2	Calculation of Body Mass Index

$$\text{Body mass index (BMI)} = \frac{\text{weight (kg)}}{\text{height}^2 \text{ (m)}}$$

Example: A 150 kg, 1.8 m tall man has a BMI of 47 (more than 100% above ideal body weight). A similar patient weighing 80 kg has a BMI of 25.

B. Physiologic Disturbances Associated with Obesity (Table 13-1)

1. Obstructive Sleep Apnea is present in 2% to 4% of middle-aged adults and 5% of obese patients (**Table 13-3**).

a. Pathogenesis. Apnea occurs when the pharyngeal airways collapse. Increased inspiratory effort and response to arterial hypoxemia and hypercarbia cause arousal, which in turn restores upper airway tone. Repeated cycles occur during sleep.

b. Risk Factors (see Table 13-3)

c. Treatment. Positive airway pressure, delivered through a nasal mask, is the initial treatment of choice for clinically significant obstructive sleep apnea. Patients with mild sleep apnea who do not tolerate positive airway pressure may benefit from nighttime application of oral appliances designed to enlarge the airway by keeping the tongue in an anterior position or by displacing the mandible forward. Nocturnal oxygen therapy is a consideration for individuals who experience severe arterial oxygen desaturation. Surgical treatment of obstructive sleep apnea includes tracheostomy (patients with severe apnea who do not tolerate positive airway pressure), palatal surgery (laser-assisted uvulopalatopharyngoplasty), and maxillofacial surgical procedures to enhance upper airway patency during sleep (genioglossal advancement).

d. Management of Anesthesia (Table 13-4)

1.) *Specialized Surgical Procedures.* A tracheostomy is mandatory before any surgery that involves the base of the tongue. Postoperatively, patients undergoing extensive corrective surgery should be managed in a monitored care setting with the inclusion of supplemental oxygen, appropriate analgesics, and pulse oximetry monitoring.

a.) *Uvulopalatopharyngoplasty* is performed with the patient supine and the head slightly elevated to enhance venous drainage. Worsening of upper airway obstruction is possible during the early postoperative period due to the residual effects

TABLE 13-3	Obstructive Sleep Apnea
Manifestations	• Frequent episodes of obstructive sleep apnea ($\geq$10 seconds, occurring $\geq$5 times/hour during sleep) or hypopnea (50% decrease in airflow or decrease sufficient to drop SaO_2 by 4%) • Snoring • Daytime somnolence (concentration and memory problems, motor vehicle accidents) • Physiologic changes; arterial hypoxemia, polycythemia, arterial hypercarbia, systemic hypertension, pulmonary hypertension
Risk Factors	• Male gender • Middle age • Obesity (BMI >30) • Alcohol (evening ingestion) • Drug-induced sleep

SAO_2, oxygen saturation.

TABLE 13-4	**Management of Anesthesia and Obstructive Sleep Apnea**

Patients are extremely sensitive to central nervous system depressant drugs.

Difficult intubation (difficult airway) is possible.

Use short-acting inhalational and intravenous anesthetic agents.

Use short-acting neuromuscular blocking agents.

Regional anesthesia may be useful.

Tracheal extubation can be used when awake.

Patients are at increased risk of hypoxemia in the postoperative period (both early and late).

Management of postoperative pain should take into account increased sensitivity to the respiratory depressant effects of opioids (including neuraxial opioids), both early and late (2–5 days postoperatively).

Consider using nonsteroidal anti-inflammatory agents.

of anesthetic drugs or upper airway edema. Acute upper airway obstruction may occur immediately following extubation. Postoperative analgesia with nonsteroidal anti-inflammatory drugs is most often recommended. The adequacy of ventilation should be assessed and monitored for 24 to 48 hours postoperatively.

2.) *Obesity Hypoventilation Syndrome* (apnea without respiratory efforts) is the long-term consequence of obstructive sleep apnea. At its extreme, obesity hypoventilation syndrome culminates in the pickwickian syndrome (obesity, daytime hypersomnolence, arterial hypoxemia, polycythemia, hypercarbia, respiratory acidosis, pulmonary hypertension, right ventricular failure).

3.) *Pulmonary Function*

  a.) **Lung Volumes.** Obesity imposes a restrictive ventilatory defect because of the weight of the thoracic cage and abdomen impeding the motion of the diaphragm and decreasing functional residual capacity (FRC), especially in the supine position. These changes are accentuated by general anesthesia and impair the ability of obese patients to tolerate apnea (i.e., during direct laryngoscopy), resulting in arterial oxygen desaturation after induction of anesthesia, often despite preoxygenation.

  b.) **Gas Exchange.** $PaCO_2$ and ventilatory response to carbon dioxide remain within a normal range in obese patients.

  c.) **Lung Compliance and Resistance.** Obesity is associated with decreases in respiratory compliance and resistance that result in rapid, shallow breathing patterns and increased work of breathing that is most marked in the supine position.

  d.) **Work of Breathing.** Normocapnia is maintained by increased minute ventilation, resulting in increased oxygen cost (work) of breathing.

4.) *Cardiovascular Issues*
   a.) **Systemic Hypertension** is present in 50% to 60% of obese patients (increased extracellular fluid volume, increased cardiac output, hyperinsulinemia). Pulmonary hypertension is common and most likely reflects the impact of chronic arterial hypoxemia or increased pulmonary blood volume (or both).
   b.) **Ischemic Heart Disease.** Obesity seems to be an independent risk factor for the development of ischemic heart disease and is more common in obese individuals with central distributions of fat.
   c.) **Congestive Heart Failure (Fig. 13-1).** Systemic hypertension causes concentric left ventricular hypertrophy and a progressively noncompliant left ventricle, which, when combined with hypervolemia, increases the risk of congestive heart failure. Obesity-induced cardiomyopathy is associated with hypervolemia and increased cardiac output.

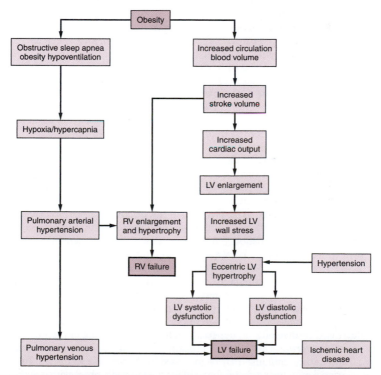

Figure 13-1 • Obesity-induced cardiomyopathy and its association with congestive heart failure (right ventricular [RV], left ventricular [LV]), systemic hypertension, and ischemic heart disease. (Adapted from Adams JP, Murphy PG: Obesity in anesthesia and intensive care. Br J Anaesth 2000;85:91–108.)

5.) *Gastric Emptying.* The notion that obese patients are at increased risk of aspiration is probably not true. Obese patients without reflux symptoms have resistance gradients between the stomach and gastroesophageal junction similar to those in nonobese individuals in both the sitting and supine positions. Gastric volume is greater in obese individuals, but gastric emptying may be more rapid, although the residual gastric volume is larger in obese individuals.

6.) *Diabetes Mellitus.* Glucose tolerance curves are often abnormal, and the incidence of diabetes mellitus is increased several fold in obese patients, as a result of the resistance of peripheral tissues to the effects of insulin in the presence of increased adipose tissue.

7.) *Hepatobiliary Disease.* Abnormal liver function tests and fatty liver infiltration are common findings in obese patients. The risk of developing gallbladder and biliary tract disease is increased threefold.

8) *Thromboembolic Disease.* The risk of deep vein thrombosis in obese patients undergoing surgery is approximately double that of nonobese individuals (polycythemia, increased abdominal pressure, immobilization).

9) *Pharmacokinetics of Drugs* is altered in obesity (increase in blood volume and cardiac output, decrease in total body water, altered protein binding) (**Table 13-5**). The idea that slow emergence of morbidly obese patients from the effects of general anesthesia reflects delayed release of the volatile anesthetic from fat stores is not accurate. Slow emergence, if real, most likely reflects a central nervous system effect. Overall, recovery times are often comparable in obese and lean individuals undergoing surgery that requires anesthesia for less than 4 hours.

C. Management of Anesthesia

1. Induction of Anesthesia. Difficulties with mask ventilation and tracheal intubation may occur (because of fat face and cheeks, short neck, large tongue, excessive palatal and pharyngeal soft tissue, restricted mouth opening, limited cervical and mandibular mobility, or large breasts). Obese patients are traditionally presumed to be at increased risk of pulmonary aspiration during the induction of anesthesia, but the risk of pulmonary aspiration is related to difficult tracheal intubation. Rapid decreases in arterial oxygenation may be seen with direct laryngoscopy and tracheal intubation.

2. Maintenance of Anesthesia. Specially designed tables may be required for safe anesthesia for bariatric surgery. Neural injuries are more common, especially in the superobese and any obese patients with diabetes. Pneumoperitoneum during laparoscopy causes physiologic changes that may be accentuated in obesity (decreased venous return, decreased cardiac output, hypercarbia, higher myocardial oxygen demand).

a. Monitoring. The technical difficulty of placing intravenous catheters and invasive monitors may be increased by the presence of obesity. Invasive arterial monitoring should be used for the morbidly obese with severe cardiopulmonary disease and for those patients in whom a poor fit of the noninvasive blood pressure cuff is seen because of the severe conical shape of the upper arms or unavailability of appropriately sized cuffs.

TABLE 13-5 Medication Dosing in Obesity

Drug	Dosing	Comments
Propofol	IBW Maintenance: TBW	Systemic clearance and V_D at steady-state correlates well with TBW. High affinity for excess fat and other well-perfused organs. High hepatic extraction and conjugation relates to TBW.
Thiopental	TBW	Increased V_D, increased blood volume, cardiac output, and muscle mass. Increased absolute dose. Prolonged duration of action.
Midazolam	TBW	Central V_D increases in line with body weight. Increased absolute dose. Prolonged sedation because larger initial doses are needed to achieve adequate serum concentrations.
Succinylcholine	TBW	Plasma cholinesterase activity increases in proportion to body weight. Increased absolute dose.
Vecuronium	IBW	Recovery may be delayed if given according to TBW because of increased V_D and impaired hepatic clearance.
Rocuronium	IBW	Faster onset and longer duration of action. Pharmacokinetics and pharmacodynamics are not altered in obese subjects.
Atracurium, cisatracurium	TBW	Absolute clearance, V_D, and elimination half-life do not change. Unchanged dose per unit body weight without prolongation of recovery because of organ-independent elimination.
Fentanyl Sufentanil	TBW TBW Maintenance: IBW	Increased V_D and elimination half time, which correlates positively with the degree of obesity. Distributes as extensively in excess body mass as in lean tissues. Dose should account for total body mass.
Remifentanil	IBW	Systemic clearance and V_D corrected per kilogram of TBW—significantly smaller in the obese. Pharmacokinetics are similar in obese and nonobese patients. Age and lean body mass should be considered for dosing.

IBW, ideal body weight; TBW, total body weight; V_D, volume of distribution.

b. Pharmacokinetics. Awakening of obese patients is more prompt after exposure to desflurane or sevoflurane than after administration of either isoflurane or propofol. Dexmedetomidine may be a useful anesthetic adjunct for patients who are susceptible to narcotic-induced respiratory depression. *c. Spinal and Epidural Anesthesia* may be technically difficult in obese patients, as bony landmarks are obscured. Local anesthetic requirements for spinal and epidural anesthesia in obese patients may be as much as 20% lower than in nonobese patients.

d. Management of Ventilation. Controlled ventilation using large tidal volumes is often applied in an attempt to offset the decreased FRC. Positive end-expiratory pressure may improve ventilation-to-perfusion matching and arterial oxygenation in obese patients, but adverse effects on cardiac output and oxygen delivery may offset these benefits.

e. Extubation is considered when obese patients are fully recovered from the depressant effects of anesthetics. Ideally, obese patients should recover in a head-up to sitting position. A history of obstructive sleep apnea or obesity hypoventilation syndrome mandates intense postoperative monitoring to ensure maintenance of a patient's upper airway and acceptable oxygenation and ventilation.

f. Postoperative Analgesia. Opioid depression of ventilation in obese patients is a concern, and the intramuscular route of administration may be unreliable owing to the unpredictable absorption of drugs. Patient-controlled analgesia or neuraxial opioids are commonly used.

g. Postoperative Complications include wound infection, hypoventilation, deep vein thrombosis, and pulmonary embolism.

D. Treatment. A weight loss of only 5 to 20 kg has been associated with a decrease in systemic blood pressure and plasma lipid concentrations and enhanced control of diabetes mellitus.

1. Lifestyle Changes include exercise and decreased calorie intake.

2. Medications. Sibutramine is an appetite suppressant that inhibits the reuptake of serotonin and norepinephrine, and orlistat is a lipase inhibitor that acts in the gastrointestinal tract and is not absorbed.

3. Surgical Treatment includes gastric restriction (gastric lap banding, gastroplasty) and procedures to induce intestinal malabsorption (biliopancreatic division, Roux-en-Y gastric bypass). Adult bariatric surgery results in significant, sustained weight loss and reduction of obesity-related co-morbidities (hypertension, diabetes). Complications include anastomotic leaks or strictures, pulmonary embolism, sepsis, gastric prolapse, and bleeding. Protein-calorie malnutrition is the most serious metabolic complication of bariatric surgery. Fat malabsorption and absorption of fat-soluble vitamins are commonly associated with biliopancreatic division. Bariatric surgery in adolescents is controversial.

E. Obesity and Obstetrics (Table 13-6). The major maternal complications reported to be associated with obesity during pregnancy include hypertension (both chronic and preeclampsia); diabetes mellitus (pregestational and gestational); respiratory disorders (asthma and sleep apnea); thromboembolic disease; increased incidence of cesarean section; and infections, primarily urinary tract infections, wound infections, and endometritis. Complications during labor, such as intrapartum fetal distress, meconium aspiration, failure to progress, abnormal presentation, shoulder dystocia, and an increased rate of instrumental delivery, are also more common in the obese parturient. The incidence of failed tracheal intubation is approximately 1 in 280 in the obstetric population, compared with 1 in 2230 in the general surgical population.

1. Anesthetic Management. A functional epidural catheter for labor analgesia is advantageous should any operative intervention be required.

TABLE 13-6	Cardiopulmonary Changes with Pregnancy and Obesity		
Parameter	Pregnancy	Obesity	Combined
Heart rate	↑	↑↑	↑↑
Stroke volume	↑↑	↑	↑
Cardiac output	↑↑	↑↑	↑↑↑
Cardiac index	↑ or ↔	↔	↔ or ↓
Hematocrit	↓↓	↑	↓
Blood volume	↑↑	↑	↑
Systemic vascular resistance	↓↓	↑	↔ or ↓
Mean arterial pressure	↑	↑↑	↑↑
Supine hypotension	Present	Present	↑↑
Left ventricular morphology	Hypertrophy	Hypertrophy and dilation	Hypertrophy and dilation
Sympathetic activity	↑	↑↑	↑↑↑
Systolic function	↔	↔ or ↓	↔ or ↓
Diastolic function	↔	↓	↓
Central venous pressure	↔	↑	↑↑
Pulmonary wedge pressure	↔	↑↑	↑↑
Pulmonary hypertension	Absent	May be present	May be present
Preeclampsia	↔	n/a	↑↑
Progesterone level	↑	↔	↑
Sensitivity to CO_2	↑	↓	↑
Tidal volume	↑	↓	↑
Respiratory rate	↑	↔ or ↑	↑
Minute volume	↑	↓ or ↔	↑
Inspiratory capacity	↑	↓	↑
Inspiratory reserve volume	↑	↓	↑
Expiratory reserve volume	↓	↓↓	↓
Residual volume	↓	↓ or ↔	↑
Functional residual capacity	↓↓	↓↓↓	↓↓
Vital capacity	↔	↓	↓
FEV_1	↔	↓ or ↔	↔
FEV_1/vital capacity	↔	↔	↔
Total lung capacity	↓	↓↓	↓
Compliance	↔	↓↓	↓
Work of breathing	↑	↑↑	↑
Resistance	↓	↑	↓

Continued

225

Parameter	Pregnancy	Obesity	Combined
V/Q mismatch	↑	↑	↑↑
DL_{CO}	↑ or ↔	↔	↔
PaO_2	↓	↓↓	↓
$PaCO_2$	↓	↑	↓

TABLE 13-6 Cardiopulmonary Changes with Pregnancy and Obesity—cont'd

↑, increase; ↓, decrease; ↔, no change (multiple arrows represent the degree of intensity); DL_{CO}, diffusion capacity of lung for carbon monoxide; FEV_1, forced expiratory volume in 1 second; V/Q, ratio of ventilation to perfusion; $PaCO_2$, partial pressure of carbon dioxide; PaO_2, partial pressure of oxygen.

Hormone-related changes during pregnancy may enhance neural blockade in the parturient. Problems with spinal block include technical difficulties, potential for high spinal blockade, profound dense thoracic motor blockade leading to cardiorespiratory compromise, and inability to prolong the blockade. Obese parturients are at increased risk of postoperative complications (e.g., hypoxemia, atelectasis, pneumonia, deep vein thrombosis, pulmonary embolism, pulmonary edema, postpartum cardiomyopathy, postoperative endometritis, wound infection and dehiscence).

II. EATING DISORDERS (Table 13-7)

A. Anorexia Nervosa is characterized by striking decreases in food intake, excessive physical activity, and weight loss of more than 25% of normal body weight with the patient's perception that they are still obese.

1. Signs and Symptoms (Table 13-8)

2. Treatment is complicated by the patient's denial of the condition. Selective serotonin reuptake inhibitors (e.g., fluoxetine) may have some value.

3. Management of Anesthesia is based on the known pathophysiologic effects evoked by starvation (hypokalemia, hypovolemia, delayed gastric emptying, cardiac dysrhythmias).

B. Bulimia Nervosa is characterized by episodes of binge eating (a sense of loss of control over eating), purging, and dietary restriction.

1. Signs and Symptoms include dry skin, evidence of dehydration, fluctuant hypertrophy of the salivary glands, and resting bradycardia. The most common laboratory findings are increased serum amylase concentrations (presumably of parotid gland origin). Metabolic alkalosis secondary to purging is commonly present with increased serum bicarbonate concentrations, hypochloremia, and occasionally hypokalemia. Dental complications, including periodontal disease, are likely.

2. Treatment is cognitive-behavioral therapy. Pharmacotherapy with tricyclic antidepressants and selective serotonin reuptake inhibitors (e.g., fluoxetine) may be helpful. Potassium supplementation may be necessary in the presence of hypokalemia caused by recurrent self-induced vomiting.

TABLE 13-7 Diagnostic Criteria for Eating Disorders

Anorexia Nervosa

Body mass index <17.5

Fear of weight gain

Inaccurate perception of body shape and weight

Amenorrhea

Bulimia Nervosa

Recurrent binge eating (twice weekly for 3 months)

Recurrent purging, excessive exercise, or fasting

Excessive concern about body weight or shape

Binge-Eating Disorder

Recurrent binge eating (2 days per week for 6 months)

Eating rapidly

Eating until uncomfortably full

Eating when not hungry

Eating alone

Feeling guilty after a binge

No purging or excessive exercise

Adapted from Becker AE, Grinspoon SK, Klibanski A, et al: Eating disorders. N Engl J Med 1999;340:1092–1098

TABLE 13-8 Signs and Symptoms of Anorexia Nervosa

Unexplained weight loss

Decreased cardiac mass and contractility

Cardiomyopathy

Sudden death (ventricular arrhythmias)

Amenorrhea

Decreased body temperature

Orthostatic hypotension (altered autonomic nervous system function)

Bradycardia

Osteoporosis

Slowed gastric emptying

Impaired cognitive functioning

Hypokalemia (self-induced vomiting, laxative abuse)

Fatty liver infiltration

C. Binge-Eating Disorders resemble bulimia nervosa, but in contrast to patients with bulimia nervosa, these individuals do not purge and periods of dietary restriction are less striking. The diagnosis of binge-eating disorders should be suspected in morbidly obese patients, particularly obese patients with continued weight gain or marked weight cycling.

III. MALNUTRITION AND VITAMIN DEFICIENCIES

A. Malnutrition is a medically distinct syndrome that is responsive to caloric support provided by enteral or total parenteral nutrition (TPN) (hyperalimentation).

Malnourished patients are identified by the presence of serum albumin concentrations less than 3 g/dL and transferrin levels less than 200 mg/dL. Critically ill patients often experience negative caloric intake complicated by hypermetabolic states caused by increased caloric needs produced by trauma, fever, sepsis, and wound healing.

1. Treatment. It is often recommended that patients who have lost more than 20% of their body weight be treated nutritionally before undergoing elective surgery.

a. Enteral Nutrition. When the gastrointestinal tract is functioning, enteral nutrition can be provided by means of nasogastric or gastrostomy tube feedings. Complications of enteral feedings are infrequent but may include hyperglycemia leading to osmotic diuresis and hypovolemia (exogenous insulin administration is a consideration).

b. Total Parenteral Nutrition is indicated when the gastrointestinal tract is not functioning. When daily caloric requirements exceed 2000 calories or prolonged nutritional support is required, a catheter is traditionally placed in the subclavian vein to permit infusion of hypertonic parenteral solutions (approximately 1900 mOsm/L) in a daily volume of approximately 40 mL/kg. Potential complications of TPN are numerous (**Table 13-9**).

TABLE 13-9	Other Complications of Total Parenteral Nutrition/ Peripheral Parenteral Nutrition	
Hypokalemia	Hypomagnesemia	Hypocalcemia
Hypophosphatemia	Venous thrombosis	Infection/sepsis
Bacterial translocation from the gastrointestinal tract	Osteopenia	Elevated liver enzymes
Renal dysfunction	Hyperchloremic metabolic acidosis	Fluid overload
Nonketotic hyperosmolar hyperglycemic coma		Refeeding syndrome*

*Hemolytic anemia, respiratory distress, tetany, paresthesia, and cardiac arrhythmias. More common in patients with anorexia or alcoholism and in rapid refeeding, and associated with low phosphorus, potassium, and magnesium.

B. Vitamin Deficiencies (**Table 13-10**)

IV. INBORN ERRORS OF METABOLISM (Table 13-11)

A. **Porphyrias** are a group of inborn errors of metabolism characterized by the overproduction of porphyrins (essential for many vital physiologic functions, including oxygen transport and storage) and their precursors. The synthetic pathway involved in the production of porphyrins is determined by a sequence of enzymes. A defect in any of these enzymes results in accumulation of the preceding intermediaries and produces a form of porphyria (**Fig. 13-2**). Heme is the most important porphyrin (hemoglobin and cytochrome P-450), and its production is controlled by aminolevulinic acid (ALA) synthetase, an inducible enzyme.

1. **Classification (Table 13-12; Fig. 13-2).** Only acute forms of porphyria are relevant to the management of anesthesia, as they are the only forms of porphyria that may result in life-threatening reactions in response to certain drugs (**Table 13-13**).

2. **Acute Porphyrias.** Acute attacks are most commonly precipitated by events that decrease heme concentrations, thus increasing the activity of ALA synthetase and stimulating the production of porphyrinogens (**Fig. 13-2**). Enzyme-inducing drugs are the most important triggering factors for the development of acute porphyrias.

   a. Signs and Symptoms. Acute attacks are characterized by severe abdominal pain, autonomic nervous system instability (tachycardia, hypertension), electrolyte disturbances, dehydration, skeletal muscle weakness, seizures, and other neuropsychiatric manifestations ranging from mild disturbances to fulminating life-threatening events. Complete and prolonged remissions are likely between attacks. Many individuals with the genetic defect never develop symptoms. Patients may experience their first symptoms in response to inadvertent administration of triggering drugs during the perioperative period. ALA synthetase concentrations are increased during all acute attacks of porphyria.

   b. Triggering Drugs (Table 13-13)

   c. Types of Porphyria

      1.) Acute Intermittent Porphyria produces the most serious symptoms (systemic hypertension, renal dysfunction) and is the one most likely to be life threatening.

      2.) Variegate Porphyria is characterized by neurotoxicity and cutaneous photosensitivity in which bullous skin eruptions occur on exposure to sunlight as a result of the conversion of porphyrinogens to porphyrins.

      3.) Hereditary Coproporphyria. Acute attacks of hereditary coproporphyria are less common than acute intermittent porphyria or variegate porphyria. Neurotoxicity and cutaneous hypersensitivity are characteristic but less severe.

      4.) Porphyria Cutanea Tarda. ALA synthetase activity is not important, and drugs capable of precipitating attacks of other forms of porphyria do not provoke an attack of porphyria cutanea tarda. Signs and symptoms most often appear as photosensitivity in men older than 35 years of age. Anesthesia is not a hazard, although the

TABLE 13-10	Vitamin Deficiencies		
Vitamin	Laboratory Test	Causes of Deficiency	Signs of Deficiency
Thiamine (B_1) (beriberi)	Urinary thiamine	Chronic alcoholism caused by decreased intake of thiamine	Low SVR, high CO, polyneuropathy (demyelination, sensory deficit, paresthesia), exaggerated decreased response to hemorrhage, change in body position, positive pressure ventilation
Riboflavin (B_2)	Urinary riboflavin	Almost always caused by dietary deficiency, photodegradation of milk, other dairy products	Magenta tongue, angular stomatitis, seborrhea, cheilosis
Pantothenic acid (B_3)	Urinary pantothenic acid	Liver, yeast, egg yolks, and vegetables	Nonspecific and include gastrointestinal disturbance, depression, muscle cramps, paresthesia, ataxia, and hypoglycemia
Niacin (B_5) (pellagra)	Urinary niacin metabolite	Nicotinic acid is synthesized from tryptophan; carcinoid tumor uses tryptophan to form serotonin instead of nicotinic acid, making these patients more susceptible.	Mental confusion, irritability, peripheral neuropathy, achlorhydria, diarrhea, vesicular dermatitis, stomatitis, glossitis, urethritis, and excessive salivation
Pyridoxine (B_6)	Plasma B_6	Alcoholism, isoniazid	Seborrhea, glossitis, convulsions, neuropathy, depression, confusion, microcytic anemia
Folate (B_9)	Serum folate	Alcoholism, sulfasalazine, pyrimethamine, triamterene	Megaloblastic anemia, atrophic glossitis, depression, $\uparrow$ homocysteine
Cyanocobalamin (B_{12})	Serum B_{12}	Gastric atrophy (pernicious anemia), terminal ileal disease, strict vegetarianism	Megaloblastic anemia, loss of vibratory and position sense, abnormal gait, dementia, impotence, loss of bladder and bowel control, $\uparrow$ homocysteine, $\uparrow$ methylmalonic acid

TABLE 13-10	Vitamin Deficiencies—cont'd		
Vitamin	**Laboratory Test**	**Causes of Deficiency**	**Signs of Deficiency**
Biotin	Serum biotin	Liver, soy, beans, yeast, and egg yolks; egg white contains the protein avidin, which strongly binds the vitamin and reduces its bioavailability	Mental changes (depression, hallucinations), paresthesia, anorexia, nausea; scaling, seborrheic, and erythematous rash may occur around the eyes, nose, and mouth, as well as on the extremities
Ascorbic acid (C) (scurvy)	Serum ascorbic acid	Smoking, alcoholism	Capillary fragility, petechial hemorrhage, joint and skeletal muscle hemorrhage, poor wound healing, catabolic state, loosened teeth and gangrenous alveolar margins, low potassium, iron
A	Plasma vitamin A	Dietary lack of leafy vegetables and animal liver or malabsorption	Loss of night vision, conjunctival drying, corneal destruction, anemia
D (rickets)	Plasma 25-dihydroxy vitamin D	Decreased vitamin D leads to less calcium absorption balanced by parathormone activity that increases due to low calcium, leading to increased osteoclastic activity and bone resorption	Thoracic kyphosis could lead to hypoventilation, normal to low serum calcium, low serum phosphate, high plasma alkaline phosphatase
E	Plasma α-tocopherol	Occurs only with fat malabsorption or genetic abnormalities of vitamin E metabolism/transport	Peripheral neuropathy, spinocerebellar ataxia, skeletal muscle atrophy, retinopathy
K	Prothrombin time	Formed by intestinal bacteria that are eliminated by prolonged antibiotic therapy or failure of fat absorption	Bleeding

CO, cardiac output; SVR, systemic vascular resistance.

TABLE 13-11	Inborn Errors of Metabolism
Porphyria	
Gout	
Pseudogout	
Hyperlipidemia	
Carbohydrate metabolism disorders	
Amino acid disorders	
Mucopolysaccharidoses	
Gangliosidoses	

choice of drugs should take into consideration the likely presence of coexisting liver disease.

5.) *Erythropoietic Uroporphyria.* In contrast to porphyrin synthesis in the liver, porphyrin synthesis in the erythropoietic system is responsive to changes in hematocrit and tissue oxygenation. Hemolytic anemia, bone marrow hyperplasia, and splenomegaly are often present. Repeated infections are common, and photosensitivity is severe. The urine of affected patients turns red when exposed to light. Neurotoxicity and abdominal pain do not occur.

6.) *Erythropoietic Protoporphyria,* a less debilitating form of erythropoietic porphyria, is characterized by photosensitivity. Administration of barbiturates does not affect the course of the disease. Survival to adulthood is common.

d. Management of Anesthesia. Most patients with porphyria can be safely anesthetized assuming that appropriate precautions are taken (short-acting drugs to limit exposure and reduce enzyme induction, avoidance of repeated or prolonged use). Exposure to multiple potential enzyme-inducing drugs may be more dangerous than exposure to any one drug.

1.) *Preoperative Evaluation* includes a careful family history, examination for skin lesions, and notation of the presence of peripheral and/ or autonomic neuropathy. If an acute attack is suspected, evaluation and treatment of fluid and electrolyte disorders should be undertaken. If prolonged fasting is anticipated, administration of a glucose-saline infusion should be considered (caloric restriction has been linked to the precipitation of acute porphyria attacks).

2.) *Regional Anesthesia.* There is no absolute contraindication to the use of regional anesthesia, but it is essential to perform a neurologic examination prior to the block to minimize the likelihood that worsening of any preexisting neuropathy would be erroneously attributed to the regional anesthetic. Autonomic nervous system blockade induced by the regional anesthetic could unmask cardiovascular instability (autonomic neuropathy, hypovolemia, or both). There is no evidence that any local anesthetic has ever induced an acute attack of porphyria or neurologic damage in porphyric individuals.

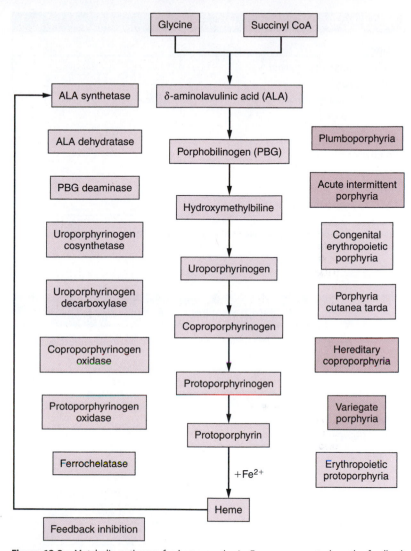

Figure 13-2 • Metabolic pathways for heme synthesis. Enzymes are noted on the feedback inhibition loop of the sequence, and the type of porphyria associated with the enzyme deficiency is designated on the right. Examples of acute porphyrias are indicated by the boxes. CoA, coenzyme A. (Adapted from James MFM, Hift RJ: Porphyrias. Br J Anaesth 2000;85:143–153.)

TABLE 13-12	Classification of Porphyrias
Acute	
Acute intermittent porphyria	
Variegate porphyria	
Hereditary coproporphyria	
Plumboporphyria	
Nonacute	
Porphyria cutanea tarda	
Erythropoietic porphyrias	
Erythropoietic uroporphyria	
Erythropoietic protoporphyria	

Adapted from James MFM, Hift RJ: Porphyrias. Br J Anaesth 2000;85:143–153.

TABLE 13-13	Recommendations Regarding the Use of Anesthetic Drugs in the Presence of Acute Porphyrias
Drug	**Recommendation**
Inhaled Anesthetics	
Nitrous oxide	Safe
Isoflurane	Probably safe*
Sevoflurane	Probably safe*
Desflurane	Probably safe*
Intravenous Anesthetics	
Propofol	Safe
Ketamine	Probably safe*
Thiopental	Avoid
Thiamylal	Avoid
Methohexital	Avoid
Etomidate	Avoid
Analgesics	
Acetaminophen	Safe
Aspirin	Safe
Codeine	Safe
Morphine	Safe
Fentanyl	Safe
Sufentanil	Safe
Ketorolac	Probably avoid[†]
Phenacetin	Probably avoid[†]
Pentazocine	Avoid

234

TABLE 13-13	Recommendations Regarding the Use of Anesthetic Drugs in the Presence of Acute Porphyrias—cont'd
Drug	**Recommendation**
Neuromuscular Blocking Drugs	
Succinylcholine	Safe
Pancuronium	Safe
Atracurium	Probably safe*
Cisatracurium	Probably safe*
Vecuronium	Probably safe*
Rocuronium	Probably safe*
Mivacurium	Probably safe*
Opioid Antagonists	
Naloxone	Safe
Anticholinergics	
Atropine	Safe
Glycopyrrolate	Safe
Anticholinesterases	
Neostigmine	Safe
Local Anesthetics	
Lidocaine	Safe
Tetracaine	Safe
Bupivacaine	Safe
Mepivacaine	Safe
Ropivacaine	No data
Sedatives and Antiemetics	
Droperidol	Safe
Midazolam	Probably safe*
Lorazepam	Probably safe*
Cimetidine	Probably safe*
Ranitidine	Probably safe*
Metoclopramide	Probably safe*
Ondansetron	Probably safe*
Cardiovascular Drugs	
Epinephrine	Safe
α-Agonists	Safe
β-Agonists	Safe
β-Antagonists	Safe
Diltiazem	Probably safe*
Nitroprusside	Probably safe*
Nifedipine	Probably avoid†

*Although safety is not conclusively established, the drug is unlikely to provoke acute porphyria.
†Use only if expected benefits outweigh the risks.
Adapted from James MFM, Hift RJ: Porphyrias. Br J Anaesth 2000;85:143–153.

3.) *General Anesthesia.* The total dose of drugs administered and the length of exposure may influence the risk of triggering a porphyric crisis in vulnerable patients (**Table 13-13**).

4.) *Cardiopulmonary Bypass.* Clinical experience does not support an increased incidence of porphyric crises in these patients when undergoing cardiopulmonary bypass.

5.) *Treatment of a Porphyric Crisis* includes removal of any known triggering factors, adequate hydration and carbohydrates, correction of electrolyte disturbances, sedation, treatment of pain, nausea and vomiting, β-adrenergic blockers to control tachycardia and hypertension, and anticonvulsants to control seizures. Hematin (3 to 4 mg/kg intravenously [IV] over 20 minutes) is the only specific form of therapy for an acute porphyric crisis. Somatostatin decreases the rate of formation of ALA synthetase and combined with plasmapheresis may effectively decrease pain and induce remission.

B. Gout is a disorder of purine metabolism characterized by hyperuricemia with recurrent episodes of acute arthritis owing to deposition of urate crystals in joints. The incidence of systemic hypertension, ischemic heart disease, and diabetes mellitus is increased in patients with gout.

1. Treatment consists of decreasing serum concentrations of uric acid (probenecid, allopurinol) and colchicine to relieve joint pain, presumably by modifying leukocyte migration and phagocytosis.

2. Management of Anesthesia focuses on prehydration to facilitate continued renal elimination of uric acid. Sodium bicarbonate alkalinizes the urine and facilitates excretion of uric acid. The increased incidence of systemic hypertension, ischemic heart disease, and diabetes mellitus in patients with gout is considered.

C. Lesch-Nyhan Syndrome is a genetically determined disorder of purine metabolism that occurs exclusively in males and is characterized by mental retardation, spasticity, and self-mutilation patterns that usually involves trauma to perioral tissues. Subsequent scarification may present difficulties with direct laryngoscopy for tracheal intubation.

D. Disorders of Carbohydrate Metabolism usually reflect genetically determined enzyme defects.

1. Glycogen Storage Disease Type 1a (von Gierke's Disease) is caused by the deficiency or lack of the enzyme glucose 6-phosphatase. Characteristics are hypoglycemia, metabolic acidosis, osteoporosis, mental retardation, growth retardation, seizures, hepatomegaly, and platelet dysfunction. Death usually occurs by age 2. Management of anesthesia includes provision of exogenous glucose, avoidance of lactate-containing solutions, and monitoring of arterial pH.

2. Glycogen Storage Disease Type 1b is deficiency of glucose 6-phosphate transport that results in glycogen accumulation in the liver, kidneys, and intestinal mucosa. Hypoglycemia and lactic acidosis ensue. Clinical signs and symptoms resemble those described for glycogen storage disease type 1a.

E. Disorders of Amino Acid Metabolism There are more than 70 known disorders of amino acid metabolism, but most are extremely rare. Classic manifestations include mental retardation, seizures, and aminoaciduria (**Table 13-14**). Metabolic acidosis, hyperammonemia, hepatic failure, and

TABLE 13-14 Disorders of Amino Acid Metabolism

Disorder	Mental Retardation	Seizures	Metabolic Acidosis	Hyper-ammonemia	Hepatic Failure	Thrombo-embolism	Other
Phenylketonuria	Yes	Yes	No	No	No	No	Friable skin
Homocystinuria	Yes/no	Yes	No	No	No	Yes	
Hypervalinemia	Yes	Yes	Yes	No	No	No	Hypoglycemia
Citrullinemia	Yes	Yes	No	Yes	Yes	No	
Branched-chain aciduria (maple syrup urine disease)	Yes	Yes	Yes	No		Yes	Hypoglycemia Neurologic deterioration during perioperative period
Methylmalonyl coenzyme amutase deficiency			Yes	Yes			Acidosis intraoperatively Avoid nitrous oxide?
Isoleucinemia	Yes	Yes	Yes	Yes	Yes	No	Hypovolemia
Methioninemia	Yes	No	No	No	No	No	Thermal instability
Histidinuria	Yes	Yes/no	No	No	No	No	Erythrocyte fragility
Neutral aminoaciduria (Hartnup's disease)	Yes/no		Yes	No	No	No	Dermatitis
Arginemia	Yes		No	Yes	Yes	No	

thromboembolism can also occur. Management of anesthesia is directed toward maintenance of intravascular volume and acid-base homeostasis.

1. Phenylketonuria is the prototype of disorders caused by abnormal amino acid metabolism. Clinical features include mental retardation and seizures. Patients are more liable to vitamin B_{12} deficiency. They may also be more sensitive to narcotics.

2. Homocystinuria. Manifestations include dislocation of the lens, osteoporosis, kyphoscoliosis, brittle light-colored hair, malar flush, and often mental retardation. Thromboembolism (caused by activation of the Hageman factor by homocysteine and increased platelet adhesiveness) can be life threatening. Efforts to reduce the risk of thromboembolism during the perioperative period should include administration of pyridoxine (decreases platelet adhesiveness), hydration, infusion of dextran, and early ambulation.

3. Maple Syrup Urine Disease (metabolic defect causes the urine to smell like maple syrup) is associated with growth retardation and delayed psychomotor development. Infection or fasting often results in acute metabolic decompensation. Glucose-containing intravenous solutions should be administered intraoperatively. Measurement of arterial pH is helpful for detecting metabolic acidosis, which may necessitate treatment with intravenous sodium bicarbonate.

4. Methylmalonyl–Coenzyme A Mutase Deficiency is an inborn error of metabolism resulting in the formation of methylmalonic acidemia. Events during the perioperative period that increase protein catabolism (fasting, bleeding into the gastrointestinal tract, stress responses, tissue destruction) predispose to acidosis. Clear fluid ingestion should be allowed up to 2 hours before scheduled induction of anesthesia. Anesthesia management involves minimizing hypovolemia and protein catabolism.

CHAPTER 14

Renal Disease

The kidneys are responsible for, or contribute to, a number of essential functions, including water conservation, electrolyte homeostasis, acid-base balance, and several neurohumoral or hormonal functions.

I. CLINICAL ASSESSMENT OF RENAL FUNCTION

Renal function can be evaluated with laboratory tests that reflect glomerular filtration rate (GFR) and renal tubular function (**Table 14-1**).

A. Glomerular Filtration Rate. Alterations in the GFR are associated with predictable changes in erythropoietic activity. Clinical manifestations of uremia generally appear when the GFR is less than 15 mL/min/1.73 m^2 (normal: $\geq$90 mL/min/1.73 m^2).

B. Blood Urea Nitrogen (BUN) concentrations vary with the GFR, dietary protein intake, co-existing disease, intravascular fluid, and increased protein catabolism (e.g., fever). BUN concentrations greater than 50 mg/dL usually reflect a decreased GFR.

C. Serum Creatinine levels can be used as an estimate of the GFR. Normal serum creatinine concentrations range from 0.6 to 1.0 mg/dL in women and 0.8 to 1.3 mg/dL in men. Serum creatinine values are slow to reflect acute changes in renal function.

D. Creatinine Clearance correlates with the GFR and is the most reliable measure of GFR. Creatinine clearance does not depend on corrections for age or the presence of a steady state. Preoperatively, patients with creatinine clearances of 10 to 25 mL/min must be considered at risk of developing prolonged or adverse responses to drugs that depend on renal excretion for their clearance from the plasma.

E. Renal Tubular Function and Integrity

1. Urine Concentrating Ability. Renal tubular dysfunction is present if the kidneys do not produce appropriately concentrated urine in the presence of a physiologic stimulus for the release of antidiuretic hormone (ADH). In the absence of diuretic therapy or glycosuria, urine specific gravity greater than 1.018 suggests that the ability of renal tubules to concentrate urine is adequate.

TABLE 14-1 Tests Used to Evaluate Renal Function	
Test	**Normal Value**
Glomerular Filtration Rate	
Blood urea nitrogen	10–20 mg/dL
Serum creatinine	0.7–1.5 mg/dL
Creatinine clearance	110–150 mL/min
Proteinuria (albumin)	<150 mg/day
Renal Tubular Function and/or Integrity	
Urine specific gravity	1.003–1.030
Urine osmolality	38–1400 mOsm/L
Urine sodium excretion	<40 mEq/L
Glucosuria	
Enzymuria	
N-Acetyl-β-glucosaminidase	
α-Glutathione-S-transferase	
Factors That Influence Interpretation	
Dehydration	
Variable protein intake	
Gastrointestinal bleeding	
Catabolism	
Advanced age	
Skeletal muscle mass	
Accurate timed urine volume measurement	

2. Proteinuria. Transient proteinuria may be associated with fever, congestive heart failure, seizure activity, pancreatitis, and exercise, and resolves with the underlying stimulus/illness. Orthostatic proteinuria is benign, occurring in up to 5% of adolescents while in the upright position and not in the recumbent position. Persistent proteinuria generally connotes significant renal disease.

3. Urinary Sodium Excretion greater than 40 mEq/L reflects decreased ability of the renal tubules to conserve sodium or drug-induced diuresis. Urine osmolarity is likely to be less than 350 mOsm/L. Drug-induced diuresis is associated with increased urinary excretion of sodium.

4. Urinalysis can detect the presence of protein, glucose, acetoacetate, blood, and leukocytes. The urine pH and solute concentrations (specific gravity) are determined, and sediment microscopy is used to determine the presence of cells, casts, micro-organisms, and crystals.

II. ACUTE RENAL FAILURE/INSUFFICIENCY (ARF)

ARF is characterized by deterioration of renal function over a period of hours to days, resulting in failure of the kidneys to excrete nitrogenous waste products and to maintain fluid and electrolyte homeostasis. ARF may be oliguric (urinary output <400 mL/day) or nonoliguric (urinary output >400 mL/day). The mortality rate of severe ARF requiring dialysis remains high. ARF is associated with a number of other systemic diseases, acute clinical conditions, drug treatments, and interventional therapies (**Table 14-2**).

A. Prerenal Azotemia predisposes patients to ischemia-induced acute tubular necrosis. Prerenal azotemia is rapidly reversible if the underlying cause (hypovolemia, congestive heart failure) is corrected. Elderly patients are susceptible to prerenal azotemia because of their predisposition to hypovolemia (poor fluid intake) and high incidence of renovascular disease. Urinary indices may help distinguish prerenal from intrinsic ARF (**Table 14-3**).

TABLE 14-2	Etiology of Acute Renal Failure
Prerenal Azotemia (Decreased Renal Blood Flow)	
Absolute decrease	
Acute hemorrhage	
Gastrointestinal fluid loss	
Trauma	
Surgery	
Burns	
Low output syndrome	
Renal artery stenosis	
Relative decrease	
Sepsis	
Hepatic failure	
Allergic reaction	
Renal Azotemia (Intrinsic)	
Acute glomerulonephritis (5% of cases)	
Interstitial nephritis (drugs, sepsis) (10% of cases)	
Acute tubular necrosis (85% of cases)	
Ischemia (50% of cases)	
Nephrotoxic drugs (antibiotics [35% of cases], anesthetic drugs?)	
Solvents (carbon tetrachloride, ethylene glycol)	
Radiographic contrast dyes	
Myoglobinuria	
Postrenal (Obstructive)	
Upper urinary tract obstruction (ureteral)	
Lower urinary tract obstruction (bladder outlet)	

Adapted from Klahr S, Miller SB: Acute oliguria. N Engl J Med 1998;338:671–675; and Thadhani R, Pascual M, Bonventre JV: Acute renal failure. N Engl J Med 1996;334:1148–1169.

TABLE 14-3	Characteristic Urinary Indices in Patients with Acute Oliguria Due to Prerenal or Renal Causes	
Index	Prerenal Causes	Renal Causes
Urinary sodium concentration (mEq/L)	<20	>40
Fractional excretion of sodium (%)	<1	>1
Urine osmolarity (mOsm/L)	>400	250–300
Urine creatinine/plasma creatinine	>40	<20
Urine/plasma osmolarity	>1.5	<1.1

Adapted from Klahr S, Miller SB: Acute oliguria. N Engl J Med 1998;338:671–675.

B. Renal Azotemia. Intrinsic renal diseases that result in ARF are categorized according to the site of injury (renal tubules, interstitium, glomerulus, renal vasculature). Injury to the renal tubules is most often ischemic or nephrotoxic (aminoglycoside antibiotics, radiographic contrast agents). Ischemia and toxins often combine to cause ARF in severely ill patients with conditions such as sepsis or AIDS. ARF due to acute interstitial nephritis is usually caused by allergic reactions to drugs.

C. Postrenal Azotemia. ARF occurs when urinary outflow tracts are obstructed (prostatic hypertrophy, cancer of the prostate or cervix). The potential for recovery is inversely related to the duration of the obstruction. Renal ultrasonography is the best diagnostic test.

D. Risk Factors for Development of ARF include co-existing renal disease, advanced age, congestive heart failure, symptomatic cardiovascular disease, and major operative procedures (cardiopulmonary bypass, abdominal aneurysm resection). Sepsis and multiple organ system dysfunction caused by trauma introduce the risk of ARF. Iatrogenic causes include inadequate fluid replacement, delayed treatment of sepsis, and administration of nephrotoxic drugs or dyes.

E. Complications Associated with ARF (Table 14-4)

    1. Diagnosis of ARF is usually made based on an acute rise in serum creatinine. Urinalysis may be helpful in diagnosing whether ARF is likely to be prerenal, intrarenal, or postrenal. The sensitivity and specificity of urinary sodium below 20 mEq/L in differentiating prerenal azotemia from acute tubular necrosis are 90% and 82%, respectively (see **Table 14-3**).

    2. Management Treatment of ARF is aimed at limiting further renal injury and correcting the water, electrolyte, and acid-base derangements. Underlying causes should be sought and terminated or reversed, if possible. Prompt and adequate correction of hypovolemia and hypotension is much more important than the type of fluid used. Vasopressors may increase renal vasoconstriction and exacerbate ARF and should be used with caution. The use of dopamine to treat or prevent ARF is not supported by the literature. The practice of trying to convert oliguric to nonoliguric ARF with diuretics is not advised. Mannitol yields better outcomes in

TABLE 14-4	Complications of Acute Renal Failure
Neurologic	Confusion
	Asterixis
	Somnolence
	Seizure
Cardiovascular	Hypertension
	Congestive heart failure
	Pulmonary edema
	Dysrhythmias
	Pericarditis
	Anemia
Gastrointestinal (GI)	Anorexia
	Nausea and vomiting
	Ileus
	GI bleeding
Infection	Respiratory tract
	Urinary tract

posttransplantation acute tubular necrosis (ATN) and in combination with forced alkaline diuresis to prevent ATN in severe crush injuries. N-acetylcysteine may reduce ARF in high-risk patients exposed to radiocontrast dye. Activated protein C and steroid replacement reduce mortality in patients with severe sepsis. Dialysis (or hemofiltration) is still the mainstay of severe ARF.

3. Prognosis for hospital-acquired ARF is poor, with current mortality rates of more than 20%, and 50% or more once dialysis is required. Only 15% of patients developing ARF will fully recover their renal function.

4. Drug Dosing in Patients with Renal Impairment. The rate of elimination of drugs excreted by the kidneys is proportional to the GFR. If the patient is oliguric, use 5 mL/min for creatinine clearance.

> *a. Loading Dose Guidelines.* If extracellular fluid volume looks normal, use a normal loading dose. If extracellular fluid is contracted, reduce the loading dose; if the extracellular fluid is expanded, use a higher loading dose.
>
> *b. Repeat Dosing.* A combination of increasing the dosing interval and decreasing the dose is often used (e.g., analgesics; **Table 14-5**).
>
> *c. Drugs Removed by Hemodialysis* are usually given at the end of the dialysis schedule to avoid the necessity of redosing.

5. Anesthetic Management. Principles are maintenance of an adequate mean systemic blood pressure and cardiac output and the avoidance of further renal insults including hypotension, hypovolemia, hypoxia, and nephrotoxic exposure. Invasive hemodynamic monitoring may be critical, as are frequent blood gas analysis and electrolyte determination. For patients undergoing renal replacement therapy, institute postoperative dialysis/hemodialysis as soon as the patient is stable.

TABLE 14-5 Renal Effects of Commonly Used Analgesics

Drug	Adjustment Method	GFR >50 mL/min	GFR 10–50 mL/min	GFR <10 mL/min
Acetaminophen	↑ interval	Q4h	Q6h	Q8h
Acetylsalicylic acid	↑ interval	Q4h	Q6–8h	Avoid
Al/remi/sufentanil	↔ dose	100%	100%	100%
Codeine	↓ dose	100%	75%	50%
Fentanyl	↓ dose	100%	75%	50%
Ketorolac*	↓ dose	100%	50%	50%
Meperidine	↓ dose	100%	75%	50%
Methadone	↓ dose	100%	100%	50%–75%
Morphine	↓ dose	100%	75%	50%

*Usually avoided because this class of drug may be associated with worsening of renal function
↓, decreases; ↑, increases; ↔, no change; Q, every.
Adapted from Schrier RW: Manual of Nephrology, 6th ed. Philadelphia, Lippincott Williams & Wilkins, 2005, p 268.

III. CHRONIC RENAL FAILURE (CRF)

CRF is progressive, irreversible deterioration of renal function that results from a wide variety of diseases (**Table 14-6**). Diabetes mellitus is the leading cause of end-stage renal disease (ESRD), followed by hypertension. Stages of CRF are summarized in **Table 14-7**.

A. Pathogenesis. Intrarenal hemodynamic changes (glomerular hypertension, glomerular hyperfiltration and permeability changes, glomerulosclerosis) are likely responsible for progression of renal disease.

1. Systemic Hypertension is a major risk factor. Administration of angiotensin-converting enzyme inhibitors (ACEIs) and/or angiotensin receptor blockers (ARBs) appears to be renoprotective (decreased proteinuria and slowed progression of glomerular sclerosis) compared with other antihypertensive regimens.

2. Dietary Factors. New guidelines call for moderate protein restriction in all patients with renal insufficiency.

3. Strict Control of Blood Glucose Concentrations can delay the onset of proteinuria and slow the progression of nephropathy, neuropathy, and retinopathy.

B. Signs and Symptoms. of CRF include general malaise, and anorexia. Volume overload (peripheral edema, dyspnea, congestive heart failure) and electrolyte or acid-base disturbances are late signs of CRF. Other symptoms include cognitive impairment, peripheral neuropathy, infertility, and increased susceptibility to infection (**Table 14-8**).

C. Diagnosis is made from signs and symptoms of fluid overload and concomitant cardiac disease and confirmed by laboratory testing.

TABLE 14-6	Causes of Chronic Renal Failure

Glomerulopathies
Primary glomerular disease
Focal glomerulosclerosis
Membranous nephropathy
Immunoglobulin A nephropathy
Membranoproliferative glomerulonephritis
Glomerulopathies associated with systemic disease
Diabetes mellitus
Amyloidosis
Postinfectious glomerulonephritis
Systemic lupus erythematosus
Wegener's granulomatosis
Tubulointerstitial disease
Analgesic nephropathy
Reflux nephropathy with pyelonephritis
Myeloma kidney
Sarcoidosis
Heredity disease
Polycystic kidney disease
Alport syndrome
Medullary cystic disease
Systemic hypertension
Renal vascular disease
Obstructive uropathy
Human immunodeficiency virus

Adapted from Tolkoff-Rubin NE, Pascual M: Chronic renal failure. Sci Am Med 1998;1–12.

D. Associated Clinical Conditions

1. Uremic Syndrome is a constellation of signs and symptoms (anorexia, nausea, vomiting, pruritus, anemia, fatigue, coagulopathy) that reflect the kidney's progressive inability to perform its excretory, secretory, and regulatory functions. BUN concentration is a useful clinical indicator of the severity of the uremic syndrome and the patient's response to therapy (dietary protein restriction). Serum creatinine concentration correlates poorly with uremic symptoms.

2. Renal Osteodystrophy is a complication of chronic renal failure. As the GFR decreases, phosphate concentrations increase and serum calcium concentrations decrease, stimulating parathyroid hormone (PTH) secretion and causing bone resorption and calcium release. Treatment of renal

TABLE 14-7 Stages of Chronic Renal Failure

Stage of Failure	Functioning Nephrons (% of Total)	Glomerular Filtration Rate (mL/min)	Signs	Laboratory Abnormalities
Normal	100	125	None	None
Decreased renal reserve	40	50–80	None	None
Renal insufficiency	10–40	12–50	Nocturia	Increased blood urea nitrogen Increased serum creatinine
Renal failure	10	<12	Uremia	Increased blood urea nitrogen Increased serum creatinine Anemia Hyperkalemia Increased bleeding time

TABLE 14-8 Manifestations of Chronic Renal Failure

Electrolyte imbalance

Hyperkalemia

Hypermagnesemia

Hypocalcemia

Metabolic acidosis

Unpredictable intravascular fluid volume status

Anemia

Increased cardiac output

Oxyhemoglobin dissociation curve shifted to the right

Uremic coagulopathies

Platelet dysfunction

Neurologic changes

Encephalopathy

Cardiovascular changes

Systemic hypertension

Congestive heart failure

Attenuated sympathetic nervous system activity due to treatment with antihypertensive drugs

Renal osteodystrophy

Pruritus

osteodystrophy is restriction of dietary phosphate, administration of oral calcium supplements, and vitamin D therapy.

3. Anemia occurs because of decreased erythropoietin production by the kidneys. Treatment is recombinant human erythropoietin (epoetin), eliminating the need for blood transfusions and avoiding the symptoms of anemia in most patients. Blood transfusions are avoided if possible, as the resultant sensitization to HLA antigens makes kidney transplantation less successful.

4. Uremic Bleeding. Patients with chronic renal failure have an increased tendency to bleed despite normal laboratory coagulation studies (platelet count, prothrombin time, plasma thromboplastin time). Treatment of uremic bleeding may include the administration of cryoprecipitate to provide factor VIII–von Willebrand factor (vWF) complex (risk of transmission of viral diseases) or administration of 1-desamino-8-D-arginine vasopressin (DDAVP, desmopressin) (**Table 14-9**).

E. Treatment of CRF includes aggressive treatment of the underlying cause (diabetes or hypertension if present), pharmacologic therapy to delay the progress, and renal replacement therapy as ESRD ensues.

1. Hypertension is treated with ACEIs or ARBs. For most patients, the first drug of choice is an ACEI, which is then titrated upward into the moderate- to high-dose range as tolerated. ARBs are the preferred choice in those with type 2 diabetes with CRF and proteinuria. β-Blockers and calcium channel blockers may also be useful.

2. Diabetes. The goal of treatment is to achieve less than 7% glycosylated hemoglobin. Euglycemia is associated with reversal of the typical lesions seen in diabetic nephropathy and a reduction in albuminuria. Dietary protein intake of 0.6 g/kg per day reduced the rate of progression of renal disease in patients with diabetes but should not be at the expense of nutrition in anorexic patients.

3. Anemia responds to treatment with erythropoietin in all stages of chronic kidney disease. Hemoglobin (Hb), rather than hematocrit, is the preferred method for assessing anemia. Anemia is defined for males as a hemoglobin level less than 13.0 g/dL, and for females as a hemoglobin level less than 12.0 g/dL regardless of age.

4. Renal Replacement Therapy is considered when GFR approaches 30 mL/min/1.73 m^2.

TABLE 14-9 Treatment of Uremic Bleeding				
Drug	**Dose**	**Onset of Effect**	**Peak Effect**	**Duration of Effect**
Cryoprecipitate	10 units IV over 30 min	<1 hr	4–12 hr	12–18 hr
DDAVP (desmopressin)	0.3 μg/kg IV or SC	<1 hr	2–4 hr	6–8 hr
Conjugated estrogen	0.6 mg/kg/day IV for 5 days	6 hr	5–7 days	14 days

SC, subcutaneously.
Adapted from Tolkoff-Rubin NE, Pascual M: Chronic renal failure. Sci Am Med 1998;1–12.

a. Hemodialysis is usually instituted by the time GFR is 15 mL/min/1.73 m^2. Objectives include adequate dialysis, adequate nutrition, maintenance of vascular access, correction of hormonal deficiencies, minimization of hospitalizations, and prolongation of life while enhancing its quality (**Table 14-10**).

  1.) *Complications Associated with Hemodialysis*
   a.) **Hypotension** during dialysis, hypersensitivity reactions to plyacrylonitrile in dialysis membranes (most common in patients on ACEIs).
   b.) **Fluid, Vitamin, and Electrolyte Balance.** Patients on hemodialysis have decreased total body potassium and tolerance of hyperkalemia. Water-soluble vitamins are removed by hemodialysis and should be replaced. Between treatments, a weight gain of 3% to 4% of body mass in 2 days is appropriate.
   c.) **Cardiovascular Disease** caused by accelerated atherosclerosis and impaired oxygen delivery during uremia accounts for nearly 50% of all deaths in patients on hemodialysis, Fluid retention is the most likely cause of systemic hypertension in most patients who present for hemodialysis. Essential hypertension may require treatment with antihypertensive drugs in addition to hemodialysis. Pericarditis may result from inadequate hemodialysis.

TABLE 14-10	Findings Suggestive of Inadequate Hemodialysis
Clinical	
Anorexia, nausea, vomiting	
Peripheral neuropathy	
Poor nutritional status	
Depressed sensorium	
Pericarditis	
Ascites	
Minimal weight gain or weight loss between treatments	
Fluid retention and systemic hypertension	
Chemical	
Decrease in blood urea nitrogen concentration during hemodialysis <65%	
Albumin concentration <4 g/dL	
Predialysis blood urea concentration <50 mg/dL (a sign of malnutrition)	
Predialysis serum creatinine concentration <5 mg/dL (a sign of malnutrition)	
Persistent anemia (hematocrit <30%) despite erythropoietin therapy	

Adapted from Ifudu O: Care of patients undergoing hemodialysis. N Engl J Med 1998;339:1054–1062.

      d.) **Bleeding** caused by to altered platelet function is partially
         correctable by hemodialysis.

      e.) **Infection.** There is increased susceptibility to infection caused
         by impaired phagocytosis and chemotaxis. All patients on
         hemodialysis are vaccinated against pneumococcus and, if
         appropriate, hepatitis B. Dose adjustments of drugs used to
         treat acquired immunodeficiency syndrome (AIDS) are not
         required for hemodialysis and isolation of patients with AIDS
         or use of a dedicated hemodialysis machine is not necessary.

    2.) *Perioperative Hemodialysis.* Patients should undergo adequate
      hemodialysis before elective surgery to minimize the likelihood
      of uremic bleeding, pulmonary edema, and impaired arterial
      oxygenation. Meperidine is avoided for postoperative analgesia
      because its metabolites may accumulate in patients with renal
      failure and result in seizures.

  b. Peritoneal Dialysis is simple to perform and may be useful in patients
  with severe vascular disease or congestive heart failure (more gradual
  fluid shifts, no need for vascular access). Peritonitis is the most common
  serious complication.

  c. Drug Clearance in Patients Undergoing Dialysis may dictate adjustment
  of dosing intervals and supplemental dosing if drugs are cleared by dialysis.

IV. ANESTHETIC MANAGEMENT OF PATIENTS WITH CHRONIC RENAL DISEASE/INSUFFICIENCY (Table 14-11)

A. Preoperative Evaluation includes evaluation of fluid status, glucose
management, and degree of anemia. Digoxin toxicity should be a concern in
patients being treated with digoxin. Antihypertensive drug therapy is
continued. Patients on hemodialysis should undergo dialysis during the
24 hours preceding elective surgery. Preoperative DDAVP may be considered.

B. Intraoperative.

  1. Induction. Hypotension on induction is common, particularly in
  patients on ACEIs. Decreased protein binding of drugs may result in the
  availability of more unbound drugs at receptor sites (see **Table 14-11**).
  Potassium release following administration of succinylcholine is not
  exaggerated in patients with chronic renal failure, but caution is indicated if
  preoperative serum potassium concentration is in the high-normal range.

  2. Maintenance of Anesthesia. There is no evidence that patients with
  co-existing renal disease are at increased risk of renal dysfunction with
  sevoflurane. Selection of nondepolarizing muscle relaxants should consider
  the clearance mechanisms of these drugs. Clearance of vecuronium and
  rocuronium are slowed, whereas clearance of mivacurium, atracurium, and
  cisatracurium from plasma is independent of renal function. Lactated
  Ringer's solution (potassium 4 mEq/L) or other potassium-containing fluids
  should not be administered to anuric patients. In anuric (dialysis) patients,
  noninvasive operations require replacement of only insensible water losses
  with 5% glucose in water (5–10 mL/kg IV). Measuring the central venous

TABLE 14-11	Drugs Used in Anesthesia Practice That Significantly Depend on Renal Elimination	
Class of Drug	Action Terminated by Renal Excretion	Action Partially Terminated by Renal Excretion
Induction agents	—	Barbiturates
Muscle relaxants	Gallamine, metocurine	Pancuronium, vecuronium
Cholinesterase inhibitors	—	Neostigmine, edrophonium
Cardiovascular drugs	Digoxin, inotropes	Atropine, glycopyrrolate, milrinone, hydralazine
Antimicrobials	Aminoglycosides, vancomycin, cephalosporin, penicillin	Sulfonamides

Adapted from Malhotra V, Sudheendra V, Diwan S: Anesthesia and the renal and genitourinary systems. In Miller RD, Fleischer LA, Johns RA, et al (eds): Miller's Anesthesia, 6th ed. Philadelphia, Elsevier Churchill Livingstone, 2005.

pressure may be useful for guiding fluid replacement. Arterial cannulation should be avoided if possible, to avoid injury to vessels that may be required for future dialysis access. Regional anesthesia is useful for placing the vascular shunts necessary for chronic hemodialysis.

3. Postoperative Management includes attention to inadequate reversal of muscle relaxant in anephric patients who show signs of skeletal muscle weakness during the postoperative period. Other considerations are sensitivity to opioids, arrhythmias related to hyperkalemia, and oxygen supplementation in anemic patients.

V. RENAL TRANSPLANTATION

A. Management of Anesthesia

1. General Anesthesia. Renal function after kidney transplantation is not influenced by the volatile anesthetic administered. Goals are maintenance of cardiac output and tissue oxygen delivery to promote renal perfusion. A high normal systemic blood pressure is desirable to maintain adequate urine flow. Atracurium, cisatracurium, and mivacurium are reasonable muscle relaxants, because of lack of dependence on renal clearance, although the transplanted kidney will clear muscle relaxants similarly to a normal kidney. Central venous pressure monitoring is useful to guide fluid infusions. Diuretics facilitate urine formation by the newly transplanted kidney. With release of the vascular clamps, potassium from the preservative solution and acid metabolites has been reported to lead to cardiac arrest. Hypotension results from the additional 300 mL capacity of the new kidney vascular bed. Treatment is fluid administration.

2. Regional Anesthesia. Blockade of the peripheral sympathetic nervous system can complicate control of systemic blood pressure.

3. Postoperative Complications

a. Acute Rejection (affecting the kidney vasculature) can be so rapid that inadequate circulation is evident almost immediately after the blood supply to the kidney is established. The only treatment is removal of the transplanted kidney; disseminated intravascular coagulation occurs. Postoperative graft hematomas can cause vascular or ureteral obstruction.

b. Delayed Graft Rejection. Signs include fever, local tenderness, and deterioration of urine output. Treatment is with high doses of corticosteroids and antilymphocyte globulin.

c. Acute Tubular Necrosis in the transplanted kidney secondary to prolonged ischemia usually responds to hemodialysis.

d. Cyclosporine Toxicity may also cause ARF. Ultrasonography and needle biopsy are performed to differentiate between the possible causes of kidney malfunction.

e. Opportunistic Infections owing to long-term immunosuppression are common after renal transplantation.

f. Cancer rates are 30 to 100 times higher in transplant recipients than in the general population.

B. Anesthetic Considerations in Renal Transplant Recipients Presenting for Surgery. Renal transplant recipients are often elderly and have co-existing cardiovascular disease and diabetes mellitus. The side effects of immunosuppressant drugs (systemic hypertension, lowered seizure thresholds, anemia, thrombocytopenia) must be considered. GFR and renal blood flow are likely to be lower than those of healthy individuals, and the activity of drugs excreted by the kidneys may be prolonged. Drugs that are potentially nephrotoxic or dependent on renal clearance are avoided. Diuretics are administered only with careful evaluation of the patient's intravascular fluid volume status.

VI. PRIMARY DISEASES OF THE KIDNEYS

A. Glomerulonephritis. Acute glomerulonephritis is usually caused by deposition of antigen-antibody complexes in the glomeruli. The source of antigens may be exogenous (poststreptococcal infection) or endogenous (collagen diseases). Clinical manifestations of glomerular diseases include hematuria, proteinuria, hypertension, edema, and increased plasma creatinine concentrations and the presence of red blood cell casts in the urine.

B. Nephrotic Syndrome is defined by daily urinary protein excretion exceeding 3.5 g associated with sodium retention, hyperlipoproteinemia, and thromboembolic and infectious complications. Diabetic nephropathy is the most common cause of nephrotic proteinuria.

1. Signs and Symptoms (Table 14-12)
2. Complications of Nephrotic Syndrome (Table 14-13)
3. Treatment of Nephrotic Syndrome (Table 14-14)

C. Goodpasture Syndrome is a combination of pulmonary hemorrhage and glomerulonephritis, occurring most often in young males. Prognosis is poor, with no known effective therapy to prevent progression to renal failure, usually within 1 year of the diagnosis.

D. Interstitial Nephritis can occur as a result of allergic reaction to drugs, including sulfonamides, allopurinol, phenytoin, and diuretics. Other less

TABLE 14-12	Features of Nephrotic Syndrome
Hypertension	
Proteinuria, hematuria	
Sodium retention	
Edema	
Hypovolemia	
Thromboembolism	
Hyperlipidemia	
Infectious complications	

TABLE 14-13	Complications of Nephrotic Syndrome
Thromboembolic	Renal vein thrombosis Pulmonary embolism Deep vein thrombosis
Infectious	Pneumococcal peritonitis
Decreased plasma protein binding	Decreased levels of vitamins and hormones
Edema	Generalized; should be treated slowly with loop diuretics and thiazides

TABLE 14-14	Treatment of Nephrotic Syndrome
Antihypertensive therapy*	
ACEI or ARB (antiproteinuric)†	
Dietary counseling‡	
Dietary restriction of sodium	
Diuretic therapy	
Albumin infusions as required	
Anticoagulant therapy	
Statin therapy	
Pneumococcal vaccine	

* A mean systemic blood pressure below 90 mm Hg reduces proteinuria independent of class of antihypertensive.
† ACEIs and ARBs have antiproteinuric effects separate from their blood pressure–lowering effects.
‡ Some authorities advise dietary protein restriction to reduce proteinuria, but the safety of this therapy has not been established, particularly in patients with heavy proteinuria.

common causes include autoimmune diseases (lupus erythematosus) and infiltrative diseases (sarcoidosis). Patients exhibit decreased urine-concentrating ability, proteinuria, and systemic hypertension.

E. Hereditary Nephritis (Alport's syndrome) is often accompanied by hearing loss and ocular abnormalities. Drug therapy has not proven successful.

F. Polycystic Renal Disease is an autosomal dominant disease that typically progresses slowly until renal failure occurs during middle age. Mild systemic hypertension and proteinuria are common. Hemodialysis or renal transplantation is eventually necessary in most of these patients.

G. Fanconi Syndrome results from inherited or acquired disturbances of proximal renal tubular function, causing hyperaminoaciduria, glycosuria, and hyperphosphaturia. Symptoms include polyuria, polydipsia, metabolic acidosis caused by loss of bicarbonate ions, and skeletal muscle weakness related to hypokalemia. Dwarfism and osteomalacia, reflecting loss of phosphate, is prominent in these patients.

H. Nephrolithiasis (Table 14-15). Renal stones passing down the ureter can produce intense flank pain, often radiating to the groin, associated with nausea and vomiting and mimicking an acute surgical abdomen. Hematuria is common and ureteral obstruction may cause signs and symptoms of renal failure.

1. Types of Stones

  a. Calcium Oxalate Stones. Causes of hypercalcemia (hyperparathyroidism, sarcoidosis, cancer) must be considered in these patients.

  b. Magnesium Ammonium Phosphate Stones may result from urinary tract infection with urea-splitting organisms that produce ammonia.

  c. Uric Acid Stones occur in persons with persistently acidic urine (pH <6.0) that decreases the solubility of uric acid. Approximately 50% of patients with uric acid stones have gout.

TABLE 14-15	Composition and Characteristics of Renal Stones		
Type of Stone	**Incidence (%)**	**Radiographic Appearance**	**Etiology**
Calcium oxalate	65	Opaque	Primary hyperparathyroidism, idiopathic hypercalciuria, hyperoxaluria, hyperuricosuria
Magnesium ammonium phosphate (struvite)	20	Opaque	Alkaline urine (usually caused by chronic bacterial infection)
Calcium phosphate	7.5	Opaque	Renal tubular acidosis
Uric acid	5	Lucent	Acid urine, gout, hyperuricosuria
Cystine	1.5	Opaque	Cystinuria

2. Treatment depends on identifying the composition of the stone and correcting the predisposing factors, such as hyperparathyroidism, urinary tract infection, or gout. Extracorporeal shock wave lithotripsy is a noninvasive treatment.

I. Renal Hypertension. Renal disease is the most common cause of secondary systemic hypertension. The sudden onset of a marked increase in systemic blood pressure or the presence of hypertension before the age of 30 years should arouse suspicion of renovascular disease. A bruit may be audible on auscultation of the abdomen over the kidneys. Systemic hypertension caused by renovascular disease does not respond well to treatment with antihypertensive drugs. Treatment of renovascular hypertension is with renal artery endarterectomy or nephrectomy.

J. Uric Acid Nephropathy occurs when uric acid crystals are precipitated in the renal collecting tubules or ureters, producing acute oliguric renal failure. The condition is particularly likely to occur in patients with myeloproliferative disorders being treated with chemotherapeutic drugs.

K. Hepatorenal Syndrome is acute oliguria manifesting in patients with decompensated cirrhosis of the liver. Associate signs include deep jaundice, ascites, hypoalbuminemia, and hypoprothrombinemia. Treatment is directed at intravascular fluid volume replacement. In some patients, a circulating toxin may be responsible for extreme renal vasoconstriction and ARF. Nevertheless, hemodialysis has not been reliable for eliminating suspected hepatic toxins.

L. Benign Prostatic Hyperplasia (BPH) is a nonmalignant enlargement of the prostate. Transurethral resection of the prostate (TURP) and open prostatectomy have been the traditional treatments for men with symptomatic BPH. Medical therapy consists of finasteride (inhibits 5α-reductase) to reduce prostate size and α-adrenergic antagonists (terazosin, doxazosin, tamsulosin) to decrease prostatic smooth muscle tone, improving urinary flow.

1. TURP Syndrome (Table 14-16) is characterized by intravascular fluid volume shifts and plasma solute effects caused by absorption of irrigation solution. Hypo-osmolality is the principal factor contributing to the neurologic and hypovolemic changes associated with TURP syndrome.

a. Intravascular Fluid Volume Expansion. Rapid intravascular fluid volume expansion caused by systemic absorption of irrigating fluids (absorption rates may reach 200 mL/min) can cause systemic hypertension and reflex bradycardia. Patients with poor left ventricular function may develop pulmonary edema. The most widely used indicator of intravascular fluid volume gain is hyponatremia.

b. Intravascular Fluid Volume Loss. Hyponatremia in association with systemic hypertension may result in water flux along osmotic and hydrostatic pressure gradients out of the intravascular space and into the lungs, with resultant pulmonary edema and hypovolemic shock.

c. Hyponatremia caused by intravascular absorption of sodium-free irrigating fluids may cause confusion, agitation, visual disturbances, pulmonary edema, cardiovascular collapse, and seizures.

d. Hypo-osmolality is the crucial physiologic derangement leading to central nervous system dysfunction during TURP. Cerebral edema caused by acute hypo-osmolality can result in increased intracranial

TABLE 14-16	Signs and Symptoms of Transurethral Resection of the Prostate Syndrome	
System	**Signs and Symptoms**	**Cause**
Cardiovascular	Hypertension, reflex bradycardia, pulmonary edema, cardiovascular collapse, hypotension, ECG changes (wide QRS, elevated ST segments, ventricular arrhythmias)	Rapid fluid absorption (reflex bradycardia may be secondary to hypertension or increased ICP); third spacing secondary to hyponatremia and hypo-osmolality; cardiovascular collapse, hyponatremia
Respiratory	Tachypnea, oxygen desaturation, Cheyne-Stokes breathing	Pulmonary edema
Neurologic	Nausea, restlessness, visual disturbances, confusion, somnolence, seizures, coma, death	Hyponatremia and hypo-osmolality causing cerebral edema and increased ICP, hyperglycinemia (inhibitory neurotransmitter, potentiates NMDA receptor activity), hyperammonemia
Hematologic	Disseminated intravascular hemolysis	Hyponatremia and hypo-osmolality
Renal	Renal failure	Hypotension, hyperoxaluria (metabolite of glycine)
Metabolic	Acidosis	Deamination of glycine to glyoxylic acid and ammonia

ECG, electrocardiogram; ICP, intracranial pressure; NMDA, N-methyl-D-aminotransferase.

pressure with resultant bradycardia and hypertension. Diuretics may accentuate hyponatremia and hypo-osmolality. No intervention is needed if the serum osmolality is near normal. When treatment is undertaken, serum osmolality should be monitored and corrected aggressively with hypertonic saline only until symptoms resolve substantially; then correction should be continued slowly (serum sodium concentrations increase 1.5 mEq/L per hour).

e. Metabolic Acidosis (mild) can occur because of absorption of irrigating solution.

f. Hyperammonemia is the result of systemic absorption of glycine and its oxidative deamination to glyoxylic acid and ammonia.

g. Hyperglycinemia. Glycine is the most likely cause of visual disturbances, including transient blindness, during TURP syndrome, reflecting the role of glycine as an inhibitory neurotransmitter in the retina. Vision returns to normal within 24 hours as serum glycine concentrations approach normal. Reassurance is the best treatment. Glycine may also exert toxic effects on the kidneys.

CHAPTER 15

Fluid, Electrolyte, and Acid-Base Disorders

Alterations of water and electrolyte content and distribution, as well as acid-base disturbances can produce multiple organ system dysfunctions during the perioperative period. Impairment of central nervous system, cardiac, and neuromuscular function is especially likely in the presence of water, electrolyte (sodium, potassium, calcium, magnesium), and acid-base disturbances. In addition, numerous perioperative events can initiate or aggravate fluid, electrolyte, and acid-base disturbances (**Table 15-1**).

I. ABNORMALITIES OF WATER AND ELECTROLYTE HOMEOSTASIS

Total body water content is categorized as intracellular fluid (ICF) and extracellular fluid (ECF), according to the location of the water relative to cell membranes (**Fig. 15-1**). The distribution and concentration of electrolytes differ greatly among fluid compartments. The electrophysiology of excitable cells is dependent on the intracellular and extracellular concentrations of sodium, potassium, and calcium. Unequal distribution of ions (more potassium inside and more sodium outside) produces electrochemical differences across the cell membrane. The normal kidney excretes urine with an osmolality that varies depending on serum osmolality. Regulators of water balance are osmolality sensors in the anterior hypothalamus that stimulate thirst and vasopressin (antidiuretic hormone). Vasopressin is released in response to an increase in serum osmolality and acts on the collecting ducts of the kidney, causing water retention. Vasopressin release plays an important role in the correction of disorders of fluid balance (**Table 15-2**).

TABLE 15-1	Etiology of Water, Electrolyte, and Acid-Base Disturbances during the Perioperative Period
Disease States	
Endocrinopathies	
Nephropathies	
Gastroenteropathies	
Drug Therapy	
Diuretics	
Corticosteroids	
Nasogastric suction	
Surgery	
Transurethral resection of the prostate	
Translocation of body water due to tissue trauma	
Resection of portions of the gastrointestinal tract	
Management of Anesthesia	
Intravenous fluid administration	
Alveolar ventilation	
Hypothermia	

A. Disorders of Sodium

1. Hyponatremia exists when water retention or water intake exceeds the ability of the kidneys to excrete dilute urine. Serum sodium declines to less than 136 mEq/L.

a. Signs and Symptoms of Hyponatremia depend on the rate at which hyponatremia develops. Symptoms are rare with serum sodium concentration higher than 125 mEq/L (**Table 15-3**).

b. Diagnosis. Hyponatremia usually co-exists with hypo-osmolality except in two circumstances. Glucose, mannitol, and glycine cause water to move from the intracellular space into the ECF with a resultant decrease in the serum sodium concentration without a change in total body sodium or total body water. In cases of severe hyperlipidemia or a paraproteinemic disorder, the measured sodium concentration will be falsely low (pseudohyponatremia). Once these two situations have been excluded, the approach to the diagnosis of hyponatremia is to first evaluate ECF volume from the clinical presentation (**Fig. 15-2**).

c. Treatment of Hyponatremia involves withholding free water and encouraging free water excretion with a loop diuretic. Administration of saline is only necessary if significant symptoms are present. Chronic symptomatic hyponatremia should be corrected slowly to avoid the risk of osmotic demyelination. Guidelines for correction of chronic symptomatic hyponatremia call for an initial correction in the serum sodium of approximately 10 mEq/L and thereafter to correct 1 to 1.5 mEq/L per hour (daily maximum increase of 12 mEq/L).

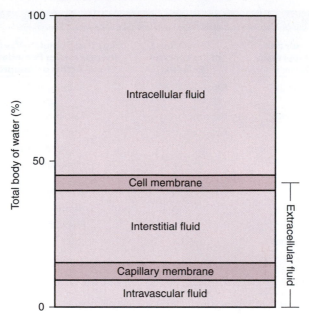

Figure 15-1 • Total body water (constituting approximately 60% of the total body weight in kilograms) is designated intracellular or extracellular fluid, depending on the location of water relative to cell membranes. Water in extracellular compartments is further subdivided into interstitial and intravascular fluid, depending on its location relative to cell membranes. Approximately 55% of total body water is intracellular, 37% is interstitial, and the remaining 8% is intravascular.

   d. Management of Anesthesia. Hyponatremia should be corrected prior to surgery whenever possible. If the surgery is urgent, then appropriate corrective treatment should continue throughout the surgery and into the postoperative period.

   1.) *Vasopressors and/or Inotropes* may be required to treat the hypotension and should be made available prior to the start of induction. Hypervolemic hyponatremic patients, particularly those with heart failure, may benefit from invasive hemodynamic monitoring.

   2.) *TURP Syndrome.* Irrigating fluid used during TURP (glycine, sorbitol, or mannitol) may be rapidly absorbed, with resulting volume overload, hyponatremia, and hypo-osmolality. This is more likely in prolonged surgery (>1 hour), if the fluid is suspended more than 40 cm above the operative field, or if the pressure in the bladder is more than 15 cm H_2O. TURP syndrome presents with cardiovascular and neurologic signs and symptoms. Treatment consists of terminating the surgical procedure, diuretics for relief of cardiovascular symptoms, and hypertonic saline administration if severe neurologic symptoms are present or the serum sodium concentration is less than 120 mEq/L.

TABLE 15-2 Factors and Drugs Affecting Vasopressin Secretion

Stimulation of Vasopressin Release	Inhibition of Vasopressin Release	Drugs That Stimulate Vasopressin Release and/or Potentiate the Renal Action of Vasopressin
Contracted ECF volume	Expanded ECF volume	Amitriptyline
Hypernatremia	Hyponatremia	Barbiturates
Hypotension	Hypertension	Carbamazepine
Nausea and vomiting		Chlorpropamide
Congestive heart failure		Clofibrate
Cirrhosis		Morphine
Hypothyroidism		Nicotine
Angiotensin II		Phenothiazines
Catecholamines		SSRIs
Histamine		
Bradykinin		

ECF, extracellular fluid; SSRIs, selective serotonin reuptake inhibitors.

2. Hypernatremia is defined as a serum sodium greater than 145 mEq/L. It is invariably accompanied by hyperosmolality and always causes cellular dehydration and shrinkage.

 a. Signs and Symptoms of Hypernatremia (Table 15-4)
 b. Diagnosis (Fig. 15-3)
 c. Treatment. The patient with euvolemic hypernatremia requires water replacement either orally or with 5% dextrose intravenously.

TABLE 15-3 Symptoms and Signs of Hyponatremia

Symptoms	Signs
Anorexia	Abnormal sensorium
Nausea	Disorientation/agitation
Lethargy	Cheyne-Stokes breathing
Apathy	Hypothermia
Muscle cramps	Pathologic reflexes
	Pseudobulbar palsy
	Seizures
	Coma
	Death

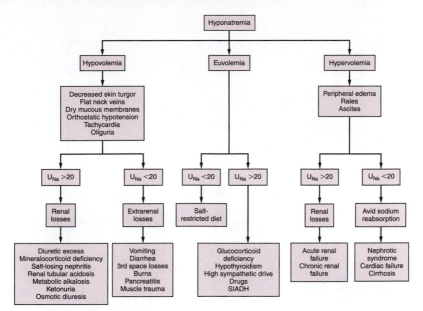

Figure 15-2 • Diagnostic algorithm for hyponatremia. Urinary sodium concentration (U_{Na}) (mEq/L) in a spot urine sample. SIADH, syndrome of inappropriate secretion of antidiuretic hormone. (Adapted from Schrier RW: Manual of Nephrology, 6th ed. Philadelphia, Lippincott Williams & Wilkins, 2006.)

Acute hypernatremia should be corrected over several hours. However, to avoid cerebral edema, chronic hypernatremia should be corrected more slowly, over 2 to 3 days. In patients with hypervolemic hypernatremia, treatment is diuresis.

d. Management of Anesthesia. Surgery should be delayed until the hypernatremia has been corrected whenever possible. Hypovolemia will

TABLE 15-4	Symptoms and Signs of Hypernatremia	
Symptoms	**Signs**
Polyuria	Muscle twitching
Polydipsia	Hyperreflexia
Orthostasis	Tremor
Restlessness	Ataxia
Irritability	Muscle spasticity
Lethargy	Focal and generalized seizures
	Death

261

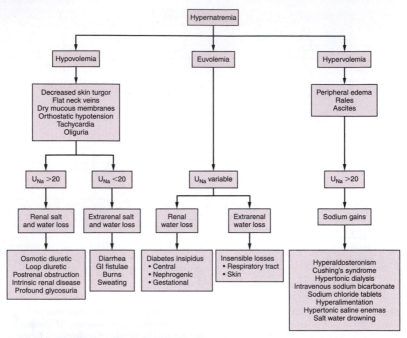

Figure 15-3 • Diagnostic algorithm for hypernatremia. GI, gastrointestinal; UNa, urinary sodium concentration (mEq/L) in a spot urine sample. (Adapted from Schrier RW: Manual of Nephrology, 6th ed. Philadelphia, Lippincott Williams & Wilkins, 2006.)

be exacerbated by induction and maintenance of anesthesia, and prompt correction of hypotension with fluids, vasopressors, and/or inotropes may be required.

B. Disorders of Potassium

1. Hypokalemia is defined as serum potassium concentration of less than 3.5 mEq/L (**Table 15-5**).

a. Signs and Symptoms of hypokalemia are generally restricted to the cardiac and neuromuscular systems and include dysrhythmias, muscle weakness, cramps, paralysis, and ileus.

b. Diagnosis is made by testing the serum potassium concentration. A spot urinary potassium will guide the diagnosis toward either renal (urinary potassium >20 mEq/L) or extrarenal causes (urinary) potassium of <20 mEq/L).

c. Treatment is dependent on the degree of potassium depletion and the underlying cause. If hypokalemia is profound or associated with life-threatening signs, potassium must be administered intravenously, and the amount depends on whether there are associated decreases in total body potassium. Typically, 20 mEq of potassium can be administered over 30 to 45 minutes and repeated as needed. Such rapid repletion requires electrocardiographic monitoring.

TABLE 15-5	Causes of Hypokalemia

Hypokalemia Due to Increased Renal Potassium Loss

Thiazide diuretics

Loop diuretics

Mineralocorticoids

High-dose glucocorticoids

High-dose antibiotics (penicillin, nafcillin, ampicillin)

Drugs associated with (aminoglycosides) magnesium depletion

Surgical trauma

Hyperglycemia

Hyperaldosteronism

Hypokalemia Due to Excessive Gastrointestinal Loss of Potassium

Vomiting and diarrhea

Zollinger-Ellison syndrome

Jejunoileal bypass

Malabsorption

Chemotherapy

Nasogastric suction

Hypokalemia Due to Transcellular Potassium Shift

β-Adrenergic agonists

Tocolytic drugs (ritodrine)

Insulin

Respiratory or metabolic alkalosis

Familial periodic paralysis

Hypercalcemia

Hypomagnesemia

Adapted from Gennari JF: Hypokalemia. N Engl J Med 1998;339: 451–458.

d. Management of Anesthesia. The decision to treat hypokalemia prior to surgery depends on the chronicity and severity of the defect. The risk of perioperative dysrhythmias in these patients remains unclear. It may be prudent to correct significant hypokalemia in patients with other risk factors for dysrhythmias such as those with congestive heart failure or on digoxin therapy. It is also important to avoid further decreases in serum potassium concentration (e.g., as a result of administration of insulin, glucose, β-adrenergic agonists, bicarbonate, and diuretics; hyperventilation; and respiratory alkalosis).

2. Hyperkalemia is defined as a serum potassium concentration greater than 5.5 mEq/L (**Table 15-6**).

TABLE 15-6	Causes of Hyperkalemia
Increased Total Body Potassium Content	
Acute oliguric renal failure	
Chronic renal disease	
Hypoaldosteronism	
Drugs that impair potassium excretion	
Triamterene	
Spironolactone	
Nonsteroidal anti-inflammatory drugs	
Drugs that inhibit the renin-angiotensin-aldosterone system	
Altered Transcellular Potassium Shift	
Succinylcholine	
Respiratory or metabolic acidosis	
Lysis of cells because of chemotherapy	
Iatrogenic bolus	
Pseudohyperkalemia	
Hemolysis of blood specimen	
Thrombocytosis/leukocytosis	

a. Signs and Symptoms of hyperkalemia are dependent on the acuity of the increase. Chronic hyperkalemia is often asymptomatic, and dialysis-dependent patients can withstand considerable variations in serum potassium concentration. Acute or significant increases in potassium manifest as cardiac and neuromuscular changes and include weakness, paralysis, nausea, vomiting, and bradycardia/asystole.

b. Diagnosis. The first step is to rule out a spuriously high potassium level secondary to hemolysis of the specimen, thrombocytosis, and leukocytosis. If hyperkalemia is associated with increased total body potassium stores, then decreased renal excretion or increased extrarenal production of potassium is likely. Urinary potassium excretion rate can aid in the differential diagnosis.

c. Treatment. Immediate treatment of hyperkalemia is required if life-threatening dysrhythmias or electrocardiograph (ECG) changes are present. This treatment consists of intravenous calcium chloride or calcium gluconate to stabilize cellular membranes, insulin with or without glucose to help redistribute potassium into cells, and sodium bicarbonate and hyperventilation to promote alkalosis and movement of potassium intracellularly. Loop diuretics and sodium polystyrene sulfonate (Kayexalate) given either orally or by enema can promote potassium elimination. Dialysis may be required to remove potassium in patients with poor renal function.

d. Management of Anesthesia. Serum potassium concentration should usually be below 5.5 mEq/L for elective surgery. Because succinylcholine increases serum potassium by approximately 0.5 mEq/L, it is best avoided. Respiratory and metabolic acidosis must be avoided because either will exacerbate the hyperkalemia and its effects. Intravenous fluids should be potassium free (avoid Ringer's lactated solution and Normosol).

C. Disorders of Calcium

1. Hypocalcemia is defined as a reduction in serum ionized calcium concentration. Binding of calcium to albumin is pH dependent, and acid-base disturbances can change the fraction and therefore the concentration of ionized calcium without changing total body calcium. Alkalosis reduces the ionized calcium concentration, so ionized calcium may be significantly reduced after bicarbonate administration or with hyperventilation.

a. Signs and Symptoms depend on the rapidity and the degree of reduction in ionized calcium. They include paresthesias, irritability, seizures, hypotension, and myocardial depression. Laryngospasm can be life threatening.

b. Diagnosis. The most common causes of hypocalcemia are caused by a decrease in parathyroid hormone secretion, end-organ resistance to parathyroid hormone, or disorders of vitamin D metabolism. These are usually seen clinically as complications of thyroid or parathyroid surgery, magnesium deficiency, and renal failure.

c. Treatment acutely is intravenous calcium and correction of metabolic or respiratory alkalosis. Treatment of hypocalcemia in the presence of hypomagnesemia is ineffective unless magnesium is also replenished. Less acute and asymptomatic hypocalcemia may be treated with oral calcium supplementation and vitamin D.

d. Management of Anesthesia. Symptomatic hypocalcemia must be treated prior to surgery. Alkalosis caused by hyperventilation or administration of bicarbonate should be avoided. Ionized calcium levels may decrease with massive transfusion of blood containing citrate or when citrate metabolism is impaired by hypothermia, liver disease, or renal failure. Sudden decreases in ionized calcium levels may occur postoperatively after thyroidectomy or parathyroidectomy and may cause laryngospasm.

2. Hypercalcemia results from increased calcium absorption from the gastrointestinal tract (milk alkali syndrome, vitamin D intoxication, granulomatous diseases such as sarcoidosis), decreased renal calcium excretion in renal insufficiency, and increased bone resorption of calcium (primary or secondary hyperparathyroidism, malignancy, hyperthyroidism, and immobilization).

a. Signs and Symptoms include confusion, hypotonia, depressed deep tendon reflexes, lethargy, abdominal pain, and nausea and vomiting, especially if the increase in serum calcium is relatively acute. Chronic hypercalcemia is often associated with polyuria, hypercalcuria, and nephrolithiasis.

b. Diagnosis includes a workup for hyperparathyroidism or cancer.

c. Treatment is correction of fluid deficits, and loop diuretics to enhance urinary excretion of sodium and calcium. Calcitonin, bisphosphonates, or mithramycin may be required in disorders associated with osteoclastic bone resorption. Dialysis may be required for life-threatening hypercalcemia. Surgical removal of the parathyroid glands may be necessary to treat primary or secondary hyperparathyroidism.

d. Management of Anesthesia includes hydration prior to induction and loop diuretics to increase urinary calcium excretion. (Avoid thiazide diuretics, which increase tubular reabsorption of calcium.)

D. Disorders of Magnesium

1. Hypomagnesemia occurs in up to 10% of hospitalized patients, particularly intensive care patients receiving parenteral nutritional or dialysis.

a. Signs and Symptoms are similar to those of hypocalcemia, including dysrhythmias, weakness, muscle twitching, tetany, apathy, and seizures.

b. Diagnosis. Hypomagnesemia caused by reduced gastrointestinal uptake or renal wasting of magnesium can be differentiated by measuring the urinary magnesium excretion rate.

c. Treatment. If cardiac dysrhythmias or seizures are present, magnesium is administered intravenously as a bolus (2 g of magnesium sulfate equals 8 mEq of magnesium), and the dose is repeated until symptoms abate.

d. Management of Anesthesia. Ventricular dysrhythmias should be anticipated and treated as necessary. Muscle relaxation should be guided by the use of a peripheral nerve stimulator because hypomagnesemia can be associated with both muscle weakness and muscle excitation.

2. Hypermagnesemia (serum magnesium concentration >2.5 mEq/L) is much less common than hypomagnesia and is usually iatrogenic—that is, as a complication of magnesium sulfate therapy for preeclampsia/eclampsia.

a. Signs and Symptoms of hypermagnesemia begin to occur at serum levels of 4 to 5 mEq/L and include lethargy, nausea and vomiting, and facial flushing. At levels above 6 mEq/L, a loss of deep tendon reflexes and hypotension are seen. Paralysis, apnea, and/or cardiac arrest are likely if the magnesium level exceeds 10 mEq/L.

b. Diagnosis of Hypermagnesemia involves determining renal function (creatinine clearance) and detecting any source of excess magnesium intake. Less common causes of hypermagnesemia include hypothyroidism, hyperparathyroidism, Addison's disease, and lithium therapy.

c. Treatment of acute clinical signs is intravenous calcium administration. Dialysis may be required.

d. Management of Anesthesia includes avoidance of acidosis and dehydration, maintenance of urine output, and recognition that response to muscle relaxants may be prolonged.

E. Acid-Base Disorders

Acid-base balance is normally regulated within the range of 7.35 to 7.45, as measured by arterial pH, to ensure an optimal pH for cellular enzyme function. Values of arterial blood pH less than 7.35 are termed acidosis or acidemia, and values greater than 7.45 are termed alkalosis or alkalemia. The major buffer system participating in regulation of body pH is the bicarbonate/carbon dioxide system. Although the respiratory system (via CO_2 regulation) can provide some defense against acid-base disorders, the kidneys have a greater ability (via bicarbonate regulation) to normalize pH.

1. The Henderson-Hasselbalch Equation describes the relationship between the pulmonary and renal regulation of pH by this buffer system:

$$pH = 6.1 + \log (\text{serum bicarbonate concentration}/0.03 \times PaCO_2).$$

Maintenance of a normal bicarbonate concentration relative to carbon dioxide tension results in an optimal ratio of approximately 20:1.

2. Identification of an Acid-Base Disturbance follows a series of steps (Figs. 15-4, 15-5, and 15-6):

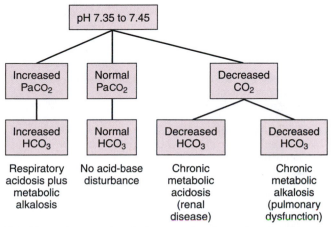

Figure 15-4 • Diagnostic approach to the interpretation of normal arterial pH based on $PaCO_2$ and bicarbonate concentration.

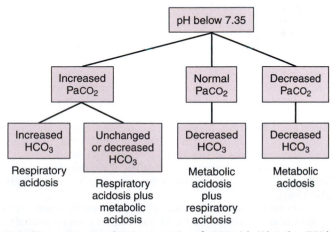

Figure 15-5 • Diagnostic approach to interpretation of an arterial pH less than 7.35 based on $PaCO_2$ and bicarbonate concentration.

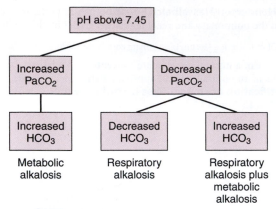

Figure 15-6 • Diagnostic approach to interpretation of an arterial pH greater than 7.45 based on PaCO₂ and bicarbonate concentration.

a. Identify whether the pH is increased or decreased. An increase identifies an alkalosis and a decrease identifies an acidosis.

b. Identify the change in $PaCO_2$ and bicarbonate from their normal levels of 40 mm Hg and 24 mEq/L, respectively.

c. If both $PaCO_2$ and bicarbonate change in the same direction (i.e., both are increased or both are decreased), then there is a primary acid-base disorder with a compensatory secondary disorder that brings the ratio of bicarbonate/carbon dioxide tension back to 20:1.

d. If bicarbonate and $PaCO_2$ change in opposite directions, there is a mixed acid-base disorder.

e. Determine the primary acid-base disorder by comparing the fractional change of the measured bicarbonate or carbon dioxide tension to the normal value.

f. There are equations and nomograms that calculate the expected change in one of the three parameters involved in acid-base determination (pH, bicarbonate, or carbon dioxide tension) for a given change in one of the other two parameters. If the actual change is markedly different from the expected change, then there is a mixed acid-base disorder.

g. Finally, calculate the anion gap to determine whether there is a hidden metabolic acidosis.

3. Signs and Symptoms. Major adverse consequences of severe systemic acidosis (pH <7.2) can occur independently of whether the acidosis is of respiratory, metabolic, or mixed origin (**Table 15-7**). Major adverse consequences of severe systemic alkalosis (pH >7.60) reflect impairment of cerebral and coronary blood flow because of arteriolar vasoconstriction (**Table 15-8**).

a. Respiratory Acidosis is present when a decrease in alveolar ventilation results in an increase in the $PaCO_2$ sufficient to decrease arterial pH to less than 7.35 (**Table 15-9**).

TABLE 15-7	Adverse Consequences of Severe Acidosis
Nervous System	
Obtundation	
Coma	
Cardiovascular System	
Impaired myocardial contractility	
Decreased cardiac output	
Decreased arterial blood pressure	
Sensitization to re-entrant cardiac dysrhythmias	
Decreased threshold for ventricular fibrillation	
Decreased responsiveness to catecholamines	
Ventilation	
Hyperventilation	
Dyspnea	
Fatigue of respiratory muscles	
Metabolism	
Hyperkalemia	
Insulin resistance	
Inhibition of anaerobic glycolysis	

Adapted from Adrogué HJ, Madias NE: Management of life-threatening acid-base disorders. N Engl J Med 1998;338:26–34.

    1.) Treatment is correction of the disorder responsible for hypoventilation.

    2.) Hypokalemia and Hypochloremia are associated with metabolic alkalosis that may accompany respiratory acidosis and may require treatment.

b. Respiratory Alkalosis is present when an increase in alveolar ventilation results in a decrease in $PaCO_2$ sufficient to increase the pH to greater than 7.45 (**Table 15-10**).

    1.) Treatment of respiratory alkalosis is directed at correcting the underlying disorder responsible for alveolar hyperventilation.

    2.) The Hypokalemia and Hypochloremia that may co-exist with respiratory alkalosis may also require treatment.

c. Metabolic Acidosis. Metabolic acid lowers blood pH, stimulating the respiratory center to lower carbon dioxide tension. Respiratory compensation does not in general fully compensate for increased acid production. "Normal anion gap" acidosis is the result of a net increase in chloride concentration, or hyperchloremic metabolic acidosis. A "high anion gap" occurs when a fixed acid is added to the extracellular space.

TABLE 15-8	Adverse Consequences of Alkalosis

Nervous System

Decreased cerebral blood flow

Seizures

Lethargy

Delirium

Tetany

Cardiovascular System

Arteriolar vasoconstriction

Decreased coronary blood flow

Decreased threshold for angina pectoris

Predisposition to refractory dysrhythmias

Ventilation

Hypoventilation

Hypercarbia

Arterial hypoxemia

Metabolism

Hypokalemia

Hypocalcemia

Hypomagnesemia

Hypophosphatemia

Stimulation of anaerobic glycolysis

Adapted from Adrogué JH, Madias NE: Management of life-threatening acid-base disorders. N Engl J Med 1998; 338:107–11.

TABLE 15-9	Causes of Respiratory Acidosis

Drug-induced ventilatory depression

Permissive hypercapnia

Upper airway obstruction

Status asthmaticus

Restriction of ventilation (rib fractures/flail chest)

Disorders of neuromuscular function

Malignant hyperthermia

Hyperalimentation solutions

TABLE 15-10	Causes of Respiratory Alkalosis

Iatrogenic (mechanical hyperventilation)

Decreased barometric pressure

Arterial hypoxemia

Central nervous system injury

Hepatic disease

Pregnancy

Salicylate overdose

Lactic acidosis, ketoacidosis, renal failure, and the acidoses associated with many poisonings are examples of acidoses with a high anion gap.

1.) *Signs and Symptoms* depend on the underlying disorder and the rate of development of the acidosis.

2.) *Diagnosis* is by analysis of arterial blood for pH, carbon dioxide tension, bicarbonate concentration, and anion gap. Common causes of metabolic acidosis are listed in **Table 15-11**.

    a.) **Metabolic Acidosis of Renal Origin** occurs if the kidneys are unable to replace the bicarbonate that is lost by buffering normal endogenous acid production (distal renal tubular acidosis) or because an abnormally high fraction of bicarbonate is lost in the urine (proximal renal tubular acidosis or acetazolamide use).

    b.) **Metabolic Acidosis of Extrarenal Origin** includes gastrointestinal bicarbonate losses, ketoacidosis, and lactic acidosis.

3.) *Treatment* of metabolic acidosis includes treatment of the cause, and in some cases administration of sodium bicarbonate for acute treatment (e.g., if the pH is less than 7.1 or the bicarbonate concentration is less than 10 mEq/L). Acute changes in pH toward normal (or alkalosis) may result in increased hemoglobin

TABLE 15-11	Causes of Metabolic Acidosis

Lactic acidosis

Diabetic ketoacidosis

Renal failure

Hepatic failure

Methanol and ethylene glycol intoxication

Aspirin intoxication

Increased skeletal muscle activity

Cyanide poisoning

Carbon monoxide poisoning

affinity for oxygen and reduce oxygen tissue oxygen delivery. The 2005 American Heart Association Guidelines for Cardiopulmonary Resuscitation and Emergency Cardiovascular Care do not recommend administering sodium bicarbonate routinely during cardiac arrest and cardiopulmonary resuscitation unless life-threatening hyperkalemia or cardiac arrest associated with a preexisting metabolic acidosis has occurred.

   4.) *Management of Anesthesia.* Elective surgery should be postponed until an acidosis has been treated. Invasive hemodynamic monitoring should be considered. Frequent laboratory measurement of acid-base parameters should be made throughout the perioperative period.

d. Metabolic Alkalosis is an increase in pH, an increase in plasma bicarbonate concentration, and a compensatory increase in carbon dioxide tension. Common causes of metabolic alkalosis are noted in **Table 15-12**.

   1.) *Treatment* rarely requires administration of an acid; usually volume replacement is all that is needed.

   2.) *Management of Anesthesia.* Management is directed at judicious volume replacement and adequate supplementation with chloride, potassium, and magnesium as needed.

TABLE 15-12   Causes of Metabolic Alkalosis
Hypovolemia
Vomiting
Nasogastric suction
Diuretic therapy
Bicarbonate administration
Hyperaldosteronism
Chloride-wasting diarrhea

CHAPTER 16

Endocrine Disease

I. DIABETES MELLITUS

Diabetes mellitus results from inadequate supply of insulin and/or inadequate tissue response to insulin with increased circulating glucose levels and eventual microvascular and macrovascular complications. Type 1a diabetes is caused by autoimmune destruction of pancreatic islet beta cells and complete absence or negligible circulating insulin levels. Type 1b diabetes is a rare nonautoimmune disease with absolute insulin deficiency. Type 2 diabetes is not immune mediated; it is caused by a relative deficiency of insulin coupled with an insulin receptor defect or defect(s) in its postreceptor intracellular signaling pathways.

A. Signs and Symptoms

1. Type 1 Diabetes (5%–10% of all diabetes mellitus) presents before age 40. It is caused by T cell–mediated autoimmune destruction of pancreatic beta cells. Viruses (e.g., enteroviruses), dietary proteins, and drugs/chemicals may initiate the autoimmune process in genetically susceptible hosts. After a long preclinical period (9–13 years), the onset of clinical disease (hyperglycemia, fatigue, weight loss, polyuria, polydipsia, blurring of vision, and volume depletion) is often sudden and severe. Diagnosis is based on a random blood glucose test result of more than 200 mg/dL and a hemoglobin (Hb) A_{1c} level greater than 7%. The presence of ketoacidosis indicates severe insulin deficiency and unrestrained lipolysis.

2. Type 2 Diabetes (90% of all diabetes mellitus) occurs typically in middle to older patients (more recently in younger patients and children due to obesity) and is caused by relative beta-cell insufficiency and insulin resistance. Three important defects in type 2 diabetes are (1) increased rate of hepatic glucose release, (2) impaired basal and stimulated insulin secretion, and (3) inefficient use of glucose by peripheral tissues (insulin resistance). Insulin resistance appears to be inherited. Acquired characteristics (obesity, sedentary lifestyle) are contributing factors.

3. The Metabolic Syndrome or insulin-resistance syndrome (**Table 16-1**) is a combination of insulin resistance with other clinical characteristics (hypertension, dyslipidemia, a procoagulant state, obesity, premature atherosclerosis, and cardiovascular disease).

TABLE 16-1	Metabolic Syndrome

At least three of the following

Fasting plasma glucose ≥110 mg/dL

Abdominal obesity (waist girth >40 [in men], 35 [in women])

Serum triglycerides ≥150 mg/dL

Serum high-density lipoprotein cholesterol <40 mg/dL (men), <50 mg/dL (women)

Blood pressure ≥130/85 mm Hg

Adapted from Expert Panel on Detection, Evaluation, and Treatment of High Blood Cholesterol in Adults: Executive Summary of The Third Report of The National Cholesterol Education Program (NCEP) Expert Panel on Detection, Evaluation, and Treatment of High Blood Cholesterol in Adults (Adult Treatment Panel III). JAMA 2001;285:2486–2497.

B. Diagnosis (Table 16-2). Normal fasting plasma glucose is 70 to 100 mg/dL. Hyperglycemia that does not meet the criteria for diabetes is classified as either impaired fasting glucose or impaired glucose tolerance. Hb A_{1c} represents the percentage of hemoglobin molecules that has been glycosylated and reflects the average plasma glucose concentration during the previous 60 to 90 days. Normal range for Hb A_{1c} is 4% to 6%. Increased risk of microvascular and macrovascular disease begins at an Hb A_{1c} of 6.5%.

C. Treatment

  1. Considerations in Type 2 Diabetes

  a. Diet. Patients with type 2 diabetes should adopt low-calorie (800 to 1500 kcal) or very low calorie (<800 kcal) diets with limits on cholesterol-raising fats and added sugars. The goal is to reduce body fat, decrease insulin resistance, and normalize plasma glucose, lipids, and lipoproteins.

  b. Oral Antidiabetic Agents (four types). These agents are used alone in or combination to maintain glucose control (fasting glucose, 90 to 130 mg/dL; peak postprandial glucose, <180 mg/dL; Hb A_{1c} <7%) in the initial stages of the disease.

  1.) Secretagogues (sulfonylureas, meglitinides) increase insulin secretion from pancreatic beta cells and enhance tissue utilization of glucose (**Table 16-3**). Hypoglycemia is the most common side effect.

TABLE 16-2	Diagnostic Criteria for Diabetes Mellitus

Symptoms of diabetes (polyuria, polydipsia, unexplained weight loss) plus a random plasma glucose concentration ≥200 mg/dL

OR

Fasting (no caloric intake for ≥8 hours) plasma glucose ≥126 mg/dL

OR

2-hour plasma glucose >200 mg/dL during an oral glucose tolerance test

TABLE 16-3	Sulfonylureas			
Drug	Initial Dose (mg/day)	Daily Dose Range (mg/day)	Duration (hr)	Doses/Day
Second Generation				
Glyburide	1.25–2.5	1.25–20	18–24	1–2
Glipizide	2.5–5.0	2.5–40	12–18	1–2
Glimepiride	1–2	4–8	24	1

2.) Biguanides (metformin) suppress excessive hepatic glucose release. Metformin is often combined with a sulfonylurea.

3.) Thiazolidinediones, or glitazones (rosiglitazone, pioglitazone), improve insulin sensitivity.

4.) α-Glucosidase Inhibitors (acarbose, miglitol) delay gastrointestinal glucose absorption.

c. Insulin Therapy in Type 2 Diabetes. An algorithm for treatment of type 2 diabetes, including oral agents, is summarized in **Fig. 16-1**. Monotherapy with oral agents eventually usually fails, and combination therapy becomes necessary. If combination therapy is ineffective, a bedtime dose of intermediate-acting insulin is added. If oral agents plus single-dose insulin therapy is ineffective, type 2 diabetics are switched to insulin exclusively. A combination of intermediate and regular insulin twice daily is commonly used for optimal control. Goals of therapy include Hb A_{1c} less than 7%, low-density lipoprotein less than 100 mg/dL, high-density lipoprotein more than 40 mg/dL in men and more than 50 mg/dL in women, triglycerides less than 200 mg/dL, and blood pressure less than 130/80.

2. Types of Insulin (Table 16-4). Insulin, usually administered two to three times daily, is always necessary to manage type 1 diabetes (and is necessary for many patients with type 2 diabetes).

a. Basal Insulins are intermediate-acting (NPH, lente, lispro protamine, aspart protamine) and given twice daily.

b. Long-Acting Insulins (ultralente and glargine) are given once daily.

c. Short-Acting Insulins (regular insulin) or rapid-acting insulins (lispro, aspart) provide glycemic control at mealtimes (prandial insulin).

3. Management of Insulin Therapy

a. Conventional Therapy involves twice-daily injections of combinations of intermediate-acting and short- or rapid-acting insulins (Humulin 70/30 insulin [70% NPH, 30% regular], Novolog 70/30 [70% insulin aspart protamine plus 30% insulin aspart], or Humalog 75/25 [75% insulin lispro protamine plus 25% insulin lispro]) (**Fig. 16-2**).

b. Intensive Insulin Therapy requires three or four daily injections or continuous infusion. Three daily injections include NPH plus short-acting (regular) or rapid-acting (lispro, aspart) insulin before breakfast, short-acting or rapid-acting insulin before dinner, and NPH insulin at bedtime (**Fig. 16-3**). Four daily injections can include a single

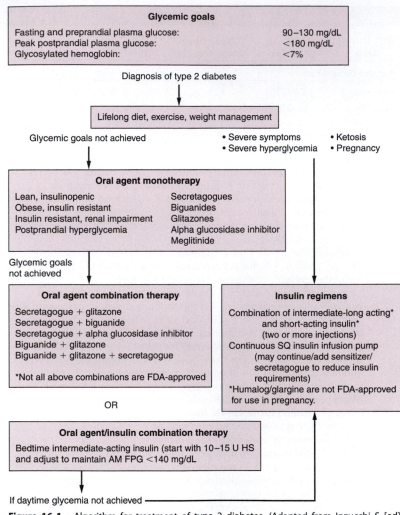

Figure 16-1 • Algorithm for treatment of type 2 diabetes. (Adapted from Inzucchi S [ed]: The Diabetes Mellitus Manual: A Primary Companion to Ellenberg and Rifkin's Sixth Edition. New York, McGraw-Hill, 2005, p 193.)

injection of NPH, lente, or insulin glargine (Lantus) at bedtime plus short-acting or rapid-acting insulin before breakfast, lunch, and dinner (**Figs. 16-4 and 16-5**).

1.) *Continuous Subcutaneous Infusion* uses regular or rapid-acting insulin with a usual range of 0.5 to 2.0 units/hour (**Fig. 16-6**). A typical total daily basal dose of insulin equals weight (kg) × 0.3, with

Insulins	Onset	Peak	Duration
Short Acting			
Human regular	30 min	2–4 hr	5–8 hr
Lispro (Humalog)	10–15 min	1–2 hr	3–6 hr
Aspart (Novolog)	10–15 min	1–2 hr	3–6 hr
Intermediate			
Human NPH	1–2 hr	6–10 hr	10–20 hr
Lente	1–2 hr	6–10 hr	10–20 hr
Long Acting			
Ultralente	4–6 hr	8–20 hr	24–48 hr
Glargine (Lantus)	1–2 hr	Peakless	~ 24 hr

TABLE 16-4 Insulin

the hourly rate obtained by dividing by 24. Basal rates vary during a 24-hour period, with lower rates required at bedtime, higher rates between 3:00 and 9:00 AM, and intermediate rates during the day.

  c. Ideal Glycemic Goals for type 1 diabetics include the following: before meals, 70 to 120 mg/dL; after meals, less than 150 mg/dL; at bedtime, 100 to 130 mg/dL; and at 3:00 AM more than 70 mg/dL.

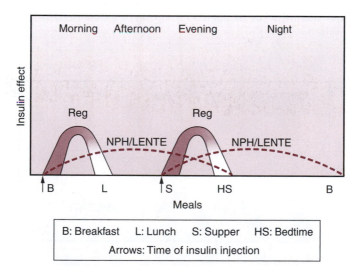

Figure 16-2 • Insulin effect from two daily doses of NPH plus regular insulin. (Adapted from Hirsch IB, Farkas-Hirsch R, Skyler JS: Intensive insulin therapy for treatment of type I diabetes. Diabetes Care 1990;13.)

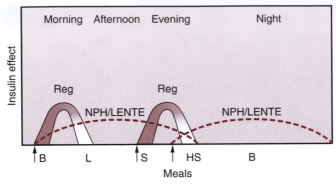

Figure 16-3 • Insulin effect of the three injections per day regimen (NPH and regular in morning, regular before supper, NPH at bedtime).

D. Complications of Diabetes and Diabetes Therapy

1. Hypoglycemia is the most common and dangerous complication of insulin therapy. β-Blockers may exacerbate hypoglycemia by inhibiting adipose tissue lipolysis, which provides alternate fuel during hypoglycemia. The diagnosis in adults requires a plasma glucose level less than 50 mg/dL. Symptoms are adrenergic (sweating, tachycardia, palpitations, restlessness, pallor) and neuroglycopenic (fatigue, confusion, headache, somnolence, convulsions, coma). Treatment is oral sugar in the form of sugar cubes, glucose tablets, or soft drinks (in unconscious patients, glucose 0.5 g/kg intravenously [IV] or glucagon 0.5 to 1.0 mg IV, intramuscularly [IM], or subcutaneously [SC]).

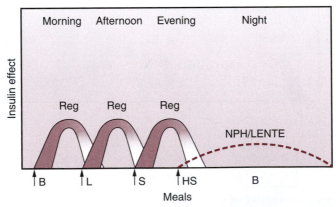

Figure 16-4 • Insulin effect of the four injections per day regimen of short-acting insulin before each meal and NPH at bedtime.

278

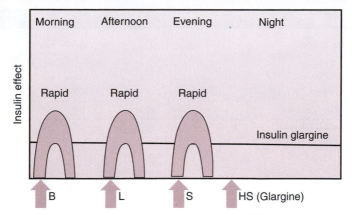

Figure 16-5 • Insulin effect of multiple-dose regimen: three premeal doses of rapid-acting insulin (lispro/aspart) plus basal insulin (glargine). B, breakfast; HS, bedtime; L, lunch; S, supper.

2. Diabetic Ketoacidosis (DKA) occurs more commonly in type 1 diabetics and may be precipitated by infection or acute illness, insulin omission, and the new onset of diabetes mellitus (**Table 16-5**).

   a. Characteristics

      1.) Increased Ketoacid Production and metabolic acidosis are hallmarks of DKA. Acidosis is associated with an increased anion gap ($Na^+ - [\,Cl^- + HCO_3^-\,]$ normal: 8–14 mEq/L).

      2.) Hyperglycemia

      3.) Osmotic Diuresis and Hypovolemia

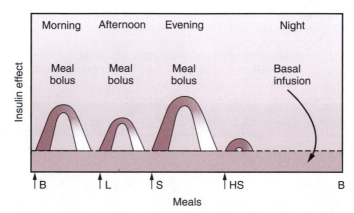

Figure 16-6 • Insulin effect of continuous subcutaneous infusion of short-/rapid-acting insulin before meals and snacks.

TABLE 16-5	Diagnostic Features of DKA
Glucose (mg/dL)	≥ 300
pH	≤ 7.3
HCO_3^- (mEq/L)	≤ 18
SOsm (mOsm/L)	<320
Ketones	$++-+++$

DKA, diabetic ketoacidosis; SOsm, serum osmolarity.

4.) *Total Body Deficits in Water, Potassium, and Phosphorus,* even if laboratory values are normal.
5.) *Hyponatremia*
b. *Treatment*
1.) *Normal Saline* (large volumes may be needed)—rehydration will lower plasma glucose by 30% to 50%.
2.) *Insulin.* Intravenous loading dose of 0.1 U/kg regular insulin and insulin infusion of 0.1 U/kg/hr should be given until normal acid-base status is achieved. This may paradoxically require administration of glucose if hyperglycemia is corrected before acid-base status is normal.
3.) *Electrolyte Supplementation*
4.) *Sodium Bicarbonate* should be given for a pH of less than 7.1.
3. Hyperglycemic Hyperosmolar Syndrome (Table 16-6) is severe hyperglycemia, hyperosmolarity, and dehydration, usually in elderly type 2 diabetics with an acute illness (infection, myocardial infarction, cerebrovascular accident, pancreatitis, intestinal obstruction, endocrinopathy, renal failure, burns).
a. *Signs and Symptoms* include polyuria, polydipsia, hypovolemia, hypotension, tachycardia, organ hypoperfusion, obtundation (caused by hyperosmolarity), and aketotic metabolic acidosis.
b. *Treatment*
1.) If the plasma osmolarity is more than 320 mOsm/L, large volumes (1000–1500 mL/hr) of 0.45% normal saline should be administered

TABLE 16-6	Diagnostic Feature of Hyperglycemic Hyperosmolar Syndrome
Glucose (mg/dL)	≥ 600
pH	≥ 7.3
HCO_3^- (mEq/L)	≥ 15
SOsm (mOsm/L)	≥ 350

SOsm, serum osmolarity.

until the osmolarity is less than 320 mOsm/L, at which time large volumes (1000–1500 mL/hr) of 0.9% normal saline are administered.

   2.) *Insulin.* An intravenous bolus of 15 units of regular insulin is administered, followed by a 0.1-U/kg per hour infusion. The infusion is decreased to 2 to 3 U/hr when the glucose decreases to 250 to 300 mg/dL.

   3.) *Electrolyte Supplementation*

4. Microvascular Complications

   a. Diabetic Nephropathy. End-stage renal disease develops in 30% to 40% of type 1 diabetics and 5% to 10% of type 2 diabetics.

   1.) *Clinical Progression.* Renal function remains normal for approximately 15 years. Proteinuria is the earliest laboratory manifestation, followed within 5 years by increases in blood urea nitrogen and creatinine. Renal failure occurs in 3 to 5 years.

   2.) *Treatment.* Antihypertensive treatment (low-sodium diet, low-dose diuretics, and one of several antihypertensive agents, including a β_1-antagonist, angiotensin-converting enzyme inhibitor [ACEI], angiotensin II receptor blocker, calcium channel blocker, and/or an α_1-blocker) can slow progression. If end-stage renal disease develops, four treatment options are available: hemodialysis, peritoneal dialysis, continuous ambulatory peritoneal dialysis, and kidney or combined kidney/pancreas transplantation.

   b. Peripheral Neuropathy develops in more than 50% of patients who have had diabetes for longer than 25 years. Distal symmetrical diffuse sensorimotor polyneuropathy is most common, appearing in the toes or feet and progressing proximally in a "stocking glove" distribution. Significant morbidity results from foot ulcers, recurrent infections, foot fractures (Charcot's joint), and subsequent amputations. Treatment of peripheral neuropathy includes optimal glucose control, nonsteroidal anti-inflammatory agents, antidepressants, and anticonvulsants for pain control.

   c. Retinopathy results from hemorrhages, exudates, and growth of abnormal vessels and fibrous tissue. Visual impairment ranges from minor changes in color vision to total blindness. Strict glycemic control and blood pressure control can reduce the risk of development and progression of retinopathy.

5. Macrovascular Complications

   a. Cardiovascular Disease is a major cause of morbidity and the leading cause of mortality in diabetics. Dyslipidemia is the major contributor to the initiation and development of atherosclerotic lesions. Statin therapy (3-hydroxy-3-methylglutaryl coenzyme A reductase inhibitors) should be considered for all diabetics. Prevention of coronary artery disease in diabetics includes aggressive management of elevated lipids, elevated glucose, and hypertension, as well as aspirin for thrombolysis. Medical management of symptomatic coronary artery disease includes β_1-blockers, ACEIs, nitrates, calcium channel blockers, statins, fibrates, antiplatelet drugs, and possibly thrombolysis, stent placements, or, in severe cases, coronary artery bypass.

6. Diabetic Autonomic Neuropathy (DAN) can affect any part of the autonomic nervous system and depends on the duration of diabetes and the degree of metabolic control. Cardiovascular autonomic neuropathy is characterized by abnormalities in heart rate and central/peripheral vascular dynamics. In DAN, counterregulatory hormone responses are impaired and warning signs of hypoglycemia may be absent.

E. Management of Anesthesia. Hyperglycemia appears to increase the risk of ischemic myocardial injury by decreasing coronary collateral blood flow and coronary vasodilator reserve, impairing coronary microcirculation, and causing endothelial dysfunction. Acute hyperglycemia causes dehydration, impaired wound healing, an increased rate of infection, worsening central nervous system/spinal cord injury with ischemia, and hyperviscosity with thrombogenesis. Tight control of serum glucose in the perioperative period is a primary goal.

1. Preoperative Evaluation should include evaluation for possible cardiac and renal disease, control of hypertension, management of insulin and glucose control, and examination for limited joint mobility (especially neck) that may affect endotracheal intubation.

a. Management of Insulin in the Preoperative Period

1.) Two thirds of the usual bedtime dose of insulin should be given the night before surgery and half the usual NPH dose on the day of surgery. Regular insulin should be held the morning of surgery.

2.) A 5% dextrose with 0.45% normal saline ($D_5\frac{1}{2}$ NS) intravenous infusion at 100 mL/hr should be initiated preoperatively.

3.) Insulin Pump. The overnight rate should be decreased by 30%. On the morning of surgery, the pump can be kept at the basal rate, replaced with a intravenous insulin infusion at the same rate, or the patient can be given subcutaneous glargine and the pump discontinued in 60 to 90 minutes.

4.) If the patient uses glargine and lispro or aspart for daily glycemic control, the patient should take two thirds of the glargine dose plus the entire lispro or aspart dose the night before surgery and hold all morning insulin.

5.) Oral Hypoglycemics should be discontinued 24 to 48 hours preoperatively.

6.) For major surgery, if serum glucose is higher than 270 mg/dL, surgery should be delayed for rapid control. If serum glucose is higher than 400 mg/dL, surgery should be postponed and the metabolic state restabilized.

2. Intraoperative Management. Goals are to minimize hyperglycemia (serum glucose 120 to 180 mg/dL) and avoid hypoglycemia. Management should be with continuous intravenous infusion of insulin. Subcutaneous insulin should not be used. Intraoperative serum glucose levels should be monitored at least hourly. $D_5\frac{1}{2}$ NS should also be infused to provide carbohydrate and inhibit hepatic glucose production and protein catabolism.

3. Postoperative Care includes aggressive insulin therapy. Tight glucose control (80–110 mg/dL) is associated with better outcomes, possibly because of better neutrophil and macrophage function, beneficial changes to mucosal/skin barriers, enhanced erythropoiesis, reduced cholestasis, improved respiratory muscle function, and decreased axonal degeneration.

II. INSULINOMA

Insulinomas are insulin-secreting tumors of pancreatic beta cells manifested clinically as fasting hypoglycemia. The principal anesthetic challenge during excision of an insulinoma is maintenance of a normal blood glucose concentration. Profound hypoglycemia can occur, particularly during manipulation of the tumor, and marked hyperglycemia can follow successful surgical removal of the tumor. Frequent (every 15 minutes) monitoring of glucose is mandatory.

III. THYROID DISEASE

A. Anatomy and Physiology. Thyroid hormones T_4 (thyroxine) and T_3 (triiodothyronine) stimulate virtually all metabolic processes, synthetic and catabolic. They influence growth and maturation of tissues, enhance tissue function, and stimulate protein synthesis and carbohydrate and lipid metabolism. Thyroid hormone increases myocardial contractility, decreases systemic vascular resistance, and increases intravascular volume.

B. Diagnosis

1. **Hyperthyroidism and Hypothyroidism.** Free T_4 (FT_4) is elevated in 90% of patients with hyperthyroidism and is low in 85% of patients with hypothyroidism. The thyroid-stimulating hormone (TSH) level is now the single best test of thyroid hormone action at the cellular level. A low TSH level with normal levels of FT_3 and FT_4 is diagnostic of subclinical hyperthyroidism. An elevated TSH level with normal levels of FT_3 and FT_4 is diagnostic of subclinical hypothyroidism. Radioactive iodine uptake is sometimes used to confirm hyperthyroidism. Other tests include detection of antibodies directed toward thyroid antigens.

2. **Thyroid Nodules.** Thyroid scans using ^{123}I or technetium-99m evaluate nodules as "warm" or normal, "hot" or hyperfunctioning, or "cold" or hypofunctioning. Ultrasonography is 90% to 95% accurate for determining whether a lesion is cystic, solid, or mixed.

C. Hyperthyroidism.

1. **Signs and Symptoms of Hyperthyroidism (Table 16-7)**

2. **Graves' Disease** is characterized by a classic triad of hyperthyroidism, exophthalmos, and dermopathy. It appears to be a systemic autoimmune disease with thyroid-stimulating antibodies (long-acting thyroid stimulator [LATS]), binding to TSH receptors in the thyroid. Graves' ophthalmopathy includes upper lid retraction, a wide-eyed stare, muscle weakness, proptosis, and an increase in intraocular pressure. Steroids, bilateral tarsorrhaphies, external radiation, or surgical decompression may be necessary in these cases.

   a. *Diagnosis* of Graves' disease is confirmed by elevated thyroid hormone levels and radioactive iodine uptake. The TSH level is often low, and thyroid-stimulating antibodies are increased.

3. **Toxic Multinodular Goiters** usually arise from long-standing simple goiters and can produce extreme thyroid enlargements with signs and symptoms of airway obstruction. Hypermetabolism is usually less severe than with Graves' disease, and there is no associated opthalmopathy or dermopathy. The diagnosis is confirmed by a thyroid scan and, occasionally, thyroid biopsy.

4. A solitary Toxic Nodule (toxic adenoma) is diagnosed with the same tests used for multinodular goiters.

5. Treatment for hyperthyroidism are the antithyroid drugs propylthiouracil (PTU) or methimazole (Tapazole), which interfere with thyroid hormone synthesis and peripheral conversion of T_4 to T_3. Iodide in high concentration inhibits release of hormones from the thyroid gland, and it is usually reserved for preparing hyperthyroid patients for surgery, managing patients with actual or impending thyroid storm, or treating patients with severe thyrocardiac disease. β-Adrenergic antagonists may relieve signs and symptoms (anxiety, sweating, heat intolerance, tremors, tachycardia). Ablative therapy with radioactive ^{131}I or surgery is recommended for patients with refractory Graves' disease and in patients with toxic multinodular goiter or a toxic adenoma. Surgery (subtotal thyroidectomy, total thyroidectomy) results in prompt control of disease and a lower incidence of hypothyroidism than radioactive iodine.

6. Management of Anesthesia. Euthyroidism should be established preoperatively (may require 6–8 weeks of therapy). In emergency cases, the use of an intravenous β-blocker, ipodate, cortisol, or dexamethasone and PTU is usually necessary. The anesthesiologist should be prepared to manage thyroid storm. Controlled studies demonstrate no clinically significant increase in anesthetic requirements.

a. Thyroid Storm and malignant hyperthermia can present with similar signs and symptoms (hyperpyrexia, tachycardia, hypermetabolism). Treatment includes rapid alleviation of thyrotoxicosis, fluid resuscitation, cooling measures to counter fever, medications to control heart rate, and glucocorticoids. Antithyroid drugs (PTU 200–400 mg every 8 hours) may be given through a nasogastric tube, orally, or rectally. If circulatory shock is present, an intravenous direct vasopressor (phenylephrine) is indicated.

D. Hypothyroidism

1. Signs and Symptoms (Table 16-7)

2. Diagnosis of primary hypothyroidism is confirmed by reduced thyroid hormone levels and elevated TSH level.

3. Treatment is usually L-thyroxine (levothyroxine sodium). Alternative hormone preparations include thyroid extract USP, L-triiodothyronine (liothyronine sodium), and liotrix, a combination of T_4 and T_3 in a 4:1 ratio.

4. Management of Anesthesia. Patients with subclinical hypothyroidism usually present no anesthetic problems. Patients with mild to moderate disease should probably receive daily L-thyroxine (100–200 μg/day) in the preoperative period. In an overtly hypothyroid patient, the potential for severe cardiovascular instability intraoperatively and myxedema coma in the postoperative period is high. If emergency surgery can be delayed for 24 to 48 hours, intravenous thyroid replacement therapy (L-thyroxine 300–500 μg or L-triiodothyronine 25–50 μg IV) is indicated. Other anesthetic considerations are summarized in **Table 16-8**.

E. Myxedema Coma is a rare severe form of hypothyroidism characterized by delirium or unconsciousness, hypoventilation, hypothermia (80% of patients), bradycardia, hypotension, and a severe dilutional hyponatremia. Treatment is with L-thyroxine or L-triiodothyronine, intravenous hydration with

TABLE 16-7	Signs and Symptoms of Hyper- and Hypothyroidism
Hyperthyroidism	**Hypothyroidism**
Hypermetabolism	Hypometabolism
Anxiety, restlessness, hyperkinesis	Fatigue, lethargy, listlessness, apathy
Warm, moist skin	Dry, thickened, pale, cool skin
Increased sweating	Decreased sweating
Flushed face	Large tongue, hoarse voice
Fine hair, fragile nails	Dry hair
Upper eyelid retraction	Periorbital edema
Heat intolerance	Cold intolerance
Proximal muscle weakness	Prolonged deep tendon reflexes
Sleep disturbance	Menorrhagia
Tremor	Hypercholesterolemia, hypertriglyceridemia
Weight loss, diarrhea	Weight gain, constipation
Tachycardia, arrhythmias, palpitations	Ventricular arrhythmias
Increased cardiac output, cardiomegaly	Reduced myocardial contractility
Normal or high T_3 and T_4, reduced TSH	Decreased T_3 and T_4, increased TSH

glucose-containing saline solutions, temperature regulation, ventilatory support, and hydrocortisone for possible adrenal insufficiency.

F. Euthyroid Sick Syndrome occurs in critically ill patients with significant nonthyroidal illness who demonstrate abnormal thyroid function tests (low levels of T_3 and T_4 and a normal TSH). No treatment for thyroid function is necessary.

G. Cretinism is extreme hypothyroidism that occurs during fetal life, infancy, and early childhood resulting in growth failure and mental retardation. The diagnosis must be made and treatment administered within a few weeks after birth to prevent organ damage.

H. Goiter. A goiter results from compensatory hypertrophy and hyperplasia of follicular epithelium secondary to a reduction in thyroid hormone output. The

TABLE 16-8	Anesthetic Considerations in Patients with Hypothyroidism

- Administer dexamethasone or cortisol; decreased adrenal function is associated with hypothyroidism.
- Phosphodiesterase inhibitors (milrinone) may be the most effective inotrope because they do not depend on β-receptors, which may be reduced in number and sensitivity.
- Avoid or reduce preoperative sedation.
- Invasive monitoring depends on cardiovascular status.
- Administer dextrose-containing IVs to avoid hypoglycemia.
- Provide controlled ventilation to avoid hypoventilation.

etiology may be a deficient intake of iodine, a dietary (i.e., cassava) or pharmacologic (i.e., phenylbutazone, lithium) goitrogen, or a defect in the hormonal biosynthetic pathway.

I. Thyroid Tumors. Surgical resection of benign nodules or carcinomas rarely creates problems for the anesthesiologist. However, the anesthetic management of a patient for surgical removal of a large thyroid mass that compromises the airway presents a major challenge. Awake intubation may be needed. Airway obstruction caused by extrinsic compression may occur with cessation of spontaneous respiration. Computed tomography (CT) scan and/or echocardiography may further delineate the thyroid mass.

J. Complications of Thyroid Surgery include recurrent laryngeal nerve injury and hypoparathyroidism caused by damage to the blood supply of the parathyroid glands (anxiety circumoral numbness, tingling fingertips, muscle cramps, positive Chvostek's sign, and Trousseau's sign may point to hypocalcemia). Respiratory compromise as a result of tracheal compression caused by hematoma formation can also occur.

IV. PHEOCHROMOCYTOMA

Pheochromocytomas are catecholamine-secreting tumors that arise independently or as part of the multiple endocrine neoplastic syndromes (**Table 16-9**). Patients with von Recklinghausen's disease, tuberous sclerosis, and Sturge-Weber syndrome have increased risk of pheochromocytoma.

A. Signs and Symptoms. Hypertension, headache, sweating, pallor, and palpitations are classic signs and symptoms. Hypertensive crises mimic the hemodynamic responses of acute catecholamine administration. Cardiomyopathy, cardiac hypertrophy, and electrocardiography (ECG) abnormalities and arrhythmias can occur. The presentation of a pheochromocytoma may mimic thyrotoxicosis, malignant hypertension, diabetes mellitus, malignant carcinoid syndrome, or gram-negative septicemia. Hyperglycemia, but rarely frank diabetes, occurs in most patients due to catecholamine stimulation of glycogenolysis and inhibition of insulin release.

B. Diagnosis relies on demonstration of excess catecholamine secretion. The most sensitive test for high-risk patients (familial pheochromocytoma or classic symptoms) is a finding of plasma-free normetanephrine greater than 400 pg/mL and/or metanephrine greater than 220 pg/mL. A pheochromocytoma is excluded if normetanephrine is less than 112 pg/mL and metanephrine is less than 61 pg/mL. Determination of elevated urinary free catecholamine levels and their metabolites (i.e., metanephrine, normetanephrine, vanillylmandelic acid) is easy to perform and readily available and is sufficient for patients with a low probability of having a pheochromocytoma. Results of these tests are equivocal in 5% to 10% of patients, in which case a clonidine suppression test may be used (lowers plasma catecholamines in patients without pheochromocytoma but not in patients with pheochromocytoma). A positive glucagon stimulation test is the safest and most specific provocative test (causes tumor release of catecholamines of at least three times baseline or >2000 pg/mL within 1 to 3 minutes) but should be limited to patients with diastolic blood pressure of less than 100 mm Hg. Tumor location can be predicted by the pattern of catecholamine production (**Table 16-10**). CT and magnetic resonance imaging

TABLE 16-9 Multiple Endocrine Neoplasia

Syndrome	Manifestations
MEN type 2a (Sipple syndrome)	Medullary thyroid cancer Parathyroid adenoma Pheochromocytoma
MEN type 2b	Medullary thyroid cancer Mucosal adenomas Marfan appearance Pheochromocytoma
Von Hippel–Lindau syndrome	Hemangioblastoma of the central nervous system Pheochromocytoma

MEN, multiple endocrine neoplasia.

(MRI) are the optimal noninvasive anatomic adrenal imaging studies. ^{131}I-MIBG scintigraphy localizes tumors via ^{131}I-MIBG uptake in catecholamine-secreting tumors.

C. Treatment is surgical excision whenever possible. α-Methylparatyrosine (inhibits the rate-limiting step of the catecholamine synthetic pathway) may decrease catecholamine production by 50% to 80%. Usual doses range from 250 mg twice daily to 3 to 4 g/day. It is especially useful for malignant and inoperable tumors. Side effects include extrapyramidal reactions and crystalluria.

D. Management of Anesthesia (Table 16-11)

    1. Preoperative Management. Most pheochromocytomas secrete predominantly norepinephrine. The therapeutic goal is normotension, resolution of symptoms, elimination of ST-T changes on the electrocardiogram, and elimination of arrhythmias.

        a.* α-*Blockade (phenoxybenzamine, a noncompetitive α$_1$-antagonist, or alternatively prazocin, an α$_1$-competitive blocker) is used to lower blood pressure, increase intravascular volume, prevent paroxysmal hypertensive episodes, allow resensitization of adrenergic receptors, and decrease myocardial dysfunction. Because of its prolonged effect on α-receptors,

TABLE 16-10 Pattern of Catecholamine Production and Tumor Site

	Adrenal	Extra-adrenal	Adrenal + Extra-adrenal
Norepinephrine	61%	31%	8%
Epinephrine	100%	—	—
Norepinephrine + epinephrine	95%	—	5%

Adapted from Kaser H: Clinical and diagnostic findings in patients with chromaffin tumors: Pheochromocytomas, pheochromoblastomas. Recent Results Cancer Res 1990;118:97–105.

TABLE 16-11	Anesthetic Considerations in Pheochromocytoma
Preoperative	• α-Blockade; phenoxybenzamine, prazosin α-methylparatyrosine • β-Blockade for tachycardia (propranolol, metoprolol, atenolol) • Calcium channel blockers, ACEIs
Intraoperative	• Avoid fear, stress, pain, shivering, hypoxia, hypercarbia (stimulate catecholamine release) • Catecholamine release during induction, intubation, surgical incision, abdominal exploration, and tumor manipulation • Monitoring: arterial catheter, CVP or PA catheter, Foley catheter • Significant fluid administration possible to prevent hypotension after tumor removal • All anesthetics are used • Drugs to avoid: morphine and atracurium (histamine release can provoke catecholamine release), atropine, pancuronium, and succinylcholine (may stimulate the sympathetic nervous system), halothane (sensitizes the myocardium to catecholamine-induced arrhythmias), droperidol, chlorpromazine, metoclopramide, and ephedrine (hypertensive responses) • Intraoperative hypertension: treat with sodium nitroprusside or phentolamine • Antiarrhythmics to have available: lidocaine, esmolol, amiodarone • Intraoperative blood salvage
After tumor removal	• Hypotension caused by catecholamine decrease: fluids, decrease anesthetic depth; vasopressors if these measures fail • Hypoglycemia caused by increased insulin levels: monitor glucose, use dextrose-containing intravenous fluids • Glucocorticoid therapy if bilateral adrenalectomy
Postoperative	• Hypertension may persist for several days; consider persistent hypertension or residual tumor • Hypotension is most common cause of death • Hypoglycemia may persist • ICU monitoring for at least 24 hours

CVP, central venous pressure; ICU, intensive care unit; PA, pulmonary arterial;

it has been recommended to discontinue phenoxybenzamine 24 to 48 hours before surgery or alternatively to administer only one half to two thirds of the morning dose preceding surgery to avoid vascular unresponsiveness immediately following removal of the tumor. Hypertension usually occurs with manipulation of the tumor.

b. β-*Adrenergic Blockade* (propranolol, atenolol, metoprolol) is prescribed if tachycardia (i.e., heart rates >120 bpm) or other arrhythmias result following α_2-blockade from phenoxybenzamine. Esmolol has a fast onset and short elimination half-life and can be administered intravenously in the immediate preoperative period. A nonselective β-blocker should never be administered prior to α-blockade because blockade of vasodilatory β_2-receptors results in unopposed α-agonism, resulting in vasoconstriction and hypertensive crises.

c. α-*Methylparatyrosine* in combination with phenoxybenzamine during the preoperative period may facilitate intraoperative hemodynamic management.

d. Calcium Channel Blockers (Nifedipine, Diltiazem, Verapamil) and ACEIs (Captopril) have all been used to control preoperative hypertension. An α_1-blocker plus a calcium channel blocker is an effective combination for resistant cases.

V. ADRENAL GLAND DYSFUNCTION

The adrenal cortex is responsible for the synthesis of three groups of hormones: glucocorticoids (cortisol essential for life), mineralocorticoids (aldosterone), and androgens. These hormones are involved in blood pressure regulation, gluconeogenesis, sodium and potassium regulation, inhibition of inflammation, and fluid balance. The adrenal medulla synthesizes norepinephrine and epinephrine. Adrenal medulla insufficiency is not known to occur.

A. Hypercortisolism (Cushing's Syndrome) is categorized as adrenocorticotropic hormone (ACTH)–dependent Cushing's syndrome (high ACTH concentrations stimulate the adrenal cortex to produce excess cortisol) and ACTH-independent Cushing's syndrome (excess production of cortisol by abnormal adrenocortical tissues causes the syndrome and suppresses secretion of corticotropic-releasing hormone [CRH] and ACTH). Cushing's disease is defined as Cushing's syndrome caused by high secretion of ACTH by pituitary adenomas.

1. Diagnosis. Symptoms and signs include weight gain, moon facies, facial telangiectasias, hypertension, glucose intolerance, oligomenorrhea or amenorrhea in premenopausal women, decreased libido in men, spontaneous ecchymoses, and skeletal muscle wasting and weakness. Diagnosis is confirmed by demonstrating cortisol hypersecretion based on 24-hour urinary secretion of cortisol. Determining whether a patient's hypercortisolism is ACTH dependent or ACTH independent requires reliable measurements of plasma ACTH using immunoradiometric assays. A high-dose dexamethasone suppression test distinguishes Cushing's disease from ectopic ACTH syndrome (complete resistance present).

2. Treatment for patients with Cushing's disease is transsphenoidal microadenomectomy of the pituitary adenoma. Pituitary radiation and bilateral total adrenalectomy are necessary in some patients. Surgical removal of the adrenal gland is the treatment for adrenal adenoma or carcinoma.

3. Management of Anesthesia

a. Preoperative Evaluation of systemic blood pressure, electrolyte balance, and the blood glucose concentration are especially important. Osteoporosis is a consideration when positioning patients for the operative procedure.

b. Intraoperative. Etomidate may transiently decrease the synthesis and release of cortisol by the adrenal cortex. Mechanical ventilation is recommended caused by skeletal muscle weakness. A continuous infusion of cortisol (100 mg/day IV) may be initiated intraoperatively to avoid acute adrenal insufficiency following tumor removal. Transient diabetes insipidus and meningitis may occur after microadenomectomy.

B. Primary Hyperaldosteronism (Conn's Syndrome) is excess secretion of aldosterone from a functional tumor (aldosteronoma) independent of a physiologic stimulus.

1. Signs and Symptoms are systemic hypertension (headache, sodium retention, increased extracellular fluid volume) or hypokalemia (polyuria, nocturia, skeletal muscle cramps, skeletal muscle weakness, metabolic alkalosis). Hypomagnesemia and abnormal glucose tolerance may be present.

2. Diagnosis. Spontaneous hypokalemia in patients with systemic hypertension is highly suggestive of aldosteronism. A plasma aldosterone concentration less than 9.5 ng/dL at the end of a saline infusion rules out primary aldosteronism.

3. Treatment is supplemental potassium and administration of a competitive aldosterone antagonist, such as spironolactone. Definitive treatment for an aldosterone-secreting tumor is surgical excision. Bilateral adrenalectomy may be necessary if multiple aldosterone-secreting tumors are found.

4. Management of Anesthesia

> *a. Preoperative* goals are correction of hypokalemia and treatment of hypertension.

> *b. Intraoperative.* Hypokalemia may modify responses to nondepolarizing muscle relaxants. Bilateral mobilization of the adrenal glands to excise multiple functional tumors, however, may introduce the need for exogenous administration of cortisol. A continuous intravenous infusion of cortisol, 100 mg every 24 hours, may be initiated on an empirical basis if transient hypocortisolism caused by surgical manipulation is a consideration.

C. Hypoaldosteronism. Hyperkalemia in the absence of renal insufficiency suggests the presence of hypoaldosteronism. Hyporeninemic hypoaldosteronism typically occurs in patients more than 45 years old with chronic renal disease and/or diabetes mellitus. Indomethacin-induced prostaglandin deficiency is a reversible cause of this syndrome. Treatment of hypoaldosteronism includes liberal sodium intake and daily administration of fludrocortisone.

D. Adrenal Insufficiency (AI)

1. Signs and Symptoms. In primary disease (Addison's disease), the adrenal glands are unable to elaborate sufficient quantities of glucocorticoid, mineralocorticoid, and androgen hormones. The most common cause is autoimmune disease. Addison's disease is characterized by fatigue, weakness, anorexia, nausea and vomiting, cutaneous and mucosal hyperpigmentation, cardiopenia secondary to chronic hypotension, hypovolemia, hyponatremia, and hyperkalemia. Secondary adrenal insufficiency is caused by inadequate pituitary CRH or ACTH production. Unlike Addison's disease, there is only a glucocorticoid deficiency with secondary disease. The most common cause is iatrogenic (pituitary surgery, pituitary irradiation, use of synthetic glucocorticoids).

2. Diagnosis. Critically ill patients with cortisol levels less than 20 μg/dL have AI. The classic definition of AI includes a baseline plasma cortisol below 20 μg/dL and a cortisol level below 20 μg/dL following an ACTH stimulation test. Absolute AI is characterized by a low baseline cortisol level and a positive ACTH stimulation test. Relative AI has a higher baseline cortisol level but a positive ACTH stimulation test.

3. Treatment. The most common cause of AI is exogenous steroids (**Table 16-12**). For patients with a history of long-term steroid use, it may take 6 to 12 months after discontinuation of steroids for the adrenal glands to recover. Preoperative glucocorticoid coverage should be provided for patients with a positive ACTH stimulation test, with Cushing's syndrome and AI, or who are at risk for AI because of prior glucocorticoid therapy. Patients with known or suspected adrenal suppression or AI should receive their baseline therapy plus supplementation in the perioperative period. Supplementation is individualized based on the surgery (see **Table 16-12**).

4. Management of Anesthesia. Therapy includes glucocorticoid replacement and correction of water and sodium deficits. Glucocorticoid replacement may include intravenous hydrocortisone, methylprednisolone, or dexamethasone. Volume deficits may be substantial (2 to 3 L), and 5% glucose in normal saline is the fluid of choice. Hemodynamic support with vasopressors such as dopamine may be necessary. Metabolic acidosis and hyperkalemia usually resolve with fluids and steroids. Acute AI should be considered in the differential diagnosis of hemodynamic instability only after more common etiologies have been treated or ruled out (hypovolemia, anesthetic overdose, cardiopulmonary disorders, surgical mechanical problems). Etomidate inhibits the synthesis of cortisol transiently in normal patients and should be avoided. Patients with untreated AI presenting for emergency surgery may require invasive monitoring.

5. Intensive Care Unit Management. The incidence of AI in high-risk, critically ill patients with hypotension, shock, and sepsis is approximately 30% to 40%. All patients suspected of having AI should be tested for serum cortisol and have an ACTH stimulation test, especially if the stress level is uncertain.

VI. PARATHYROID GLAND DYSFUNCTION

A. Hyperparathyroidism is present when the secretion of parathormone is increased. Serum calcium concentrations may be increased, decreased, or unchanged. Hyperparathyroidism is classified as primary, secondary, or ectopic.

1. Primary Hyperparathyroidism results from excessive secretion of parathormone because of a benign parathyroid adenoma, carcinoma of a

TABLE 16-12 Steroid (Hydrocortisone) Supplementation	
Superficial surgery Dental, biopsies	None
Minor surgery Inguinal hernia, colonoscopy	25 mg IV
Moderate surgery Cholecystectomy, colon	50–75 mg IV, taper 1–2 days
Severe surgery Cardiovascular, liver, Whipple	100–150 mg IV, taper 1–2 days
Intensive care unit Sepsis, shock	50–100 mg q6–8h for 2 days to 1 wk, taper

parathyroid gland, or hyperplasia of the parathyroid glands. Hyperparathyroidism caused by an adenoma or hyperplasia is the most common presenting symptom of multiple endocrine neoplasia 1 syndrome.

a. Diagnosis. Hypercalcemia (serum calcium concentration >5.5 mEq/L and ionized calcium concentration >2.5 mEq/L) is the hallmark of primary hyperparathyroidism. Measurement of serum parathormone concentrations is not always sufficiently reliable to confirm the diagnosis of primary hyperparathyroidism.

b. Signs and Symptoms (Table 16-13)

c. Treatment

   1.) Medical Management is saline infusion (150 mL/hr) and loop diuretics (furosemide 40 to 80 mg IV every 2 to 4 hours). Bisphosphonates such as disodium etidronate are administered intravenously for life-threatening hypercalcemia. Hemodialysis can lower serum calcium concentrations, as can calcitonin, but the effects of this hormone are transient. Mithramycin inhibits the osteoclastic activity of parathormone, producing prompt lowering of serum calcium concentrations. The toxic effects (thrombocytopenia, hepatotoxicity, nephrotoxicity) limit its use.

   2.) Surgical Management is the definitive treatment, resulting in normalization of serum calcium concentration within 3 to 4 days.

TABLE 16-13	Signs and Symptoms of Hypercalcemia Caused by Hyperparathyroidism
Organ System	**Signs and Symptoms**
Neuromuscular	Skeletal muscle weakness
Renal	Polyuria and polydipsia Decreased glomerular filtration rate Kidney stones
Hematopoietic	Anemia
Cardiac	Prolonged PR interval Short QT interval Systemic hypertension
Gastrointestinal	Vomiting Abdominal pain Peptic ulcer Pancreatitis
Skeletal	Skeletal demineralization Collapse of vertebral bodies Pathologic fractures
Nervous system	Somnolence Decreased pain sensation Psychosis
Ocular	Calcifications (band keratopathy) Conjunctivitis

Postoperative complications include hypocalcemic tetany, hypomagnesemia, and acute arthritis.

3.) *Management of Anesthesia.* There is no evidence that any specific anesthetic drugs or techniques are necessary in patients with primary hyperparathyroidism undergoing elective surgical treatment of the disease.

2. Secondary Hyperparathyroidism reflects an appropriate compensatory response of the parathyroid glands to secrete more parathormone to counteract a disease process that produces hypocalcemia (e.g., chronic renal disease). Secondary hyperparathyroidism seldom produces hypercalcemia, and treatment is directed at controlling the underlying disease.

3. Ectopic Hyperparathyroidism is caused by secretion of parathormone (or a substance with similar endocrine effects) by tissues other than the parathyroid glands. Carcinoma of the lung, breast, pancreas, or kidney and lymphoproliferative disease are the most likely ectopic sites for parathormone secretion.

B. Hypoparathyroidism is present when secretion of parathormone is absent or deficient or peripheral tissues are resistant to the effects of the hormone (**Table 16-14**). Pseudohypoparathyroidism is a congenital disorder in which the release of parathormone is intact but the kidneys are unable to respond to the hormone. Affected patients manifest mental retardation, calcification of the basal ganglia, obesity, short stature, and short metacarpals and metatarsals.

1. Diagnosis. A serum calcium concentration less than 4.5 mEq/L and an ionized calcium concentration less than 2.0 mEq/L indicate hypoparathyroidism.

TABLE 16-14   Etiology of Hypoparathyroidism
Decreased or Absent Parathormone
Accidental removal of parathyroid glands during thyroidectomy
Parathyroidectomy to treat hyperplasia
Idiopathic (DiGeorge syndrome)
Resistance of Peripheral Tissues to Effects of Parathormone
Congenital
Pseudohypoparathyroidism
Acquired
Hypomagnesemia
Chronic renal failure
Malabsorption
Anticonvulsive therapy (phenytoin)
Unknown
Osteoblastic metastases
Acute pancreatitis

2. Signs and Symptoms. Signs and symptoms of hypoparathyroidism depend on the rapidity of the onset of hypocalcemia.

a. Acute Hypocalcemia may manifest as perioral paresthesias, restlessness, and neuromuscular irritability, as evidenced by a positive Chvostek sign or Trousseau sign. A positive Chvostek sign consists of facial muscle twitching produced by manual tapping over the area of the facial nerve at the angle of the mandible. A positive Trousseau sign is carpopedal spasm produced by 3 minutes of limb ischemia produced by a tourniquet. Inspiratory stridor reflects neuromuscular irritability of the intrinsic laryngeal musculature.

b. Chronic Hypocalcemia is associated with fatigue and skeletal muscle cramps, and, possibly, prolonged QT interval on the electrocardiogram. Neurologic changes include lethargy, cerebration deficits, and personality changes. Chronic hypocalcemia is associated with formation of cataracts, calcification involving the subcutaneous tissues and basal ganglia, and thickening of the skull. Chronic renal failure is the most common cause of chronic hypocalcemia.

3. Treatment of acute hypocalcemia is infusion of calcium (10 mL of 10% calcium gluconate IV) until signs of neuromuscular irritability disappear. For treatment of asymptomatic hypoparathyroidism, treatment is oral calcium and vitamin D.

4. Management of Anesthesia. Goals are to prevent further decreases in the serum calcium concentrations (avoid hyperventilation, rapid infusion of blood) and to treat the adverse effects of hypocalcemia.

VII. PITUITARY GLAND DYSFUNCTION

The pituitary gland, located in the sella turcica at the base of the brain, consists of the anterior pituitary and posterior pituitary. The anterior pituitary secretes six hormones under control of the hypothalamus (**Table 16-15**).

A. Acromegaly is caused by excessive secretion of growth hormone in adults, most often by an adenoma in the anterior pituitary gland. Failure of plasma growth hormone concentrations to decrease 1 to 2 hours after ingestion of 75 to 100 g of glucose or growth hormone concentrations greater than 3 ng/mL are presumptive evidence of acromegaly. Radiographic or CT evidence of enlargement of the sella turcica is characteristic of anterior pituitary adenomas.

1. Signs and Symptoms (Table 16-16)

2. Treatment. Transsphenoidal surgical excision of pituitary adenomas is the preferred initial therapy. When adenomas have extended beyond the sella turcica, surgery or radiation is no longer feasible; medical treatment with suppressant drugs (bromocriptine) may be an option.

3. Management of Anesthesia for patients with acromegaly should consider potential changes in the upper airway (distorted facial anatomy, enlargement of the tongue and epiglottis, narrowed glottic opening, nasal turbinate enlargement) that can predispose to difficult intubation and should anticipate the possible need to insert a smaller-diameter tracheal tube. When placing a catheter in the radial artery, it is important to consider the possibility of inadequate collateral circulation at the wrist. Monitoring

TABLE 16-15 Hypothalamic and Related Pituitary Hormones

Hypothalamic Hormone	Action	Pituitary Hormone or Organ Affected	Action
Corticotropin-releasing hormone	Stimulatory	Corticotropin	Stimulates secretion of cortisol and androgens
Thyrotropin-releasing hormone	Stimulatory	Thyrotropin	Stimulates secretion of thyroxine and triiodothyronine
Gonadotropin-releasing hormone	Stimulatory	Follicle-stimulating hormone Luteinizing hormone	Stimulates secretion of estradiol[*] Stimulates secretion of progesterone,[*] stimulates ovulation,[*] stimulates secretion of testosterone,[†] stimulates spermatogenesis[†]
Growth hormone–releasing hormone	Stimulatory	Growth hormone	Stimulates production of insulin-like growth factor
Dopamine	Inhibitory	Prolactin	Stimulates lactation[*]
Somatostatin	Inhibitory	Growth hormone	
Vasopressin (antidiuretic hormone)	Stimulatory	Kidneys	Stimulates free-water reabsorption
Oxytocin	Stimulatory	Uterus	Stimulates uterine contractions[*]
		Breasts	Stimulates milk ejection[*]

[*]Actions in females.
[†]Actions in males.
Adapted from Vance ML: Hypopituitarism. N Engl J Med 1994;330:1651–1662.

blood glucose concentrations is useful if diabetes mellitus or glucose intolerance accompanies acromegaly.

B. Diabetes Insipidus reflects the absence of vasopressin (antidiuretic hormone [ADH]) caused by destruction of the posterior pituitary (neurogenic diabetes insipidus) or failure of renal tubules to respond to ADH (nephrogenic diabetes insipidus). Neurogenic and nephrogenic diabetes insipidus are differentiated based on the response to desmopressin, which concentrates urine in the presence of neurogenic, but not nephrogenic, diabetes insipidus.

1. Treatment is intravenous infusion of electrolyte solutions if oral intake cannot offset polyuria. Chlorpropamide potentiates the effects of ADH on

TABLE 16-16	Manifestations of Acromegaly
Parasellar	
Enlarged sella turcica	
Headache	
Visual field defects	
Rhinorrhea	
Excess growth hormone	
Skeletal overgrowth (prognathism)	
Soft-tissue overgrowth (lips, tongue, epiglottis, vocal cords)	
Connective tissue overgrowth (recurrent laryngeal nerve paralysis)	
Peripheral neuropathy (carpal tunnel syndrome)	
Visceromegaly	
Glucose tolerance	
Osteoarthritis	
Osteoporosis	
Hyperhydrosis	
Skeletal muscle weakness	

renal tubules and may be useful for treating nephrogenic diabetes insipidus. Treatment of neurogenic diabetes insipidus is with ADH administered intramuscularly every 2 to 4 days or by intranasal administration of DDAVP.

2. Management of Anesthesia for patients with diabetes insipidus includes monitoring the urine output and serum electrolyte concentrations during the perioperative period.

C. Syndrome of Inappropriate Secretion of Antidiuretic Hormone (SIADH) can occur in many pathologic processes (intracranial tumors, hypothyroidism, porphyria, carcinoma of the lung).

1. Diagnosis. Inappropriately increased urinary sodium concentrations and osmolarity in the presence of hyponatremia and decreased serum osmolarity are highly suggestive of inappropriate ADH secretion. Abrupt decreases in serum sodium concentrations, especially less than 110 mEq/L, can result in cerebral edema and seizures.

2. Treatment is restricted oral fluid intake (approximately 500 mL/day), antagonism of the effects of ADH on the renal tubules by administration of demeclocycline, and intravenous infusions of sodium chloride. In patients manifesting acute neurologic symptoms caused by hyponatremia, intravenous infusions of hypertonic saline sufficient to increase serum sodium concentrations 0.5 mEq/L/hr are recommended. Overly rapid correction of chronic hyponatremia has been associated with central pontine myelinolysis.

CHAPTER 17

Hematologic Disorders

ERYTHROCYTE DISORDERS

Disease states may be related to abnormal concentrations (anemia, polycythemia) or structures of hemoglobin (Hb). Oxygen-carrying capacity and adequacy of tissue oxygen delivery are often the most important clinical manifestations of these derangements.

I. ANEMIA

A. Physiology. In adults, anemia is usually defined as Hb concentrations less than 11.5 g/dL (hematocrit, 36%) for women and less than 12.5 g/dL (hematocrit, 40%) for men. Adverse effects of anemia are decreased tissue oxygen delivery due to decreases in arterial content of oxygen (CaO_2). Compensatory mechanisms for anemia are (1) rightward shift of the oxyhemoglobin dissociation curve (release of oxygen from Hb to tissues—see **Fig. 17-1**), (2) increased cardiac output, and (3) increased release of erythropoietin to stimulate red blood cell (RBC) production.

B. Symptoms include fatigue and decreased exercise tolerance.

C. Anesthetic Considerations. Generally accepted minimum Hb concentration for elective anesthesia and surgery is 10 g/dL. Transfusion is not based on absolute Hb concentration, but on risks of anemia (depends on age, co-existing disease) versus those of transfusion (infectious disease, transfusion reaction, immunosuppression). In chronic anemia, cardiac output does not increase below Hb concentration of about 7 g/dL. In patients undergoing anesthesia who have chronic anemia, conditions that interfere with tissue oxygen delivery (decreased cardiac output, respiratory alkalosis, hypothermia) should be avoided. Normovolemic hemodilution and intraoperative blood salvage should be considered.

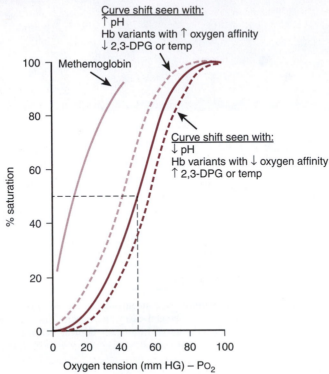

Figure 17-1 • Normal oxyhemoglobin dissociation curve and factors that result in displacement of O_2 dissociation. 2,3-DPG, 2,3-diphosphoglycerate; Hb, hemoglobin.

II. DISORDERS AFFECTING RED CELL STRUCTURE.

The mature RBC at rest takes the shape of a flexible biconcave disk. It lacks a nucleus or mitochondria, and intracellular energy requirements are supplied by glucose metabolism. Without a nucleus or protein metabolic pathway, the cell has a limited life span of 100 to 120 days.

A. Hereditary Spherocytosis (HS): Clinical Manifestations. HS is usually an autosomal dominant disease. These cells show abnormal osmotic fragility and shortened circulation half-life. Hemolytic anemia can range from mild to severe. Hemolytic crises (hemolysis, jaundice, rare aplastic crisis) sometimes occur. The primary anesthetic consideration is the occurrence of episodic anemia.

B. Hereditary Elliptocytosis. An autosomal dominant abnormality in one of the membrane proteins, spectrin or glycophorin, makes the erythrocyte less pliable. Heterozygous patients rarely experience hemolysis, but homozygous or compound heterozygous patients may have significant hemolysis and anemia.

C. Acanthocytosis is a defect in membrane structure in patients with a congenital lack of lipoprotein-β (abetalipoproteinemia) and with severe cirrhosis or pancreatitis. The membrane has a spiculated appearance. Hemolysis and anemia are the primary issues.

D. Paroxysmal Nocturnal Hemoglobinuria is a clonal disorder of hematopoietic cells involving abnormalities in or reductions of a membrane protein (glycosylphosphatidyl glycan). Patients often present with hemolytic anemia and are at increased risk of venous thrombosis due to activation of coagulation by abnormal complement activation.

III. DISORDERS AFFECTING RED CELL METABOLISM

The stability of the RBC membrane and the solubility of intracellular Hb depend on four glucose-supported metabolic pathways (**Fig. 17-2**). Anesthetic concerns involve avoiding triggering events for hemolysis and management of chronic anemia.

A. The Embden-Meyerhof Pathway (nonoxidative or anaerobic pathway) generates adenosine triphosphate necessary for membrane function and maintenance of cell shape and pliability. Defects in anaerobic glycolysis are associated with increased cell rigidity and decreased survival, as well as hemolytic anemia. There are no characteristic morphologic changes. The severity of hemolysis is highly variable.

B. The Phosphogluconate Pathway counteracts environmental oxidants and prevents globin denaturation. Lack of either of the two key enzymes, glucose-6-phosphate dehydrogenase (G6PD) or glutathione reductase, results in membrane damage and hemolysis.

    1. Glucose-6-Phosphate Dehydrogenase (G6PD) Deficiency is one of the most prevalent disease-causing mutations and is encoded on the X chromosome. Manifestations are (1) chronic hemolytic anemia, (2) acute episodic hemolytic anemia, or (3) no apparent hemolysis. Events exacerbating anemia include infections, drugs (methylene blue), and fava bean ingestion.

    2. Pyruvate Kinase Deficiency (the most common erythrocyte enzyme defect causing hemolytic anemia) is more likely than G6PD deficiency to cause a chronic hemolytic anemia. Splenectomy decreases the rate of RBC destruction. Severity ranges from mild hemolysis without anemia to life-threatening, transfusion-requiring hemolytic anemia present at birth. Other clinical signs are chronic jaundice, pigmented gallstones, and splenomegaly.

C. The Methemoglobin Reductase Pathway maintains heme iron in its ferrous state. Mutation of the methemoglobin reductase enzyme results in an inability to counteract oxidation of Hb to methemoglobin (which will not transport oxygen). Patients with type I enzyme deficiency accumulate small amounts of methemoglobin in circulating red cells, whereas type II patients have severe cyanosis and mental retardation.

D. The Luebering-Rapaport Pathway produces 2,3-DPG (also known as 2,3-bisphosphoglycerate). A single enzyme, bisphospheroglyceromutase, mediates both the synthase activity, resulting in 2,3-DPG formation, and the phosphatase activity that converts 2,3-DPG to 3-phosphoglycerate, returning it to the glycolytic pathway. Severe phosphate depletion results in a reduced 2,3-DPG production response.

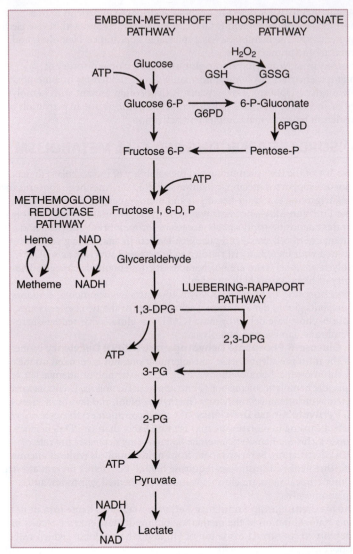

Figure 17-2 • Diagrammatic representation of the four most common disorders affecting the red cell metabolism. 6PGD, 6-phosphogluconate dehydrogenase; ATP, adenosine triphosphate; G6PD, glucose-6-phosphate dehydrogenase; GSH, glutathione reductase; GSSG, oxidized glutathione; NAD, nicotinamide adenine dinucleotide; NADH, reduced form of nicotinamide adenine dinucleotide.

IV. THE HEMOGLOBIN MOLECULE

Each heme group can bind an oxygen molecule. The respiratory motion (i.e., uptake and release of oxygen) involves a specific change in the molecular structure of Hb. Oxygen binding by one of the heme groups increases the affinity of the other groups for oxygen. Inherited defects in Hb structure can interfere with this respiratory motion. Some defects restrict the molecule to either a low- or high-affinity state, and others either change heme iron from ferrous to ferric or reduce the solubility of the Hb molecule. Hb S (sickle cell disease) results in reduced solubility and precipitation of the abnormal Hb.

A. Disorders of Hemoglobin Resulting in Hemolysis

1. Sickle S Hemoglobin. In the deoxygenated state, Hb S undergoes conformational changes exposing a hydrophobic region of the molecule. These regions aggregate, distorting and damaging the erythrocyte membrane, causing deformation and a shortened life span. Sickle cell anemia (homozygous Hb S disease) presents early in life as severe hemolytic anemia and vaso-occlusive disease involving the marrow, spleen, kidney, and central nervous system. Other clinical manifestations are painful crises (bone and joint pain, recurrent splenic infarction [functional asplenia], renal medullary infarcts [chronic renal failure], and acute chest syndrome [new pulmonary infiltrate and at least one of the following: chest pain, fever higher than 38.5°C, tachypnea, wheezing, or cough]) and eurologic complications (stroke).

>   *a. Anesthetic Considerations.* Risk factors for perioperative complications include age, frequency of hospitalizations and/or transfusions for episodes of crisis, and evidence of organ damage. There is no benefit in aggressive preoperative transfusion to decrease the ratio of Hb S to normal Hb, compared with the goal of achieving a preoperative hematocrit of 30%. Anesthetic technique does not affect the risk. Avoiding dehydration, acidosis, and hypothermia during anesthesia should reduce perioperative sickling. Acute chest syndrome may develop typically 2 to 3 days into the postoperative period.

2. Sickle C Hemoglobin, much less prevalent than Hb S, causes the erythrocyte to lose water via enhanced activity of the potassium-chloride co-transport system and is associated with a mild-to-moderate hemolytic anemia. The presence of both Hb S and Hb C (Hb SC) produces a tendency toward sickling and associated complications approaching that of Hb SS disease. Transfusions may reduce the incidence of sickle complications in this subset.

3. Hemoglobin Sickle–β-Thalassemia. Clinical presentation is largely determined by whether it is associated with reduced amounts of Hb A (sickle cell–β+ thalassemia) or complete absence of Hb A (sickle cell-β_{zero} thalassemia). In the latter, patients experience acute vaso-occlusive crises, acute chest syndrome, and other sickling complications at rates approaching those of Hb SS. Anesthetic considerations are the same as those for homozygous sickle S Hb.

B. Unstable Hemoglobins.
Structural changes can destabilize Hb molecules and reduce their solubility or make them more susceptible to oxidation. Destabilizing mutations typically impair globin folding or heme-globin binding that holds the heme moiety within the globin pocket. Once freed

from the pocket, heme binds nonspecifically to other regions of the globin chains, causing them to form a precipitate containing globin chains and chain fragments and heme (Heinz body). Heinz bodies reduce red cell deformability and favor their removal by splenic macrophages. Anesthetic management involves transfusion for severe hemolysis and avoidance of oxidizing agents.

V. DISORDERS OF HEMOGLOBIN RESULTING IN REDUCED OR INEFFECTIVE ERYTHROPOIESIS: MACROCYTIC/MEGALOBLASTIC ANEMIA

Disruption of the red cell maturation sequence by vitamin deficiencies, chemotherapy, or preleukemic states results in macrocytic anemias and megaloblastic bone marrow morphology.

A. Folic Acid and Vitamin B_{12} Deficiencies are primary causes of macrocytic anemia in adults. Marrow precursors appear much larger than normal and are unable to complete cell division. The marrow becomes megaloblastic, and macrocytic red cells are released into the circulation.

B. Other Causes include alcoholism, tropical and nontropical sprue (malabsorption), and chronic nitrous oxide exposure.

C. Macrocytic Anemia caused by folate or vitamin B_{12} deficiency may result in Hb levels less than 8 to 10 g/dL, a mean red cell volume of 110 to 140 fL (normal = 90 fL), a normal reticulocyte count, and increased levels of lactate dehydrogenase and bilirubin. Vitamin B_{12} deficiency is associated with bilateral peripheral neuropathy (degeneration of the lateral and posterior spinal cord columns), memory impairment, and depression.

D. Anesthetic Management is aimed at maintaining oxygen delivery to tissues. Regional techniques might be avoided because of the presence of neuropathy. Even relatively short exposures to nitrous oxide may produce megaloblastic changes.

VI. DISORDERS OF HEMOGLOBIN RESULTING IN REDUCED OR INEFFECTIVE ERYTHROPOIESIS: MICROCYTIC ANEMIA

A. Iron Deficiency Anemia is caused by chronic blood loss in nonpregnant adults. Nutritional deficiency of iron causes anemia only in infants and small children. Parturients are susceptible to iron deficiency anemia caused by increased RBC mass and the needs of the fetus for iron.

    1. Diagnosis is made by evidence of mild microcytic, hypochromic anemia (Hb 9-12 g/dL), and decreased serum ferritin concentrations.

    2. Treatment is ferrous iron salts (oral ferrous sulfate). Appropriate response to iron therapy is an increase in Hb concentration of 2 g/dL in 3 weeks or return of Hb concentrations to normal in 6 weeks. Recombinant human erythropoietin may be used to treat drug-induced anemia or to improve Hb concentrations before elective surgery.

B. Defective Production of Globin Chains: the Thalassemias. In adults, 96% to 97% of Hb consists of two α-globin and two β-globin chains (Hb A) with minor components of Hb F and A_2. An inherited defect in globin chain synthesis, thalassemia, is one of the leading causes of microcytic anemia.

1. **Thalassemia Minor** occurs in individuals who are heterozygotes for a α-globin (α-thalassemia trait) or β-globin (β-thalassemia trait) gene mutation. The anemia is usually modest (Hb 10–14 g/dL) and morbidity is rare.

2. **Thalassemia Intermedia** patients present with more severe anemia and prominent microcytosis and hypochromia. They may have hepatosplenomegaly, cardiomegaly, and skeletal changes secondary to marrow expansion. These patients have either a milder form of homozygous β-thalassemia, a combined α- and β-thalassemia defect, or β-thalassemia with high levels of Hb F.

3. **Thalassemia Major** patients develop severe, life-threatening anemia during during childhood and require long-term transfusion therapy. Complications of iron overload (cirrhosis, right-sided heart failure, and endocrinopathy) often require chelation therapy. In its most severe forms, patients exhibit three defects that markedly depress their oxygen-carrying capacity: (1) ineffective erythropoiesis, (2) hemolytic anemia, and (3) hypochromia with microcytosis. Other features of severe thalassemia include those attributable to massive marrow hyperplasia (frontal bossing, maxillary overgrowth, stunted growth, osteoporosis) and extramedullary hematopoiesis (hepatomegaly). Bone marrow transplantation is a therapeutic option.

VII. HEMOGLOBINS WITH INCREASED OXYGEN AFFINITY: HEMOGLOBIN CHESAPEAKE, J-CAPETOWN, KEMSEY, AND CRETEIL

These Hbs bind oxygen more readily than normal and deliver less oxygen to tissues at normal capillary PO_2 levels. Blood returns to the lungs still saturated with oxygen. Mild tissue hypoxia results, with increased erythropoietin production and polycythemia. Patients with mild erythrocytosis do not need treatment. Patients with high hematocrits (>55%–60%), whose blood viscosity may further compromise oxygen delivery, may require exchange transfusion and careful avoidance of hemoconcentration both pre- and intraoperatively. Hemodilution and blood loss, however, may cause critical decreases in the tissue oxygen delivery, even at hematocrits tolerated by patients with normal Hbs.

VIII. HEMOGLOBINS WITH DECREASED OXYGEN AFFINITY

A. **Methemoglobinemia.** Methemoglobin (MHb) is formed when iron in the Hb is oxidized from the ferrous (Fe^{2+}) state to the ferric (Fe^{3+}) state. The normal erythrocyte maintains MHb levels at 1% or less. MHb has high oxygen affinity and delivers little oxygen to the tissues. When MHb is 30% to 50% of the total hemoglobin, symptoms of oxygen deprivation occur, and at more than 50%, coma and death can ensue.

Methemoglobinemias result from (1) mutations that favor formation of MHb, (2) mutations impairing the methemoglobin reductase system, and

(3) toxic exposures that oxidize normal Hb iron at a rate exceeding the capacity of normal reducing mechanisms. MHb has a brownish-blue color that does not change to red on exposure to oxygen, giving patients a cyanotic appearance independent of their PaO_2.

1. Patients with MHbs are usually asymptomatic, as their MHb levels rarely exceed 30% of their total Hb.

2. Mutations impairing the methemoglobin reductase system rarely result in methemoglobinemia levels greater than 25%.

3. Exposure to chemical agents may produce an acquired methemoglobinemia that is virtually the only situation in which life-threatening amounts of MHb accumulate.

4. Emergency Treatment is 1to 2 mg/kg of intravenous methylene blue infused over 3 to 5 minutes. Methylene blue acts through the reduced nicotinamide adenine dinucleotide phosphate reductase system and accordingly requires the activity of G6PD. Patients who are G6PD deficient and patients severely affected may require exchange transfusions.

5. Anesthetic Management includes avoidance of oxidizing agents and measurement of blood pH and occasionally MHb levels (for the rare patient at risk of methemoglobinemia >30%).

IX. DISORDERS OF RED CELL PRODUCTION

A. Hypoproliferation

1. Constitutional Aplastic Anemia (Fanconi Anemia) is an autosomal recessive disorder that presents with severe pancytopenia usually in the first two decades of life and often progresses to acute leukemia.

2. Drug-Associated and Radiation-Associated Marrow Damage Anemia is a predictable side effect of chemotherapy and radiation therapy. Recovery is usually full, provided there is a sufficient infection-free period. Long-term exposure to low levels of external radiation or ingested radioisotopes and certain drugs can cause aplastic anemia (**Table 17-1**).

3. Infection-Associated Marrow Damage Anemia. Marrow damage can result from direct invasion of the marrow itself by an infectious agent (miliary TB) or by immunosuppression of stem cell growth. Aplastic anemia is seen following viral illnesses (hepatitis, Epstein-Barr virus infection, human immunodeficiency virus, rubella, parvovirus).

4. Anemia Caused by Hematologic or Other Marrow-Involving Malignancy. Anemias may be caused by any leukemia, by solid tumor metastases to the marrow (breast, lung, prostate), and by clonal expansion of other marrow constituents (myelodysplastic syndromes, myeloproliferative disorders). By contrast, clonal expansion of erythroid cells in the marrow, or erythrocytosis, may produce polycythemia vera, discussed in the next section.

5. Patients may present for surgery with anemia and thrombocytopenia that require transfusion. Immunocompromise may affect the need for and choice of antibiotic coverage.

B. Polycythemia. Sustained hypoxia causes a rise in the RBC mass and hematocrit. At a hematocrit level >50%, blood viscosity can be increased to a point at which blood flow to key organs such as the brain can be significantly reduced.

TABLE 17-1	Classes of Drugs Associated with Marrow Damage

Antibiotics (chloramphenicol, penicillin, cephalosporins, sulfonamides, amphotericin B, streptomycin)

Antidepressants (lithium, tricyclics)

Antiepileptics (Dilantin, carbamazepine, valproic acid, phenobarbital)

Anti-inflammatory drugs (phenylbutazone, nonsteroidals, salicylates, gold salts)

Antiarrhythmics (lidocaine, quinidine, procainamide)

Antithyroidal drugs (propylthiouracil)

Diuretics (thiazides, pyrimethamine, furosemide)

Antihypertensives (captopril)

Antiuricemics (allopurinol, colchicine)

Antimalarials (quinacrine, chloroquine)

Hypoglycemics (tolbutamide)

Platelet inhibitors (ticlopidine)

Tranquilizers (prochlorperazine, meprobamate)

1. Physiology. Polycythemia can be relative (reduction in plasma volume, no change in red cell mass) or absolute (increased red cell mass). Clinical signs and symptoms vary but, at hematocrit values of 55% to 60% or higher, can include headaches, easy fatigability, compromised organ perfusion, and venous and arterial thrombosis.

2. Primary Polycythemia, or Polycythemia Vera (PV), is a clonal stem cell disorder, which is nearly always caused by a mutation in the JAK-2 gene. Platelets and leukocytes may also be increased. Diagnostic criteria for PV are an elevated hematocrit or RBC mass, normal arterial oxygenation, and splenomegaly not attributable to another cause. Thrombosis (especially cerebral thrombosis) may be the presenting symptom. Treatment is regular phlebotomy to a hematocrit of 45% for men and 38% to 40% for women. Alternative treatment is administration of hydroxyurea.

   a. Anesthesia Management. PV patients are at increased risk of perioperative thrombosis and, paradoxically, hemorrhage. Bleeding associated with PV is caused by acquired von Willebrand's (vW) disease resulting from hyperviscosity-related changes in vW factor. Phlebotomy and avoidance of extreme dehydration lower the risk of both thrombosis and hemorrhage in the PV patient in the perioperative period.

3. Secondary Polycythemia Caused by Hypoxia can occur in individuals who live at high altitude, those with chronic tissue hypoxia caused by significant cardiopulmonary disease (e.g., cyanotic congenital heart disease, low cardiac output states), and inherited defects in Hb, such as high-affinity Hb and defects in 2,3-DPG amount or function (impaired delivery of oxygen causing tissue hypoxia). Anesthetic considerations include oxygen therapy, preoperative phlebotomy when indicated, and appreciation of perioperative hypercoaguability and potential for bleeding diatheses.

305

4. Secondary Polycythemia Caused by Increased Erythropoietin Production. Renal disease (hydronephrosis, polycystic renal disease, benign and malignant renal tumors) and erythropoietin-secreting tumors have been associated with secondary polycythemia. Nonrenal tumors (uterine myomas, hepatomas, cerebellar hemangiomas) sometimes secrete erythropoietin. Treatment is management of the underlying disorder and phlebotomy when necessary.

DISORDERS OF HEMOSTASIS

Disorders of hemostasis can be acquired or hereditary (**Table 17-2**). Activation of coagulation can be divided into two phases.

A. Initiation Phase. Blood is exposed to a source of tissue factor (TF), usually on subendothelial cells following damage to a blood vessel. TF binds factor VIIa in the circulating blood, catalyzing the conversion of factor X to Xa, which then generates thrombin.

B. Propagation Phase. Thrombin activates platelets and factors V and VIII, with formation of FVIIIa-IXa complex. This complex turns on a "switch" in coagulation, from the TF-VIIa catalyzed reaction to the Xase (intrinsic) pathway. This pathway is much more efficient in producing Xa, and explosive thrombin generation occurs.

Common laboratory tests of soluble coagulation (prothrombin time [PT] and activated partial thromboplastin time [PTT]) only measure the kinetics of the initiation phase. These tests are sensitive at detecting severe deficiencies in clotting factors—for example, hemophilia—and in guiding warfarin/heparin therapy; they do not necessarily predict the risk of intraoperative bleeding.

I. HEMOSTATIC DISORDERS AFFECTING COAGULATION FACTORS OF THE INITIATION PHASE

A. Factor VII Deficiency. Factor VII deficiency is a rare autosomal recessive disease with highly variable clinical severity. Only homozygous deficient patients have factor VII levels generally low enough (<15%) to have symptomatic bleeding. The unique laboratory pattern is a prolonged PT with a normal PTT.

1. Anesthetic Considerations. Treatment depends on the severity of the deficiency. Patients with mild to moderate deficiency can be treated with infusions of fresh frozen plasma (FFP). Patients with factor VII levels less than 1% require treatment with a concentrated source of factor VII, such as Proplex T (factor IX complex, with a high level of factor VII). In the case of active bleeding, activated recombinant factor VIIa should be used, beginning with a dose of 20 to 30 μg/kg, with redosing directed by PT results.

B. Congenital Deficiencies in Factors X, V, and Prothrombin (II) are autosomal recessive disorders. Severe deficiencies are rare. Patients with severe deficiencies in any of these factors demonstrate prolongations of both PT and PTT. Patients with congenital factor V deficiency may also have a prolonged bleeding time because of the relationship between factor V and platelet function in supporting clot formation.

1. Anesthetic Considerations. Deficiencies in factors X, V, and prothrombin are can be corrected with FFP, but large volumes are needed (4–6 units or

TABLE 17-2	Categorization of Coagulation Disorders
Hereditary	
Hemophilia A	
Hemophilia B	
Von Willebrand's disease	
Afibrinogenemia	
Factor V deficiency	
Factor VIII deficiency	
Hereditary hemorrhagic telangiectasia	
Protein C deficiency	
Antithrombin III deficiency	
Acquired	
Disseminated intravascular coagulation	
Perioperative anticoagulation	
Intraoperative coagulopathies	
Dilutional thrombocytopenia	
Dilution of procoagulants	
Massive blood transfusion	
Type of surgery (cardiopulmonary bypass, brain trauma, orthopedic surgery, urologic surgery, obstetric delivery)	
Drug-induced hemorrhage	
Drug-induced platelet dysfunction	
Idiopathic thrombocytopenic purpura	
Thrombotic thrombocytopenic purpura	
Catheter-induced thrombocytopenia	
Vitamin K deficiency	

800–1200 mL to increase factor level 20%–30%). Factor V is stored in platelet granules, and in a bleeding patient, platelet transfusion is an alternative way to replace factor V. For patients with severe deficiencies, several prothrombin complex concentrates (PCCs) are available, which lower the risk of volume overload but may be associated with thrombosis, thromboembolism, and disseminated intravascular coagulation (DIC).

II. HEMOSTATIC DISORDERS AFFECTING COAGULATION FACTORS OF THE PROPAGATION PHASE

Not all deficiencies causing prolongation of the PTT are associated with bleeding. Deficiencies of factor XII, high molecular weight kininogen, and prekallikrein, for example, do not increase the risk of bleeding. Patient with deficiencies in these particular factors require no special management except alteration of their coagulation testing to allow accurate measurement of physiologic factors critical to in vivo hemostasis.

A. Hemophilia A and Hemophilia B

1. Congenital Factor VIII Deficiency: Hemophilia A is an X-linked recessive genetic disorder. Clinical severity of hemophilia A is best correlated with the factor VIII activity level. Severe hemophiliacs have factor VIII activity levels less than 1% of normal (<0.01 U/mL) and are usually diagnosed during childhood because of frequent, spontaneous hemorrhages into joints, muscles, and vital organs. Factor levels only 1% to 5% of normal reduce severity of the disease, but these patients are at increased risk of hemorrhage with surgery or trauma. Patients with factor levels between 6% to 30% are only mildly affected and may go undiagnosed into adult life. They are also at risk for excessive bleeding with a major surgical procedure. Female carriers of hemophilia A can also be at risk with surgery.

a. Diagnosis. Patients with severe hemophilia A are male and have a significantly prolonged PTT (in milder disease, the PTT may be only a few seconds longer than normal). The PT is normal. Factor VIII levels are necessary to distinguish hemophilia A from hemophilia B.

b. Anesthetic Considerations. The factor VIII level must be brought to near normal (100%) for major surgery in patients with severe hemophilia A. This requires an initial infusion of 50 to 60 U/kg (3500–4000 units in a 70-kg patient) of factor VIII concentrate. Repeat infusions of 25 to 30 U/kg every 8 to 12 hours are needed to keep the plasma factor VIII level greater than 50%. In children, the half-life of factor VIII may be shorter, necessitating more frequent infusions. Peak and trough factor VIII levels should be measured to confirm the appropriate dosing level and dosing interval. Therapy must be continued for up to 2 weeks to avoid postoperative bleeding that disrupts wound healing. Longer periods of therapy (4–6 weeks) may be required in patients who undergo bone or joint surgery. Up to 30% of severe hemophilia A patients exposed to factor VIII concentrate or recombinant product develop factor VIII inhibitors.

2. Congenital Factor IX Deficiency: Hemophilia B. This disease is clinically similar to hemophilia A. Factor IX levels of less than 1% are associated with severe bleeding. Moderate disease occurs in patients with levels of 1% to 5%. Patients with factor IX levels of 5% to 40% have very mild disease. Milder hemophilia (>5% factor IX activity) may not be detected until surgery is performed or the patient has a dental extraction. Hemophilia B patients also have a prolonged PTT and a normal PT.

a. Anesthetic Considerations. Recombinant/purified product or factor IX–PCC are used to treat mild bleeding episodes or as prophylaxis for minor procedures. However, these factor preparations are associated with increased risk of thromboembolic complications. Therefore, higher doses should only be used in patients undergoing major orthopedic surgery and those with severe traumatic injuries or liver disease. Purified factor IX concentrates or recombinant IX are used over several days to treat bleeding in hemophilia B. A dose of 100 U/kg (7000 units in a 70-kg patient) is administered, followed by repeated infusions at 50% of the original dose every 12 to 24 hours to keep factor IX plasma levels above 50%. Doses of 30 to 50 U/kg will give mean factor IX levels of 20% to 40% (adequate for less severe bleeding).

3. Acquired Factor VIII or IX Inhibitors. Approximately 30% to 40% of patients with severe deficiency of factor VIII develop circulating inhibitors to factor VIII. Hemophilia B patients are less likely to develop an inhibitor to factor IX (3%–5% incidence). A severe hemophilia-like syndrome can occur in genetically normal individuals secondary to the appearance of an acquired autoantibody to either factor VIII or, very rarely, to factor IX. These patients are usually middle-aged or older with no personal or family history of abnormal bleeding and present with the sudden onset of severe, spontaneous hemorrhage.

a. Diagnosis. The presence of an inhibitor is diagnosed by a mixing study in which the patient's plasma and normal plasma are mixed in a 1:1 ratio to determine whether the prolonged PTT shortens. In classic hemophilia A with no circulating VIII inhibitor, PTT usually shortens to within 4 seconds of normal or less, while little or no correction will occur in the presence of an inhibitor. Inhibitors are measured in Bethesda Units. Factor VIII inhibitor patients fall into one of two groups. High responders (>10 Bethesda U/mL) have a marked inhibitor response after any factor infusion and dramatic anamnestic responses to therapy. Their inhibitor levels cannot be neutralized by replacement therapy. Low responders (5–10 Bethesda U/ml) develop and maintain relatively low levels of inhibitor and do not show anamnestic responses to factor VIII concentrates.

b. Anesthetic Management of hemophilia A patients with inhibitors depends on whether the patient is a high- or low-responder. Low-responders can usually be managed with factor VIII concentrates. In high-responders, treatment with factor VIII concentrates is not feasible. Major life-threatening bleeds can be treated with bypass products such as activated PCCs or recombinant factor VIIa. Because of increased risk of thrombosis with PCCs, recombinant factor VIIa is now the treatment of choice for acquired inhibitors. For active bleeding, a dose of 90 to 120 µg/kg intravenously is recommended every 2 to 3 hours until hemostasis is achieved. Usually, factor IX inhibitor patients can be managed acutely using recombinant VIIa or PCC products. Patients who develop autoantibody to factor VIII or IX with no history of hemophilia can present with life-threatening hemorrhage and may exhibit very high inhibitor levels. Treatment with recombinant factor VIIa or an activated prothrombin concentrate is required; factor VIII or IX alone will not be effective.

B. Factor XI Deficiency. The only other defect causing an isolated prolongation of the PTT and a bleeding tendency is factor XI deficiency (Rosenthal's disease).

The bleeding tendency, if present at all, is quite mild and may only be apparent following a surgical procedure. Hematomas and hemarthroses are very unusual.

1. Anesthetic Considerations. Treatment depends on the severity of the deficiency and bleeding history. Most patients' factor XI deficiency can be treated with infusions of FFP. Treatment of factor XI deficiency with active bleeding is either PCCs or recombinant factor VIIa (20–30 μg/kg, with redosing according to PT results). Management of factor XI inhibitors is comparable to that of hemophilia A and B inhibitors.

C. Congenital Abnormalities in Fibrinogen production will obviously interfere with the final step in the generation of a fibrin clot.

1. Decreased Levels of Fibrinogen (Hypofibrinogenemia, Afibrinogenemia) are rare. Patients with afibrinogenemia have a severe bleeding diathesis with both spontaneous and posttraumatic bleeding. Hypofibrinogenemic patients usually do not have spontaneous bleeding but may have difficulty with surgery. Severe bleeding can be anticipated in patients with plasma fibrinogen levels below 50 to 100 mg/dL.

2. Dysfibrinogenemia (production of abnormal fibrinogen) is a more common defect. Clinical presentation is highly variable. Patients who demonstrate both a reduced amount and a dysfunctional fibrinogen (hypodysfibrinogenemia) usually exhibit excessive bleeding. Most dysfibrinogenemic patients do not have a bleeding tendency despite abnormal coagulation tests. Some patients have a paradoxical increased risk of thrombosis.

a. Diagnosis. Laboratory evaluation includes measurement of both fibrinogen concentration and function. Both thrombin time (TT) and clotting time are sensitive to fibrinogen dysfunction. Definitive diagnosis and subclassification of dysfibrinogenemia require fibrinopeptide chain analysis and amino acid sequencing.

3. Anesthetic Considerations. Most patients have no clinical disease and do not require therapy. For those who are symptomatic or are at risk of bleeding with surgery, cryoprecipitate therapy is warranted. To increase the fibrinogen level by at least 100 mg/dL in the average-size adult, 10 to 12 units of cryoprecipitate should be infused, followed by 2 to 3 units each day. Dysfibrinogenemia patients with a thrombotic tendency require long-term anticoagulation.

D. Factor XIII Deficiency. Factor XIII is involved in clot stability. Patients with factor XIII deficiency present at birth (persistent umbilical or circumcision bleeding). Adults have a severe bleeding diathesis (recurrent soft-tissue bleeding, poor wound healing, intracranial hemorrhage, spontaneous abortion). Typically, bleeding is delayed because clots form but are weak and unable to maintain hemostasis.

1. Diagnosis. Factor XIII deficiency should be suspected in a patient with a severe bleeding diathesis who has otherwise normal coagulation screening tests (PT, PTT, fibrinogen level, platelet count, bleeding time). Clot dissolution in 5M urea can be used as a screen, and definitive diagnosis is by enzyme-linked immunosorbent assay. Patients at risk of severe hemorrhage have factor XIII levels of 1% of normal.

2. Anesthetic Considerations. Factor XIII–deficient patients can be treated with FFP, cryoprecipitate, or a plasma-derived factor XIII concentrate (Fibrogammin P). Preoperative prophylaxis is possible using intravenous injections of 10 to 20 U/kg at 4- to 6-week intervals depending on the patient's preinfusion plasma factor XIII level. Acute hemorrhage should be treated with an infusion of 50 to 75 U/kg body weight.

ARTERIAL COAGULATION

I. DISORDERS AFFECTING PLATELET NUMBER

For relatively minor procedures (catheter insertions, biopsies, lumbar puncture) the platelet count should be more than 20,000 to 30,000/μL. For major surgery, the platelet count should, if possible, be 50,000 to 100,000/μL. Each unit of apheresis platelets or 6 units of random donor platelets should increase the platelet count in a normal-sized adult by about 50,000/μL. One unit of single-donor apheresis platelets is equivalent to a random donor pool of 4 to 8 units. Random and single-donor platelets do not need to be ABO compatible. However, Rh-negative women of child-bearing age should receive platelets from Rh-negative donors or be treated with RhoGAM following transfusion of Rh-positive product. Patients with very low platelet counts (<15,000/μL) may have significant bleeding from multiple sites, including the nose, mucous membranes, gastrointestinal tract, skin, and vessel puncture sites. One sign of thrombocytopenia is a petechial rash of the skin or mucous membranes.

A. Disorders Resulting in Platelet Production Defects
1. Congenital
a. Congenital Hypoplastic Thrombocytopenia with Absent Radii (TAR Syndrome) is an autosomal recessive disorder with thrombocytopenia in the third trimester of fetal development or early after birth. Thrombocytopenia is often initially severe (<30,000/μL) but slowly improves over time, nearing the normal range by age 2.

b. Fanconi Syndrome. Hematologic manifestations do not usually appear until about age 7. The bone marrow shows reduced cellularity and reduced numbers of megakaryocytes. Treatment is rarely necessary in the neonatal period. Stem cell transplantation is curative in the majority of children.

c. May-Hegglin Anomaly typically is associated with giant platelets in circulation and Döhle bodies (basophilic inclusions) in white blood cells. One third of patients have significant thrombocytopenia and risk of bleeding.

d. Wiskott-Aldrich Syndrome is an X-linked disorder that presents with eczema, immunodeficiency, and thrombocytopenia. Circulating platelets are smaller than normal, function poorly because of granule defects, and have a reduced survival.

e. Autosomal Dominant Thrombocytopenia shows increased megakaryocyte mass and ineffective production and, in some cases, the release of macrocytic platelets into circulation. Many of these patients have nerve deafness and nephritis (Alport's syndrome).

2. Acquired. A failure in platelet production can result from marrow damage (radiation and/or chemotherapy; insecticide or benzene exposure; reactions to thiazides, alcohol, estrogens, and viral hepatitis), neoplastic marrow infiltration (multiple myeloma, acute leukemia, lymphoma), and myeloproliferative disorders. Ineffective thrombopoiesis is also seen in patients with vitamin B_{12} or folate deficiency, including patients with alcoholism and defective folate metabolism. This failure in platelet production is rapidly reversed by appropriate vitamin therapy.

a. Anesthetic Considerations. Platelet transfusions are the mainstay of therapy. Ineffective thrombopoiesis associated with either vitamin B_{12} or folate deficiency should be immediately treated with appropriate vitamin therapy. Recovery of the platelet count to normal occurs within a matter of days, making platelet transfusion unnecessary in all but the most acute situations.

B. Disorders Caused by Platelet Destruction

1. Nonimmune Destruction

a. Thrombotic Thrombocytopenic Purpura (TTP). Signs may include fever, thrombocytopenia with an otherwise negative DIC screen (normal PT, PTT, and fibrinogen levels), multiple small vessel occlusions in multiple sites (kidney, central nervous system, skin, distal extremities), and a microangiopathic hemolytic anemia with schistocytosis (mechanical fragmentation of RBCs flowing past intra-arteriolar platelet thrombi).

    1.) Diagnosis. The triad of schistocytosis, thrombocytopenia, and elevated lactate dehydrogenase (evidence of a hemolysis) is considered diagnostic. TTP can be familial, sporadic (idiopathic), a chronic relapsing condition, a complication of marrow transplantation or drug therapy (quinine, ticlopidine, mitomycin C, interferon-α, pentostatin, gemcitabine, tacrolimus, or cyclosporine), or a complication of preeclampsia. Plasma exchange may be effective treatment in some cases.

b. Hemolytic-Uremic Syndrome (HUS) is most often seen in children who present with bloody diarrhea secondary to *Escherichia coli* or related bacteria and progress to acute renal failure; thrombocytopenia and anemia are less pronounced than seen with TTP. Most young children spontaneously recover with hemodialysis support, but mortality in adults and older children is high, and they should be treated with both plasma exchange and hemodialysis, regardless of the pattern of illness.

c. HELLP Syndrome. Up to 50% of preeclamptic mothers will develop a DIC-like picture with severe thrombocytopenia (platelet counts of 20,000 to 40,000/μL) at the time of delivery. This is referred to as HELLP syndrome when the combination of red cell hemolysis (H), elevated liver enzymes (EL), and low platelet count (LP) is present. Treatment is control of hypertension and delivery of the baby. A few patients will have full-blown TTP-HUS following delivery, which is a life-threatening illness with a poor prognosis.

d. Anesthetic Considerations. In patients with nonimmune destruction, platelet and plasma transfusions are supportive. The only truly effective therapy is the treatment of the underlying cause. Surgery should be delayed whenever possible until the underlying disorder is brought under control.

2. Autoimmune Destruction.
Severity of the thrombocytopenia is highly variable. With some conditions, the platelet count falls to as low as 1000 to 2000/μL. Diagnosis can usually be made from the clinical presentation, an increase in the reticulated (RNA-containing) platelets in blood, and demonstration of an increase in marrow megakaryocytes (high rate of platelet production is required because of shortened survival of platelets in the circulation).

a. Thrombocytopenic Purpura in Adults. Adults can develop posttransfusion purpura following exposure to a blood product, most often RBCs or platelets. Usually, a potent alloantibody with PL^{A-1} specificity is readily detected in the patient's plasma.

b. Drug-Induced Autoimmune Thrombocytopenic Purpura is best known following quinine, quinidine, and sedormid exposure. Thrombocytopenia is severe (platelets <20,000/μL). Thrombocytopenia can also occur within hours of the first exposure.

c. Heparin-Induced Thrombocytopenia (HIT)

1.) *HIT type I* (nonimmune) is a modest decrease in the platelet count seen in a majority of patients within the first day of full-dose unfractionated heparin (UH) therapy. It is caused by passive heparin binding to platelets, with modest shortening of platelet life span. It is transient and clinically insignificant.

2.) *HIT type II* (immune), can occur in patients receiving heparin for longer than 5 days. Antibodies to the heparin-platelet complex form and induce platelet activation and aggregation. In addition, heparin-platelet complex binding to endothelial cells stimulates thrombin production. The result is increased clearance of platelets (thrombocytopenia) and venous and/or arterial thrombus formation involving severe organ damage and unusual thrombosis sites (adrenal, portal vein, skin). Incidence is higher with bovine heparin compared with porcine heparin. Patients on full-dose UH for longer than 5 days or who have previously received heparin should be monitored with every other day platelet counts. A more than 50% decrease in platelet count may signal the appearance of an HIT type II antibody and mandates stopping the heparin and substituting a direct thrombin inhibitor (lepirudin, argatroban). An acute form of HIT type II can occur in patients restarted on heparin within 20 days of a previous exposure. When an HIT antibody is already present, a patient restarted on heparin can exhibit an acute drug reaction (severe dyspnea, shaking chills, diaphoresis, hypertension, tachycardia). Such patients are at extreme risk of a fatal thromboembolism if heparin is continued.

d. Anesthetic Considerations for Drug-Induced Thrombocytopenia. Treatment is platelet transfusion if the patient is experiencing a life-threatening hemorrhage or is bleeding into a closed space such as an intracranial hemorrhage. If thrombocytopenia is related to a drug reaction, the most important step is to discontinue the drug. Corticosteroid therapy may speed recovery in patients with an idiopathic thrombocytopenic purpura (ITP). Human immunodeficiency virus–infected thrombocytopenic patients may benefit from treatment with zidovudine well before (1-2 months) surgery. Corticosteroids, intravenous immunoglobulin, and intravenous anti-D (WinRho) have also been used in patients with acquired immunodeficiency syndrome.

1.) In patients with HIT, all heparin forms must be stopped immediately. Substitution of low-molecular-weight heparin (LMWH) is not an option because there is significant antibody cross-reactivity. When continued anticoagulation is required, HIT patients should be started on a direct thrombin inhibitor (lepirudin, argatroban). Lepirudin is given as an intravenous bolus of 0.4 mg/kg, followed by a continuous infusion at 0.15 mg/kg per hour, adjusted to keep the PTT between 1.5 and 2.5 times normal. Argatroban is given as an infusion of approximately 2.0 μg/kg per minute, titrated to keep the PTT between 1.5 and 3 times normal. Oral anticoagulants should never be started until there is continuous successful coverage with a direct thrombin inhibitor. The immediate reduction in protein C levels with warfarin therapy can cause worsening thrombosis. If this occurs, warfarin should be discontinued and vitamin K given to reverse the effect.

3. Idiopathic Thrombocytopenic Purpura is thrombocytopenia unrelated to a drug, infection, or autoimmune disease. This diagnosis can only be made by excluding all other causes of nonimmune and immune destruction. Typically, thrombocytopenia must be severe before bleeding becomes a problem. ITP patients with platelet counts even as low as 2000/μL are usually not at great risk of a major organ or intracerebral bleed. Patients with chronic ITP generally show less severe thrombocytopenia, with platelet counts of 20,000 to 100,000/μL.

> *a. Anesthetic Considerations.* Severe ITP with bleeding manifestations in adults should be treated as a medical emergency with high-dose corticosteroids for the first 3 days. For emergency surgery or clinical evidence of intracranial hemorrhage, the patient should also be given intravenous immunoglobulin and platelet transfusions at least every 8 to 12 hours, regardless of the effect on the platelet count. Splenectomy should be considered in patients who develop chronic ITP. Chronic ITP in pregnancy can usually be managed without medication, modest amounts of prednisone, or intermittent use of intravenous immunoglobulin. When thrombocytopenia is severe, therapeutic options include higher-dose steroid therapy (0.5–1 mg/kg prednisone per day) and intravenous immunoglobulin during the last 2 to 3 weeks of pregnancy. Infants born to mothers with ITP may experience thrombocytopenia and should be monitored. Prophylactic cesarean section is still recommended by some obstetricians to decrease the chance of intracranial hemorrhage in infants born to mothers with ITP.

C. Qualitative Platelet Disorders

1. Congenital Disorders of Platelet Function: von Willebrand's Disease (vWD) is an inherited disorder of platelet function. Type 1 vWD symptomatic disease is seen in only 30% to 40% of offspring of parents carrying the defective gene. Double heterozygotes (type 3 vWD) can exhibit severe disease. Rarely, acquired type 2 vWD secondary to autoantibodies directed at vWF can occur. Presenting signs in symptomatic vWD include epistaxis, easy bruising, menorrhagia, and gingival and gastrointestinal bleeding. The designation of "clinically important" vWD, especially type 1 vWD, should be limited to patients who demonstrate abnormal bleeding.

> *a. Diagnosis.* Full evaluation of vWD patients requires measurements of factor VIII coagulant activity, vWF antigen, vWF activity (ristocetin

cofactor or collagen binding activity), and vWF multimer distribution by agarose gel electrophoresis. These studies are of diagnostic importance in the classification of vWD, which, in turn, is important in planning clinical management.

b. Type 1 Disease results from a defect in vWF release, rather than reduced platelet or endothelial stores. Administration of DDAVP improves vWF release in this group. Clinical severity of the disease is variable. In patients and families with repeated and severe bleeding episodes, vWF antigen and vWF activity are usually less than 15% to 25% of normal. These patients should be treated aggressively for bleeding and given prophylaxis treatment for even minor surgical procedures. A moderately low vWF level (<50%), by itself, does not make the diagnosis. The majority of such individuals will not suffer from an increased bleeding tendency and should not be labeled as having vWD.

c. Type 2 Disease results from a defect in the quality of plasma vWF causing a disproportionate decrease in the vWF activity (ristocetin cofactor activity) when compared with vWF antigen. Type 2 disease is further divided into 2A, 2B 2M, and 2D variants. While each has specific genetic derangements in vWF, clinically the differences are not significant.

d. Type 3 Disease is characterized by a virtual absence of circulating vWF antigen and very low levels of both vWF activity and factor VIII (3%–10% of normal). These patients experience severe bleeding with mucosal hemorrhage, hemarthroses, and muscle hematomas reminiscent of hemophilia A or B. However, unlike classic hemophilia, their bleeding times are very prolonged.

e. Anesthetic Considerations. Useful therapeutic agents are DDAVP (stimulates release of endogenous vWF) and blood products that contain vWF in high concentrations (cryoprecipitate). Patients with type 1 vWD are the best responders to DDAVP. Both vWF and factor VIII must be provided to reliably treat bleeding in type 3 vWD. DDAVP can be administered intravenously (IV) (0.3 μg/kg). A concentrated nasal spray of DDAVP can be self-administered (300 μg total dose) in type 1 vWD for management of menorrhagia and for tooth extractions or minor surgery. Because of the short duration of action and tachyphylaxis to DDAVP, vWF replacement is the more reliable therapy for severe bleeding and surgical prophylaxis, via the transfusion of cryoprecipitate or purified concentrates containing the vWF–factor VIII complex. The recommended doses (expressed in International Units [IU] of both vWF and factor VIII) for bleeding management and surgical prophylaxis are an initial loading dose of 40 to 75 IU/kg IV, followed by repeat doses of 40 to 60 IU/kg at 8- to 12-hour intervals. Once bleeding is controlled, a single daily dose of concentrate is sufficient.

D. Acquired Abnormalities of Platelet Function

1. Myeloproliferative Disease (i.e., polycythemia vera, myeloid metaplasia, idiopathic myelofibrosis, essential thrombocythemia, and chronic myelogenous leukemia) is commonly associated with abnormal platelet function. The bleeding time may be prolonged but is a poor predictor of abnormal bleeding. The most consistent laboratory abnormalities in bleeding patients are defects in epinephrine-induced aggregation and dense and α-granule function.

2. Dysproteinemias can be associated with defects in platelet adhesion, aggregation, and procoagulant activity. Almost one third of patients with Waldenström macroglobulinemia or IgA myeloma will have a demonstrable defect; immunoglobulin G multiple myeloma patients are less commonly affected. The concentration of the monoclonal protein spike appears to correlate with the abnormalities in platelet function.

3. Uremia. Platelet adhesion, activation, and aggregation are abnormal, and thromboxane A_2 generation is decreased. Bleeding time is prolonged, but corrected by hemodialysis. For acute bleeding episodes, DDAVP therapy can improve platelet function transiently. Infusion of conjugated estrogens (0.6 mg/kg per day) for 5 days will also shorten the bleeding time.

4. Liver Disease is associated with a multifaceted defect in coagulation. Thrombocytopenia related to hypersplenism and a failed thrombopoietin response is common. Platelet dysfunction is secondary to high levels of circulating fibrin degradation products. Reduced production of factor VII and low-grade chronic DIC with increased fibrinolysis are additional factors.

5. Inhibition by Drugs. Many drugs also affect platelet function (**Table 17-3**).

6. Anesthetic Considerations. Because the platelets are dysfunctional, absolute platelet number does not predict bleeding risk. Treatment with DDAVP may "overcome" a mild to moderate platelet defect, or platelet transfusions may be required. Normalization of the bleeding time, the platelet function analyzer, or the thromboelastogram will not guarantee adequacy of platelet function for the challenge of surgery. Hypothermia and acidosis adversely affect the function of both native and transfused platelets and should be minimized.

II. HYPERCOAGULABLE DISORDERS

A. Heritable Causes of Hypercoagulability (Table 17-4)

1. Thrombophilia Caused by Decreased Antithrombotic Proteins

a. Hereditary Antithrombin Deficiency is an autosomal dominant inherited trait. Homyzygosity is a fatal fetal defect, and heterozygotes have AT III levels between 40% to 70% of normal. Risk of venous thromboembolism is increased 20-fold in these patients.

b. Hereditary Protein C (PC) and Protein S (PS) Deficiencies interfere with mechanisms that limit rates of thrombin generation. This results in an overabundance of thrombin and clinically the same effect as antithrombin deficiency. Synthesis of PC and PS are both vitamin K dependent, and PC-deficient individuals are at particular risk of thrombosis if warfarin therapy is initiated without protective previous anticoagulation by heparin.

2. Thrombophilia Caused by Increased Prothrombotic Proteins

a. Factor V_{Leiden} is an abnormal factor V that is resistant to the normal cleavage and inactivation by activated protein C (APC). Accordingly, factor V_{Leiden} has prolonged action, fostering increased thrombin generation. Heterozygotes for the gene for factor V_{Leiden} have a 5- to 7-fold increased risk of DVT, while the risk of homozygous carriers is increased up to 80-fold. Up to one in 20 patients undergoing routine surgery may have increased risk attributable to this gene.

TABLE 17-3 Drugs That Inhibit Platelet Function

Strong Association

Aspirin (and aspirin-containing medications)

Clopidogrel/ticlopidine

Abciximab (ReoPro)

Nonsteroidal anti-inflammatory drugs: naproxen, ibuprofen, indomethacin, phenylbutazone, piroxicam, ketorolac

Mild to Moderate Association

Antibiotics, usually only in high doses

Penicillin, also carbenicillin, penicillin G, ampicillin, ticarcillin, nafcillin, mezlocillin

Cephalosporins

Nitrofurantoin

Volume expanders: dextran, hydroxyethyl starch

Heparin

Fibrinolytic agents: EACA, aprotinin

Weak Association

Oncologic drugs: daunorubicin, mithramycin

Cardiovascular drugs: β-blockers, calcium channel blockers, nitroglycerin, nitroprusside, quinidine

Alcohol

EACA, epsilon aminocaproic acid.

TABLE 17-4 Major Hereditary Conditions Linked to Hypercoagulability

	Prevalence in Healthy Controls	Prevalence in Patients with First DVT (%)	DVT Likelihood by Age 60 (%)
Antithrombin deficiency*	0.2	1.1	62
Protein C deficiency*	0.8	3	48
Protein S deficiency*	1.3	1.1	33
Factor V_{Leiden}*	3.5	20	6
Prothrombin 20210A*	2.3	18	<5

* All numbers pertain to heterozygous state.
DVT, deep venous thrombosis.

b. Prothrombin G20210A Gene Mutation. This gene leads to increased levels of prothrombin. Alone, it has only modest effects on DVT risk. The importance of this thrombophilia resides in the frequency of the gene, rather than its potency.

B. Acquired Causes of Hypercoagulability

1. Myeloproliferative Disorders are associated with an increased incidence of thrombophlebitis, pulmonary embolism (PE), and arterial occlusions, although the pathogenesis of the thrombosis in these patients is not clear.

2. Malignancies. Patients with certain adenocarcinomas (pancreas, colon, stomach, ovaries) may first present with a single or multiple episodes of deep venous thrombosis or migratory superficial thrombophlebitis. The pathogenesis appears to be a combination of release of procoagulant factor(s) by the tumor, endothelial damage by tumor invasion, and blood stasis.

3. Pregnancy and Oral Contraceptive Use increase the risk of thrombosis five- to six-fold. The risk of PE is highest during the third trimester of pregnancy and immediate postpartum period and is a leading cause of maternal death. Antithrombin III–deficient women are at the greatest risk and should be anticoagulated throughout pregnancy. Factor V_{Leiden} and the prothrombin G20201A mutation are associated with much less risk, and these patients do not need to be anticoagulated unless they have a history of a PE or recurrent DVT. Women who take oral contraceptives and who also smoke, have a history of migraine headaches, or carry an inherited hypercoagulable defect are at increased risk (30-fold) of venous thrombosis, PE, and cerebrovascular thrombosis.

4. Nephrotic Syndrome Patients are at risk of thromboembolic disease, including renal vein thrombosis. The reasons are unclear but may include lower than normal levels of antithrombin III or PC, factor XII deficiency, platelet hyperactivity, abnormal fibrinolytic activity, and higher than normal levels of other coagulation factors. Hyperlipidemia and hypoalbuminemia have also been proposed as possible etiologic factors.

5. Antiphospholipid Antibodies (e.g., lupus anticoagulant) are associated with increased tendency for both venous and arterial thrombosis. The term *anticoagulant* is, therefore, a clinical misnomer. The mechanism of action is not known; the antibodies may activate endothelial cells to increase the expression of vascular adhesion molecule-1 and E-selectin, increasing binding of white blood cells and platelets to the endothelial surface, leading to thrombus formation.

6. Anesthetic Considerations for Venous Hypercoagulability. Current antithrombotic strategies range from simple management (early ambulation) to the combination of subcutaneous heparin with elastic stockings followed by conversion to outpatient warfarin with laboratory monitoring.

a. Drugs for DVT Prophylaxis include heparin (unfractionated or LMWH), warfarin, direct thrombin inhibitors (hirudin), and factor Xa inhibitors (fondaparinux). Administration of heparin confers a 60% to 70% risk reduction. Graded compression elastic stockings have a 40% to 45% risk reduction, and intermittent pneumatic compression shows a risk reduction that approaches that of heparin when used as the only prophylactic method.

b. Regional Anesthesia. Although studies have shown that regional anesthesia decreases DVT, risk remains unacceptably high even when regional anesthesia is combined with early ambulation and intraoperative antiembolism stockings. With routine antithrombotic prophylaxis, the advantages of regional over general anesthesia are unclear, raising the question whether, for patients receiving pharmacologic perioperative thromboprophylaxis, neuraxial anesthesia still reduces the risks of DVT. As a result, postoperative prophylactic anticoagulation with drugs like warfarin and subcutaneous heparin is now the standard of care for high-risk operations.

c. Vena Caval Filters can be used to prevent recurrent pulmonary emboli in patients who have an absolute contraindication to anticoagulation or have a major bleeding complication.

7. Anesthetic Considerations for Patients on Long-Term Anticoagulation. Most anticoagulated patients are managed on warfarin. After discontinuing warfarin, the INR does not start to fall for about 29 hours, and then decreases with a half-life of approximately 22 hours. In high-risk patients, bridging therapy with unfractionated heparin (UH) or LMWH should be considered approximately 60 hours after the last dose of warfarin. LMWH should be given once or twice daily for 3 days before surgery, with the last dose no less than 18 hours preoperatively for a twice-daily regimen and 30 hours for a once-daily regimen. UH should be discontinued 6 hours or more before surgery. The effects of warfarin are delayed, and therefore warfarin should be resumed as soon as possible after surgery except in patients at high bleeding risk; consideration can be given to bridging therapy until the INR becomes therapeutic.

C. Acquired Hypercoagulability of the Arterial Vasculature

1. Atrial Fibrillation (AF). Patients with AF, particularly those with valvular disease, a dilated atrium, and evidence of heart failure or a previous embolus require moderate-dose warfarin therapy indefinitely. Patients with acute anterior wall infarctions who, because of a wall motion abnormality, are likely to form a mural thrombus need to receive warfarin for 2 to 3 months, after which there is little risk of embolism.

2. Antiphospholipid Antibodies. See "Acquired Causes of Hypercoagulability."

CHAPTER 18

Skin and Musculoskeletal Diseases

Diseases of the skin and musculoskeletal system manifest with obvious clinical signs, but less visible systemic effects of many of these disorders are also important.

I. EPIDERMOLYSIS BULLOSA

Epidermolysis bullosa is a group of genetic diseases of mucous membranes and skin, particularly the oropharynx and esophagus.

A. Signs and Symptoms. Epidermolysis bullosa is characterized by bulla formation (blistering) caused by separation within the epidermis followed by fluid accumulation. Bulla formation is typically initiated when lateral shearing forces are applied to the skin. Pressure applied perpendicular to the skin is not as great a hazard.

B. Treatment of epidermolysis bullosa is symptomatic and supportive, often including corticosteroids.

C. Management of Anesthesia (Table 18-1)

II. PEMPHIGUS

Pemphigus refers to a group of chronic autoimmune blistering (vesiculobullous) diseases that may involve extensive areas of the skin and mucous membranes. Cutaneous pemphigus closely resembles the oral manifestations of epidermolysis bullosa dystrophica (eating is painful; malnutrition may develop). Pemphigus may be associated with underlying malignancy, especially lymphoreticular cancer.

A. Treatment of pemphigus is with corticosteroids. Mycophenolate mofetil, rituximab, azathioprine, methotrexate, and cyclophosphamide have also been

TABLE 18-1	Anesthesia Considerations in Epidermolysis Bullosa

- Consider preoperative treatment (corticosteroids).
- Avoid trauma to skin and mucous membranes (e.g., hold IVs in place with gauze wrap; pad blood pressure cuffs; gel pad should be placed under patient).
- Minimize upper airway instrumentation, avoid esophageal stethoscopes.
- Endotracheal intubation appears safe (laryngeal involvement is rare).
- Succinylcholine appears safe.
- Avoid oropharyngeal suctioning.
- Regional anesthesia techniques may be useful.

used successfully for early treatment of pemphigus. Immune globulin has replaced high-dose corticosteroids as a rescue therapy.

B. Management of Anesthesia is similar to that of patients with epidermolysis bullosa. Preoperative evaluation must consider current drug therapy. Electrolyte derangements and dehydration may be present because of chronic fluid losses through bullous skin lesions. Airway management may be difficult because of bullae in the oropharynx. Airway manipulation, including direct laryngoscopy and endotracheal intubation, can result in acute bulla formation, upper airway obstruction, and bleeding.

III. PSORIASIS

Psoriasis is a common chronic dermatologic disorder affecting 1% to 3% of the world's population characterized by accelerated epidermal growth resulting in inflammatory erythematous papules covered with loosely adherent scales (chronic plaque psoriasis). An asymmetrical arthropathy occurs in approximately 5% to 8% of patients.

A. Treatment of psoriasis is directed at slowing the rapid proliferation of epidermal cells (coal tar, salicylic acid, topical corticosteroids, calcipotriene ointment, tazarotene). Systemic therapy with methotrexate or cyclosporine and biologic therapy with etanercept (a tumor necrosis factor inhibitor), infliximab (a monoclonal antibody to tumor necrosis factor), alefacept (an immunomodulatory fusion protein), or efalizumab (a monoclonal antibody to CD11a) may be required for severe cases. Toxic effects of these drugs include cirrhosis, renal failure, hypertension, and pneumonitis.

B. Management of Anesthesia includes evaluation of the drugs being used for the treatment of psoriasis, including topical corticosteroids and chemotherapeutic drugs. Patients with psoriasis often have a marked increase in skin blood flow that can contribute to altered thermoregulation.

IV. MASTOCYTOSIS

Mastocytosis is a rare disorder of mast cell proliferation that can occur in a cutaneous form (urticaria pigmentosa) or in a systemic form.

A. Signs and Symptoms reflect degranulation of mast cells with anaphylactoid responses characterized by pruritus, urticaria, and flushing. These changes may be accompanied by hypotension (sometimes life threatening) and tachycardia. H_1-receptor and H_2-receptor antagonists are not always protective, and the incidence of bronchospasm is low. Bleeding is unusual in these patients even though mast cells contain heparin.

B. Management of Anesthesia is usually uneventful, but there are reports of life-threatening anaphylactoid reactions with even minor surgical procedures (epinephrine should be immediately available). Preoperative administration of H_1- and H_2-receptor antagonists may be considered. Monitoring serum tryptase concentration during the perioperative period may be useful for detecting the occurrence of mast cell degranulation.

V. ATOPIC DERMATITIS

Atopic dermatitis is the cutaneous manifestation of the atopic state (dry, scaly, eczematous, pruritic patches on the face, neck, and flexor surfaces of the arms and legs). Pruritus is the primary symptom. Systemic antihistamines and corticosteroids are effective. Pulmonary manifestations of the atopic state (asthma, hay fever, otitis media, sinusitis) affect anesthetic management.

VI. URTICARIA

Urticaria may be characterized as acute urticaria, chronic urticaria, or physical urticaria (**Table 18-2**) Anesthesia management is avoidance of triggering drugs and events, H_1- and H_2-receptor antagonists and corticosteroids when appropriate, and in the case of cold urticaria, warming of intravenous (IV) fluids and IV injectable agents, and increasing the ambient temperature in the operating room.

VII. ERYTHEMA MULTIFORME

Erythema multiforme is a recurrent disease of the skin and mucous membranes characterized by lesions ranging from edematous macules and papules to vesicular or bullous lesions that may ulcerate.

A. Stevens-Johnson Syndrome (erythema multiforme major) is a severe manifestation associated with multisystem dysfunction (fever, tachycardia, tachypnea). Drugs associated with the onset of this syndrome include antibiotics, analgesics, and certain over-the-counter medications. Corticosteroids are used in the management of severe cases. Anesthetic considerations are similar to those encountered in anesthetizing patients with epidermolysis bullosa.

VIII. SCLERODERMA

Scleroderma (systemic sclerosis) is characterized by inflammation, vascular sclerosis, and fibrosis of the skin and viscera. In some patients, the disease evolves into the CREST syndrome (*c*alcinoses, *R*aynaud's phenomenon, *e*sophageal hypomotility, *s*clerodactyly, *t*elangiectasia). Prognosis is poor and related to the extent of visceral involvement. No drugs or treatments have proved safe and effective in changing the course of disease.

TABLE 18-2 Features of Common Types of Chronic Urticaria

Type of Urticaria	Age Range (yr)	Clinical Features	Angioedema	Diagnostic Test
Chronic idiopathic	20–50	Pink or pale edematous papules or wheals; wheals often annular; pruritus	Yes	
Symptomatic dermatographism	20–50	Linear wheals with a surrounding bright-red flare at sites of stimulation; pruritus	No	Light stroking of skin causes wheal.
Physical urticarias				
Cold	10–40	Pale or red swelling at sites of contact with cold surfaces or fluids; pruritus	Yes	Application of ice pack causes a wheal within 5 min of removing the ice (cold stimulation test).
Pressure	20–50	Swelling at sites of pressure (soles, palms, waist) lasting ≥2–24 hr; painful, pruritus	No	Application of pressure perpendicular to skin produces persistent red swelling after a latent period of 1–4 hr.
Solar	20–50	Pale or red swelling at site of exposure to ultraviolet or visible light; pruritus	Yes	Radiation by a solar simulator for 30–120 sec causes wheals in 30 min.
Cholinergic	10–50	Monomorphic pale or pink wheals on trunk, neck, and limbs; pruritus	Yes	Exercise or hot shower elicits wheals.

Adapted from Greaves MW: Chronic urticaria. N Engl J Med 1995;332:1767–1772.

A. Signs and Symptoms (Table 18-3)

B. Anesthesia Considerations include the possibility of difficult intubation, difficult IV access, intravascular volume depletion caused by chronic hypertension, and risk of regurgitation and pulmonary aspiration. Patients are sensitive to the respiratory depressant effects of opioids, and postoperative ventilatory support may be required in patients with severe pulmonary disease. Renal dysfunction affects the selection of anesthetic drugs. Measures to minimize peripheral vasoconstriction include maintenance of the operating room temperature at more than 21°C and administration of warmed IV fluids. The eyes should be protected to prevent corneal abrasions.

IX. PSEUDOXANTHOMA ELASTICUM

Pseudoxanthoma elasticum is a rare hereditary disorder of elastic tissue (degeneration and calcification) leading to loss of visual acuity, gastrointestinal hemorrhage, systemic hypertension, and ischemic heart disease.

A. Management of Anesthesia is based on an appreciation of the abnormalities associated with this disease. Cardiovascular derangements are probably the most important considerations. There are no specific recommendations regarding the choice of anesthetic drugs or techniques.

X. EHLERS-DANLOS SYNDROME

Ehlers-Danlos syndrome consists of a group of inherited connective tissue disorders caused by abnormal production of procollagen and collagen. The only form of this syndrome associated with an increased risk of death is the type IV

TABLE 18-3	Signs and Symptoms of Scleroderma
Skin and Musculoskeletal	• Contractures (fingers, mouth) • Proximal muscular weakness
Nervous System	• Nerve compression by thickened connective tissue • Trigeminal neuralgia • Keratoconjunctivitis sicca
Cardiovascular System	• Dysrhythmias • Conduction abnormalities • Congestive heart failure • Peripheral vasospasm (Raynaud's phenomenon)
Lungs	• Pulmonary fibrosis • Pulmonary hypertension • Cor pulmonale • Arterial hypoxemia
Kidneys	• Renal artery stenosis • Accelerated systemic hypertension
Gastrointestinal	• Dysphagia • Xerostomia • Hypomotility • Reflux

(vascular) syndrome. This form may be complicated by rupture of large blood vessels or disruption of the bowel.

A. Signs and Symptoms are joint hypermobility, skin fragility or hyperelasticity, bruising and scarring, musculoskeletal discomfort, and susceptibility to osteoarthritis. The gastrointestinal tract, uterus, and vasculative have a lot of type III collagen, accounting for such complications as spontaneous rupture of the bowel, uterus, or major arteries. Dilation of the trachea is often present. Patients may exhibit extensive ecchymoses with minimal trauma though a specific coagulation defect has not been identified.

B. Management of Anesthesia (Table 18-4)

XI. POLYMYOSITIS AND DERMATOMYOSITIS

Polymyositis and dermatomyositis are multisystem diseases of unknown etiology, manifesting as inflammatory myopathies. Dermatomyositis has characteristic skin changes (upper lid discoloration, periorbital edema, malar rash, atrophic changes over extensor surfaces of joints) in addition to muscle weakness.

A. Signs and Symptoms (Table 18-5)

B. Diagnosis is considered when proximal skeletal muscle weakness, an increased serum creatine kinase concentration, and a characteristic skin rash are present.

TABLE 18-4	Anesthesia Considerations in Ehlers-Danlos Syndrome

- Avoid intramuscular injections or instrumentation of the nose or esophagus (bleeding propensity).
- Hematoma formation may be excessive at instrumentations sites.
- Extravasation of IV fluids may go undetected because of skin laxity.
- Maintain low airway pressures during positive pressure ventilation to avoid pneumothorax.
- Regional anesthesia should be avoided.
- Surgical complications are bleeding and wound dehiscence.

TABLE 18-5	Signs and Symptoms of Polymyositis

- Proximal skeletal muscle weakness (neck, shoulders, hips); difficulty climbing stairs
- Dysphagia and aspiration (paresis of pharyngeal muscles)
- Ventilatory insufficiency (paresis of respiratory muscles)
- Increased serum creatine kinase
- Heart block
- Left ventricular dysfunction
- Myocarditis
- Associated with systemic lupus erythematosus, scleroderma, rheumatoid arthritis

C. **Treatment** is usually corticosteroids. Immunosuppressive therapy (methotrexate, azathioprine, cyclophosphamide, mycophenolate, cyclosporine) may be effective. Intravenous immunoglobulin may be useful in refractory cases.
D. **Management of Anesthesia** considers the vulnerability of patients with polymyositis to pulmonary aspiration. Responses to nondepolarizing muscle relaxants and succinylcholine are normal.

XII. SYSTEMIC LUPUS ERYTHEMATOSUS (Table 18-6)

Systemic lupus erythematosis (SLE) is a multisystem chronic inflammatory disease, usually of young women, characterized by antinuclear antibody production. SLE can be drug-induced or naturally-occuring. The natural history of SLE is highly variable, but the presence of nephritis and hypertension is associated with a worse prognosis. Pregnancy, especially in patients with nephritis and hypertension, is associated with a substantial risk of disease exacerbation and poor fetal outcome. Corticosteroids are the principal treatment for severe manifestations of lupus.

XIII. TUMORAL CALCINOSIS

Tumoral calcinosis is a rare genetic disorder that presents as metastatic calcifications adjacent to large joints. The principal anesthetic consideration is that rare involvement of the hyoid bone, hypothyroid ligament, or cervical intervertebral joints may lead to difficult intubation.

XIV. MUSCULAR DYSTROPHY

Muscular dystrophy is a group of hereditary diseases characterized by painless degeneration and atrophy of skeletal muscles.
A. **Pseudohypertrophic Muscular Dystrophy (Duchenne's Muscular Dystrophy)** is the most common and severe form of childhood progressive muscular dystrophy. The disease is caused by an X-linked recessive gene and becomes apparent in 2- to 5-year-old boys (waddling gait, frequent falling, difficulty climbing stairs). Serum creatine kinase concentrations are 20 to 100 times normal.

TABLE 18-6	Manifestations of Systemic Lupus Erythematosis
Dermatitis, malar rash	
Symmetrical arthritis	
Pericarditis, myocarditis, heart failure	
Pleuritis, restrictive lung disease	
Nephritis, hypertension	
Congitive dysfunction, psychological changes, cerebritis	
Antiphospholipid antibodies	
Myopathy	

1. Cardiopulmonary Dysfunction. Degeneration of cardiac muscle invariably accompanies this muscular dystrophy. Chronic weakness of the respiratory muscles and a decreased ability to cough result in loss of pulmonary reserve and accumulation of secretions.

2. Management of Anesthesia (Table 18-7)

B. Limb-Girdle Muscular Dystrophy is a slowly progressive but relatively benign disease with only shoulder or hip muscles involved.

C. Facioscapulohumeral Muscular Dystrophy is characterized by a slowly progressive wasting of facial, pectoral, and shoulder girdle muscles that begins during adolescence. There is no involvement of cardiac muscle, and serum creatine kinase concentration is seldom increased.

D. Nemaline Rod Muscular Dystrophy is an autosomal dominant disease characterized by slowly progressive or nonprogressive symmetrical dystrophy of skeletal and smooth muscle. Micrognathia and dental malocclusion are common. Restrictive lung disease may result from the myopathy and/or scoliosis. Cardiac failure resulting from dilated cardiomyopathy has been described.

 1. Anesthesia Considerations include possible difficult intubation, exaggerated respiratory depression, regurgitation risk (bulbar palsy), unpredictable response to muscle relaxants (succinylcholine appears safe), and myocardial depression.

E. Oculopharyngeal Dystrophy is a rare variant of muscular dystrophy characterized by progressive dysphagia and ptosis. These patients may be at risk of aspiration during the perioperative period, and their sensitivity to muscle relaxants may be increased.

F. Emery-Dreifuss Muscular Dystrophy is an X-linked recessive disorder characterized by development of skeletal muscle contractures that precede the onset of skeletal muscle weakness. Cardiac involvement may be life threatening and present as congestive heart failure, thromboembolism, or bradycardia. In contrast to the other muscular dystrophies, female carriers of this disorder may have cardiac impairment.

TABLE 18-7	Anesthetic Considerations in Pseudohypertrophic Muscular Dystrophy
Patient is at increased risk of aspiration (weak laryngeal reflexes, gastrointestinal hypomotility).	
Succinylcholine is contraindicated (rhabdomyolysis, hyperkalemia, cardiac arrest).	
Response to nondepolarizing muscles relaxants is prolonged.	
Volatile agents may be associated with rhabdomyolysis.	
Increased incidence of malignant hyperthermia is seen (dantrolene should be available).	
Regional anesthesia is acceptable.	
Monitors should be used to detect malignant hyperthermia and cardiac dysfunction.	
Anticipate postoperative pulmonary dysfunction.	

XV. MYOTONIC DYSTROPHY

Myotonic dystrophy designates a group of hereditary degenerative diseases of skeletal muscle characterized by persistent contracture (myotonia) after voluntary contraction of a muscle or following electrical stimulation. Peripheral nerves and the neuromuscular junction are not affected.

A. Myotonia Dystrophica is the most common and most serious form of myotonic dystrophy affecting adults. Death from pneumonia or heart failure often occurs by the sixth decade of life. Treatment is symptomatic and may include use of phenytoin.
  1. Signs and Symptoms (Table 18-8)
  2. Management of Anesthesia (Table 18-9)

B. Myotonia Congenita does not involve other organ systems, does not progress, and does not result in a decreased life expectancy. Patients respond to phenytoin, mexiletine, or quinine therapy. The response to succinylcholine administration is abnormal.

C. Paramyotonia Congenita is characterized by generalized myotonia that is exacerbated by exercise and cold. Treatment is similar to that of myotonia congenita.

TABLE 18-8 Signs and Symptoms of Myotonia Dystrophy
Facial muscle weakness (expressionless facies)
Ptosis
Dysarthria
Dysphagia/slowed gastric emptying/pulmonary aspiration
Inability to relax hand grip
Mental retardation
Endocrine dysfunction (gonadal atrophy, diabetes mellitus, hypothyroidism, adrenal insufficiency)
Central sleep apnea
Cardiomyopathy (dysrhythmias, cardiac conduction abnormalities)

TABLE 18-9 Anesthesia Considerations in Patients with Myotonia Dystrophica
Exaggerated myocardial depression can be produced by volatile agents.
Succinylcholine produces prolonged muscle contraction.
Response to nondepolarizing muscle relaxants is normal.
Reversal of neuromuscular blockade does not usually cause muscle contraction.
Sensitive to respiratiory-depressant drugs.
Postoperative shivering may induce myotonia.

D. Schwartz-Jampel Syndrome is a rare childhood disorder of progressive skeletal muscle stiffness; myotonia; and ocular, facial, and skeletal abnormalities, including micrognathia. Tracheal intubation is predictably difficult. These children may be susceptible to malignant hyperthermia.

XVI. PERIODIC PARALYSIS

Periodic paralysis is a spectrum of diseases characterized by intermittent acute attacks of skeletal muscle weakness or paralysis associated with hypokalemia or hyperkalemia (**Table 18-10**). Muscle strength is normal between attacks.

A. Management of Anesthesia. A principal goal is avoidance of events that precipitate skeletal muscle weakness (hypothermia, electrolyte abnormalities, carbohydrate loading in hypokalemic paralysis patients). Shorter-acting neuromuscular blockers are preferable if skeletal muscle relaxation is required. Succinylcholine is acceptable in patients with hypokalemic paralysis but should be avoided in patients with hyperkalemic paralysis.

XVII. MYASTHENIA GRAVIS

Myasthenia gravis is a chronic autoimmune disorder caused by a decrease in functional acetylcholine receptors at the neuromuscular junction because of their destruction or inactivation by circulating antibodies. The hallmarks of the disease are weakness and rapid exhaustion of voluntary muscles with repetitive use followed by partial recovery with rest. Skeletal muscles innervated by cranial nerves (ocular, pharyngeal, and laryngeal muscles) are especially vulnerable, as reflected by the appearance of ptosis, diplopia, and dysphagia, often the initial symptoms of the disease. Other conditions that cause weakness of the cranial and somatic musculature must be considered in the differential diagnosis of myasthenia gravis (**Table 18-11**).

TABLE 18-10	Clinical Features of Familial Periodic Paralysis		
Type	**Serum Potassium Concentration during Symptoms (mEq/L)**	**Precipitating Factors**	**Other Features**
Hypokalemic	<3.0	Large carbohydrate meal, strenuous exercise, glucose infusion, stress, menstruation, pregnancy, anesthesia, hypothermia	Cardiac dysrhythmias Electrocardiographic signs of hypokalemia
Hyperkalemic	>5.5	Exercise, potassium infusion, metabolic acidosis, hypothermia	Skeletal muscle weakness may be localized to tongue and eyelids

A. Classification (**Table 18-12**)
B. Signs and Symptoms (**Table 18-13**)
C. Treatment (**Table 18-14**)
D. Management of Anesthesia (**Table 18-15**)

XVIII. MYASTHENIC SYNDROME (EATON-LAMBERT SYNDROME)

Myasthenic syndrome is a disorder of neuromuscular transmission that resembles myasthenia gravis (**Table 18-16**). This syndrome has been described in patients with small-cell carcinoma of the lung, as well as in patients without cancer.

TABLE 18-11	Differential Diagnosis of Myasthenia Gravis	
Condition	**Symptoms and Characteristics**	**Comments**
Congenital myasthenic syndromes	Rare, early onset, not autoimmune	Electrophysiologic and immunocytochemical tests required for diagnosis
Drug-induced myasthenia gravis:		
Penicillamine	Triggers autoimmune myasthenia gravis	Recovery within weeks of discontinuing the drug
Nondepolarizing muscle relaxants Aminoglycosides Procainamide	Increased sensitivity	Recovery after drug discontinuation
Eaton-Lambert syndrome	Small cell lung cancer, fatigue	Incremental response on repetitive nerve stimulation, antibodies to calcium channels
Hyperthyroidism	Exacerbation of myasthenia gravis	Thyroid function abnormal
Graves' disease	Diplopia, exophthalmos	Thyroid-stimulating immunoglobulin present
Botulism	Generalized weakness, ophthalmoplegia	Incremental response on repetitive nerve stimulation, mydriasis
Progressive external ophthalmoplegia	Ptosis, diplopia, generalized weakness in some cases	Mitochondrial abnormalities
Intracranial mass compressing cranial nerves	Ophthalmoplegia, cranial nerve weakness	Abnormalities on computed tomography or magnetic resonance imaging

TABLE 18-12	Classification of Myasthenia Gravis
Type I	Limited to extraocular muscles
Type IIa	Slowly progressive, spares muscles of respiration; response to anticholinesterase therapy is good
Type IIb	Severe, rapidly progressive, may involve muscles of respiration, response to anticholinesterase therapy may not be good
Type III	Abrupt onset, rapid deterioration (within 6 months), high mortality rate
Type IV	Severe muscle weakness resulting from progression of type I or type II disease.

Myasthenic syndrome is an acquired autoimmune disease with immunoglobulin G antibodies to voltage-sensitive calcium channels that produces a deficiency of these channels at the motor nerve terminal. Anticholinesterase drugs are not effective therapy in patients with myasthenic syndrome.

XIX. RHEUMATOID ARTHRITIS

Rheumatoid arthritis, the most common chronic inflammatory arthritis, affects approximately 1% of adults (females > males), and is characterized by morning stiffness, symmetrical polyarthropathy, and significant systemic involvement (**Table 18-17**). Involvement of the proximal interphalangeal and metacarpophalangeal joints of the hands and feet distinguish rheumatoid arthritis from osteoarthritis (which typically affects weight-bearing joints and distal interphalangeal joints). The course of the disease is characterized by exacerbations and remissions.

A. Signs and Symptoms
1. **Joint Involvement.** Joints of the hands, wrists, knees, and feet are symmetrically affected. Temporomandibular joint involvement can produce marked limitation of mandibular motion. Cervical spine involvement may include atlantoaxial subluxation and consequent separation of the

TABLE 18-13	Signs and Symptoms of Myasthenia Gravis
Ptosis and diplopia (most common initial complaints)	
Dysphagia, dysarthria, drooling	
Asymmetrical skeletal muscle weakness with exercise	
Lack of muscle atrophy	
Myocarditis (cardiomyopathy, atrial fibrillation, heart block)	
Hyperthyroidism (in 10% of patients)	
Occasionally isolated respiratory failure	
Associated rheumatologic disease (rheumatoid arthritis, SLE, pernicious anemia)	
Muscle weakness may be aggravated by aminoglycoside antibiotics	

TABLE 18-14	Treatment of Myasthenia Gravis
Anticholinesterase drugs	• Pyridostigmine 60 mg PO (onset of effect in 30 minutes, and peak effect in 2 hours) • Treatment effects may wane after weeks or months of therapy
Thymectomy	• Induces remission or decreases doses of immunosuppressive drugs required • If vital capacity <2 L, preoperative plasmapheresis may help improve likelihood of adequate spontaneous ventilation postoperatively • Full benefit of thymectomy make take months to occur
Immunosuppressive therapy	• Corticosteroids, azathioprine, cyclosporine, mycophenolate • Used when muscle weakness not adequately controlled by anticholinesterase drugs
Short-term immunotherapy	• Plasmapheresis (removes antibodies, benefit is transient) • Immunoglobulin

atlanto-odontoid articulation. Cricoarytenoid arthritis with hoarseness is common.

2. Systemic Involvement. In the cardiovascular system, rheumatoid arthritis may manifest as pericarditis, myocarditis, coronary artery arteritis, accelerated coronary atherosclerosis, cardiac valve fibrosis, and formation of rheumatoid nodules in the cardiac conduction system. Patients may

TABLE 18-15	Anesthesia Management in Patients with Myasthenia Gravis
Preoperative	Avoid opioids.
Muscle relaxants	Increased sensitivity to nondepolarizing muscle relaxants. Initial dose should be titrated to response according to peripheral nerve stimulator. Patients may be resistant to succinylcholine.
Induction	Use short-acting IV drugs. Consider intubation without muscle relaxants.
Maintenance	Administer nitrous oxide plus volatile agents (decreases dose of muscle relaxants needed). Short or intermediate-acting muscle relaxants are used; decrease initial dose by half to two thirds.
Postoperative	May require postoperative ventilation (higher risk with disease duration >6 years, presence of COPD, daily dose of pyridostigmine >750 mg, vital capacity <2.9 L).

COPD, chronic obstructive pulmonary disease.

TABLE 18-16 Comparison of Myasthenic Syndrome and Myasthenia Gravis

Parameter	Myasthenic Syndrome	Myasthenia Gravis
Manifestations	Proximal limb weakness (legs more than arms), exercise improves strength, muscle pain common, reflexes absent or decreased	Extraocular, bulbar, and facial muscle weakness, fatigue with exercise; muscle pain uncommon; reflexes normal
Gender	Males more often than females	Females more often than males
Co-existing pathology	Small-cell lung cancer	Thymoma
Response to muscle relaxants	Sensitive to succinylcholine and nondepolarizing muscle relaxants. Poor response to anticholinesterases	Resistant to succinylcholine, sensitive to nondepolarizing muscle relaxants. Good response to anticholinesterases

demonstrate a neuropathy (mononeuritis multiplex), skin ulcerations, and purpura. Pulmonary manifestations include pleural effusion, pulmonary nodules, and pulmonary fibrosis. Costochondral involvement may produce restrictive lung changes with decreased lung volumes and vital capacity. Anemia and dry eyes and dry mouth (Sjögren's syndrome) are also seen.

3. Treatment goals are relief of pain, preservation of joint function and strength, prevention of deformities, and attenuation of systemic complications. Drug therapy is used to provide analgesia, control inflammation, and produce immunosuppression.

   a. Nonsteroidal Anti-Inflammatory Drugs (NSAIDs) and aspirin are important for symptomatic relief of rheumatoid arthritis but have little role in changing the underlying disease process.

   b. Corticosteroids decrease joint swelling, pain, and morning stiffness but are often associated with significant long-term side effects (osteoporosis, osteonecrosis, increased susceptibility to infection, myopathy, hyperglycemia, poor wound healing).

   c. Disease-Modifying Antirheumatic Drugs include methotrexate, sulfasalazine, leflunomide, antimalarials, D-penicillamine, azathioprine, and minocycline. These drugs generally take 2 to 6 months to achieve their effects. Cytokines play a central role in the pathogenesis of rheumatoid arthritis. Drugs such as infliximab (Remicade) and etanercept (Enbrel), which are tumor necrosis factor inhibitors, are effective therapies, although long-term toxicities such as infection (tuberculosis) and demyelinating syndromes are a concern. Anakinra, an interleukin-1 receptor antagonist, is effective but with a slower onset of action. Gold is extremely effective therapy but is not commonly used because of frequent toxicities.

   d. Surgery. Indications for surgery include intractable pain, impairment of joint function, and the need for joint stabilization.

334

		Ankylosing
TABLE 18-17	**Comparison of Rheumatoid Arthritis and Ankylosing Spondylitis**	
Parameter	**Rheumatoid Arthritis**	**Ankylosing Spondylitis**
Family history	Rare	Common
Gender	Female (30–50 years old)	Male (20–30 years old)
Joint involvement	Symmetrical polyarthropathy	Asymmetrical oligoarthropathy
Sacroiliac involvement	No	Yes
Vertebral involvement	Cervical	Total (ascending)
Cardiac changes	Pericardial effusion, aortic regurgitation, cardiac conduction abnormalities, cardiac valve fibrosis, coronary artery arteritis	Cardiomegaly, aortic regurgitation, cardiac conduction abnormalities
Pulmonary changes	Pulmonary fibrosis, pleural effusion	Pulmonary fibrosis
Eyes	Keratoconjunctivitis sicca	Conjunctivitis, uveitis
Rheumatoid factor	Positive	Negative
HLA-B27	Negative	Positive

4. Management of Anesthesia. Compromise of the airway may occur at the cervical spine, temporomandibular joints, and cricoarytenoid joints. Atlantoaxial subluxation (confirmed by radiographic examination) may predispose to cervical cord compression with neck motion. Awake, sedated endotracheal intubation by fiberoptic laryngoscopy may be indicated if preoperative evaluation suggests that direct visualization of the glottic opening will be difficult. Postoperative ventilatory support might be needed in patients with rheumatoid pulmonary involvement. The effect of aspirin or NSAIDs on platelet function must be considered. Corticosteroid supplementation may be indicated in patients undergoing long-term treatment with these drugs. Postextubation laryngeal obstruction may occur in patients with cricoarytenoid arthritis.

XX. SPONDYLOARTHROPATHIES

Spondyloarthropathies are a group of nonrheumatic arthropathies that include ankylosing spondylitis, reactive arthritis (Reiter's syndrome), juvenile chronic polyarthropathy, psoriatic arthritis, and enteropathic arthritis. These diseases are characterized by involvement of the spine and absence of rheumatoid nodules or detectable circulating rheumatoid factor (see **Table 18-17**). There are predilections for new bone formation (joint ankylosis) and ocular inflammation.

A. Ankylosing Spondylitis is a chronic, usually progressive, inflammatory disease involving the articulations of the spine and adjacent soft tissues.

Cardiomegaly, aortic regurgitation, cardiac conduction abnormalities, pulmonary fibrosis, and unilateral uveitis may be present.

1. **Treatment** consists of exercises designed to maintain joint mobility and posture plus anti-inflammatory drugs (indomethacin, diclofenac). Topical corticosteroid eyedrops are used to treat uveitis.

2. **Management of Anesthesia.** Awake fiberoptic tracheal intubation may be needed due to cervical spine disease. Restrictive lung disease from costochondral rigidity and flexion deformity of the thoracic spine must be appreciated. Sudden or excessive increases in systemic vascular resistance are poorly tolerated if significant aortic regurgitation is present. Neurologic monitoring is a consideration for patients undergoing corrective spinal surgery. Regional anesthesia is acceptable but may be technically difficult because of limited joint mobility and closed interspinous spaces.

B. **Reactive Arthritis** is an aseptic arthritis that occurs after an extra-articular infection, especially infection with *Chlamydia, Salmonella,* and *Shigella* species. Management consists of antibiotic treatment for the initial infection and NSAIDs or sulfasalazine for symptomatic relief of the arthritis.

C. **Juvenile Chronic Polyarthropathy** is similar to that of adult rheumatoid arthritis. An acute form of polyarthritis (fever, rash, lymphadenopathy, splenomegaly in young children who are negative for rheumatoid factor and HLA-B27) is designated Still's disease.

D. **Enteropathic Arthritis** is an inflammatory polyarthritis, most often involving the large joints of the lower extremities that may develop in patients with Crohn's disease or ulcerative colitis.

XXI. OSTEOARTHRITIS

Osteoarthritis is a degenerative process that affects articular cartilage and involves minimal inflammatory reaction in the joints, commonly the knees, hips, and spine. Degenerative changes are most significant in the mid to lower cervical spine and in the lower lumbar area.

A. **Treatment** includes physical therapy and exercise programs to maintain muscle function. Pain relief can also be achieved by application of heat, simple analgesics such as acetaminophen, and anti-inflammatory drugs. Systemic corticosteroids have no place in the treatment of osteoarthritis. Joint replacement surgery may be recommended when pain from osteoarthritis is persistent and disabling or significant limitation of joint function is present.

XXII. PAGET'S DISEASE

Paget's disease of bone is characterized by excessive osteoblastic and osteoclastic activity, resulting in abnormally thick but weak bones. Bone pain is the most common symptom.

A. **Complications** involve bones (fractures and neoplastic degeneration), joints (arthritis), and the nervous system (nerve compression, paraplegia). Hypercalcemia and renal calculi may also occur.

B. **Treatment** of Paget's disease is calcitonin and bisphosphonates.

XXIII. MARFAN SYNDROME

Marfan syndrome, a connective tissue disorder, is associated with skeletal abnormalities (high-arched palate, pectus excavatum, kyphoscoliosis, hyperextensibility of the joints), ocular changes (lens dislocation, myopia, retinal detachment), and cardiovascular abnormalities (aortic dilation, dissection, or rupture; mitral valve prolapse; heightened risk of endocarditis; cardiac conduction abnormalities).

A. Management of Anesthesia. Preoperative evaluation concentrates on cardiopulmonary abnormalities. It is prudent to avoid any sustained increase in systemic blood pressure to help avoid the risk of aortic dissection.

XXIV. KYPHOSCOLIOSIS

Kyphoscoliosis is a spinal deformity characterized by anterior flexion (kyphosis) and lateral curvature (scoliosis) of the vertebral column.

A. Signs and Symptoms. Restrictive lung disease and pulmonary hypertension progressing to cor pulmonale are associated with kyphoscoliosis.

B. Management of Anesthesia. Pulmonary function tests reflect the magnitude of restrictive lung disease. Arterial blood gases are helpful for detecting unrecognized hypoxemia or acidosis that could cause pulmonary hypertension. No specific anesthetic drug or drug combination can be recommended as optimal for patients with kyphoscoliosis. Nitrous oxide may increase pulmonary vascular resistance. Controlled hypotension may be used to help minimize intraoperative blood loss during extensive spine surgery. A "wake-up test" or monitoring of somatosensory and/or motor evoked potential is often employed to detect spinal cord compression/ischemia that can occur during spine straightening surgery, and these may influence the choice of anesthetic agents (total IV anesthesia is a common choice). Postoperative mechanical ventilation may be necessary in some patients with severe kyphoscoliosis.

XXV. DWARFISM

Dwarfism can occur in two forms: proportionate dwarfism in which the limbs, trunk, and head size are in the same relative proportions as a normal adult and disproportionate dwarfism in which the limbs, trunk, and head size are not in the usual proportions of a normal adult.

A. Achondroplasia is the most common cause of disproportionate dwarfism and occurs more often in females. The anticipated height of achondroplastic males is 132 cm (52 inches) and of females is 122 cm (48 inches).

1. Central Sleep Apnea in achondroplastic dwarfs may be a result of brainstem compression caused by foramen magnum stenosis. Pulmonary hypertension leading to cor pulmonale is the most common cardiovascular disturbance that develops in dwarfs.

2. Management of Anesthesia is influenced by potential airway difficulties, cervical spine instability, and the potential for spinal cord trauma with neck extension. A history of obstructive sleep apnea may predispose to development of upper airway obstruction after sedation or induction of anesthesia. Hyperextension of the neck during direct laryngoscopy should be avoided because of the likely presence of foramen magnum stenosis. Weight rather than age is the best guide for selecting the proper-size endotracheal tube. IV access may be technically difficult. Regional anesthesia might be considered for cesarean section but may be technically difficult because of kyphoscoliosis and a narrow epidural space and spinal canal.

B. Russell-Silver Syndrome is a form of dwarfism characterized by intrauterine growth retardation, dysmorphic facial features (including mandibular and facial hypoplasia), limb asymmetry, congenital heart defects, and a constellation of endocrine abnormalities, including hypoglycemia, adrenocortical insufficiency, and hypogonadism.

1. Management of Anesthesia. Preoperative evaluation should consider the serum glucose concentration, especially in neonates at risk of hypoglycemia. Intravenous infusions containing glucose may be indicated preoperatively. Intubation may be difficult, and an endotracheal tube smaller than the predicted size may be needed.

XXVI. BACK PAIN

Low back pain is the most common musculoskeletal complaint requiring medical attention (**Table 18-18**).

A. Acute Low Back Pain improves within 30 days in 90% of patients. NSAIDs are often effective for analgesia for acute back pain. Pain arising from inflammation initiated by mechanical or chemical insult to a nerve root may be responsive to epidural administration of corticosteroids. A herniated disc should be considered in patients with radiculopathy (L4–5, L5–S1) that is suggested by pain radiating down a leg or by symptoms reproduced by straight leg raising. Surgical intervention is indicated in patients with persistent radiculopathy/neurologic deficits.

B. Lumbar Spinal Stenosis is narrowing of the spinal canal or its lateral recesses because of hypertrophic degenerative changes in spinal structures, most often in

TABLE 18-18 Causes of Low Back Pain
Mechanical Low Back or Leg Pain (97%)
Idiopathic low back pain (lumbar sprain or strain) (70%)
Degenerative processes of discs and facets (age-related) (10%)
Herniated disc (4%)
Spinal stenosis (3%)
Osteoporotic compression fractures (4%)
Spondylolisthesis (2%)
Traumatic fracture (<1%)
Congenital disease (<1%)
Severe kyphosis
Severe scoliosis
Spondylolysis

TABLE 18-18	Causes of Low Back Pain—cont'd

Nonmechanical Spinal Conditions (1%)

Cancer (0.7%)
- Multiple myeloma
- Metastatic cancer
- Lymphoma and leukemia
- Spinal cord tumors
- Retroperitoneal tumors
- Primary vertebral tumors

Infection (0.01%)
- Osteomyelitis
- Paraspinal abscess
- Epidural abscess

Inflammatory arthritis
- Ankylosing spondylitis
- Psoriatic spondylitis
- Reiter's syndrome
- Inflammatory bowel disease

Visceral Disease (2%)

Disease of pelvic organs
- Prostatitis
- Endometriosis
- Pelvic inflammatory disease

Renal disease
- Nephrolithiasis
- Pyelonephritis
- Perinephric abscess

Aortic aneurysm

Gastrointestinal disease
- Pancreatitis
- Cholecystitis
- Penetrating ulcer

Percentages indicate the estimated incidence of these conditions in adult patients. Adapted from Deyo RO, Weinstein JN: Low back pain. N Engl J Med 2001;344:363–370.

elderly patients with chronic back pain and sciatica. The diagnosis is confirmed by magnetic resonance imaging or myelography. Surgical decompression and fusion are needed for those with progressive functional deterioration.

XXVII. OTHER MUSCULOSKELETAL SYNDROMES

A. Rotator Cuff Tear is the most common pathologic entity involving the shoulders. As many as half of individuals older than 55 years of age have arthrographically detectable rotator cuff tears.

    1. Treatment. Corticosteroid injection into the subacromial space may provide symptomatic relief. Arthroscopic release or manipulation under anesthesia may be used in an attempt to restore shoulder motion.

    2. Anesthesia Management. Brachial plexus anesthesia via the interscalene approach with continuous infusion of local anesthetic can provide anesthesia for shoulder surgery and postoperative analgesia.

B. Floppy Infant Syndrome is a term used to describe infants who have weak, hypotonic skeletal muscles. A diminished cough reflex and difficulty swallowing predispose to aspiration, and recurrent pneumonia is common.

    1. Management of Anesthesia, such as for skeletal muscle biopsy to confirm the diagnosis, is influenced by increased sensitivity to nondepolarizing muscle relaxants, hyperkalemia and cardiac arrest after administration of succinylcholine, and susceptibility to malignant hyperthermia.

C. Tracheomegaly is characterized by marked dilation of the trachea and bronchi because of a congenital defect in elastin and smooth muscle fibers in the tracheobronchial tree or their destruction after radiotherapy.

D. Alcoholic Myopathy. Acute and chronic forms of proximal skeletal muscle weakness commonly occur in alcoholic patients. Distinguishing alcoholic myopathy from alcoholic neuropathy is based on proximal, rather than distal, skeletal muscle involvement, an increased serum creatine kinase concentration, myoglobinuria in acute cases, and rapid recovery after cessation of alcohol consumption.

E. Prader-Willi Syndrome manifests at birth as hypotonia, which may be associated with a weak cough, swallowing difficulties, and upper airway obstruction.

    1. Anesthesia Concerns center on hypotonia and altered metabolism of carbohydrates (hypoglycemia) and fat. Weak skeletal musculature is associated with a poor cough and an increased incidence of aspiration pneumonia. Disturbances in thermoregulation, often characterized by intraoperative hyperthermia and metabolic acidosis, occur, but a relationship to malignant hyperthermia has not been established.

F. Prune-Belly Syndrome is characterized by congenital agenesis of the lower central abdominal musculature and the presence of urinary tract anomalies.

G. Mitochondrial Myopathies are a heterogeneous group of disorders of skeletal muscle energy metabolism characterized by abnormal fatigability with sustained exercise, skeletal muscle pain, and progressive weakness.

    1. Kearns-Sayre Syndrome is a rare mitochondrial myopathy accompanied by heart block. Dilated cardiomyopathy and congestive heart failure may be present.

H. Multicore Myopathy is a heterogeneous group of diseases characterized by proximal skeletal muscle weakness and musculoskeletal abnormalities (scoliosis, high-arched palate). Cardiomyopathy may accompany this myopathy. It is important to recognize the potential relationship between multicore myopathy and malignant hyperthermia.

I. Centronuclear Myopathy is characterized by progressive muscle weakness of extraocular, facial, neck, and limb muscles. Development of scoliosis with restrictive lung disease is an important manifestation of disease severity. Management of anesthesia is influenced by the degree of skeletal muscle weakness, the presence of restrictive lung disease, and gastroesophageal reflux. Muscle relaxants are often avoided, and a nontriggering general anesthetic technique is used.

J. Meige Syndrome is an idiopathic dystonic disorder that manifests as blepharospasm and oromandibular dystonia affecting middle-aged to elderly women.

K. Spasmodic Dysphonia is a laryngeal disorder characterized by adductor or abductor dystonic spasms of the vocal cords that manifests as abnormal phonation but on rare occasions is associated with respiratory distress.

    1. Anesthesia Concerns. The presence of laryngeal stenosis may necessitate the use of smaller-than-usual tracheal tubes. The risk of pulmonary aspiration may be increased by vocal cord dysfunction caused by therapeutic interventions such as botulinum toxin injection or interruption of the recurrent laryngeal nerve.

L. Juvenile Hyaline Fibromatosis is a rare syndrome characterized by the presence of numerous dermal and subcutaneous nodules. Resistance to the effects of succinylcholine has been described in these patients.

M. Chondrodysplasia Calcificans Punctata manifests as erratic cartilage calcification resulting in bone and skin lesions, cataracts, cardiac malformations, dwarfism, kyphoscoliosis, and subluxation of the hips. Tracheal stenosis can occur, which may complicate perioperative airway management.

N. Erythromelalgia literally means red, painful extremities. Erythema, intense, burning pain, and increased temperature of the involved extremities are hallmarks of the disease. Neuraxial opioids and local anesthetics may provide some pain relief.

O. Farber's Lipogranulomatosis is associated with accumulation of ceramide in tissues (pleura, pericardium, synovial lining of joints, liver, spleen, lymph nodes). Progressive arthropathy, psychomotor retardation, and nutritional failure result. Difficult airway management is a common problem because of granuloma formation in the pharynx or larynx. Tracheal intubation is best avoided if possible because laryngeal edema or bleeding from the granulomas may occur.

P. McCune-Albright Syndrome consists of a triad of physical signs: osseous lesions (polyostotic fibrous dysplasia), melanotic cutaneous macules (café au lait spots), and sexual precocity (autonomous ovarian steroid secretion). Conductive and neural deafness occur along with endocrine dysfunction (hyperthyroidism, acromegaly, hypophosphatemia).

Q. Klippel-Feil Syndrome is characterized by a short neck resulting from a reduced number of cervical vertebrae or fusion of several vertebrae. Movement of the neck is limited and associated skeletal abnormalities include spinal stenosis and kyphoscoliosis.

R. Osteogenesis Imperfecta is an inherited disease of connective tissue that affects bones, the sclera, and the inner ear. Bones are *extremely* brittle because of defective collagen production.

341

1. Anesthetic Implications (Table 18-19)

S. Fibrodysplasia Ossificans is a rare inherited autosomal dominant disease characterized by myositis and proliferation of connective tissue. Cervical spine involvement is common, and temporomandibular joint involvement may have implications for tracheal intubation.

T. Deformities of the Sternum. Pectus carinatum (outward protuberance of the sternum) and pectus excavatum (inward concavity of the sternum) produce cosmetic problems, but functional impairment is unusual. Obstructive sleep apnea is more common in young children with pectus excavatum.

U. Macroglossia is an uncommon but potentially lethal postoperative complication that is most often associated with posterior fossa craniotomy performed in the sitting position. Possible causes are arterial compression, venous compression caused by excessive neck flexion or a head-down position, and mechanical compression of the tongue by the teeth, an oral airway, or an endotracheal tube. When the onset of macroglossia is immediate, it is easily recognized and airway obstruction does not occur because tracheal extubation is delayed. But the development of macroglossia may be delayed for 30 minutes or longer, and there is then the risk of complete airway obstruction occurring at an unexpected time during the postoperative period.

TABLE 18-19	Anesthetic Considerations in Osteogenesis Imperfecta
Brittle bones (cervical and mandibular fractures can occur with airway manipulation)	
Defective dentition (prone to damage during tracheal intubation)	
Predisposition to fractures (succinylcholine-induced fasciculations and blood pressure cuff inflations can cause fractures)	
Kyphoscoliosis and pectus excavatum (decreased vital capacity, arterial hypoxemia)	
Platelet dysfunction (desmopressin may be effective treatment)	
Increased serum thyroxine concentration and oxygen consumption	
Mild hyperthermia is not a forerunner to malignant hyperthermia	

CHAPTER 19

Infectious Diseases

I. ANTIBIOTIC RESISTANCE

In recent decades new infections have emerged at an alarming rate (Lyme disease, Legionnaire's disease, hepatitis C, AIDS, severe acute respiratory syndrome [SARS], some parasitic diseases) and some "old" infections such as tuberculosis and malaria are re-emerging with resistance to treatment. Antibiotic, often multidrug, resistance is becoming an ever more significant problem especially in treatment of gram-negative organisms.

II. SURGICAL SITE INFECTIONS

Surgical site infections (SSIs) occur at a rate of 2% to 5% for extra-abdominal surgeries and up to 20% for intra-abdominal surgeries.
  A. Types of Infection (**Table 19-1**)
  B. Who Is at Risk? (**Table 19-2**)
  C. Signs and Symptoms. SSIs usually present within 30 days of surgery with surgical site inflammation and poor healing. Fever and malaise may occur.
  D. Diagnosis (**Table 19-3**)
  E. Management of Anesthesia
    1. Preoperative. Elective surgery should be postponed until infection has resolved. Cessation of smoking for 4 to 8 weeks prior to orthopedic surgery decreases the incidence of wound-related complications. One month of preoperative abstinence from alcohol reduces postoperative morbidity in alcohol abusers. Optimization of diabetes may decrease perioperative infection. Appropriate diet and weight loss may be beneficial prior to major surgery. Topical mupirocin applied to the anterior nares has been successful in eliminating carriage of *S. aureus* and decreasing postoperative infections (may promote mupirocin resistance, however). Hair clipping should be used instead of shaving to remove hair from the surgical site. Preoperative skin cleaning with chlorhexidine may reduce the incidence of SSIs.

TABLE 19-1	Types of Surgical Site Infections and Causes
Skin, subcutaneous tissue, fascia, and muscle	*S. aureus,* including MRSA, coagulase-negative staphylococci, enterococci, coliforms, and *Clostridium perfringens.*
Organ/tissue space infection following gastrointestinal surgery	Coliforms, *P. aeruginosa, Candida* species, *Bacteroides fragilis*

TABLE 19-2	Risk Factors for SSI	
Patient-Related Factors	**Microbial Factors**	**Wound-Related Factors**
Age	Enzyme production	Devitalized tissue
Nutritional status	Polysaccharide capsule	Dead space
ASA class >2	Bind to fibronectin	Hematoma
Diabetes	Biofilm and slime	Contaminated
Smoking		Foreign material
Obesity		
Co-existing infections		
Colonization		
Immunocompromised		
Length of preoperative hospital stay		

ASA, American Society of Anesthesiologists.

TABLE 19-3	Diagnosis of Surgical Site Infections	
Type of SSI	**Time Course**	**Criteria (at Least One)**
Superficial incisional SSI	Within 30 days of surgery	Superficial pus drainage Organisms from superficial tissue or fluid Signs and symptoms (pain, redness, swelling, heat)
Deep incisional SSI	Within 30 days of surgery or within 1 yr if prosthetic implant	Deep pus drainage Dehiscence or wound opened by surgeon (for fever >38°C, pain, tenderness) Abscess (e.g., radiographically diagnosed)
Organ/space SSI	Within 30 days of surgery or within 1 yr if prosthetic implant	Pus from a drain in the organ/space Organisms from aseptically obtained culture of fluid or tissue in the organ/space Abscess involving the organ/space

SSI, surgical site infection.

2. Intraoperative

a. Prophylactic Antibiotics prevent postoperative wound infections where bacterial counts are high (colonic, vaginal surgery) or where there is insertion of an artificial device such as a hip prosthesis or heart valve. Antibiotic prophylaxis should ideally be given within 30 minutes prior to incision. Prolonged surgery (>3 hours) may necessitate a second dose. A first-generation cephalosporin (cefazolin) is effective for many types of surgery. Vancomycin is indicated for MRSA. Coverage for gram-negative organisms is important during large bowel and gynecologic surgery (ertapenem, cefotetan), particularly in high-risk patients. Some patients may require specific prophylaxis to prevent subacute bacterial endocarditis (prosthetic heart valves, congenital heart disease, previous episodes of infective endocarditis, cardiac transplantation recipients with valvopathy).

b. Physical and Physiologic Preventive Measures

1.) **Oxygen.** Administration of 80% oxygen decreases the incidence of SSI in patients undergoing colorectal resection. This treatment is controversial because high inspired oxygen tension may also have adverse effects, such as pulmonary damage.

2.) **Normothermia.** Hypothermia is associated with increased infection rates.

3.) **Analgesia.** Good postoperative analgesia is associated with increased oxygen tension at wound sites and decreased rates of infection.

4.) **Carbon Dioxide.** Mild intraoperative hypercapnia increases subcutaneous and colonic oxygen tension, which may be associated with a reduction in SSIs. Interestingly, CO_2 is itself bacteriostatic.

5.) **Supplemental Perioperative Fluid Administration** increases tissue perfusion and tissue oxygen partial pressure, but excess fluids may be associated with increased morbidity, especially pulmonary complications.

6) **Glucose.** Tight control of blood sugar (between 80 and 110 mg/dL) has been shown to decrease episodes of septicemia (by 46%) and mortality in critically ill patients, especially following cardiac surgery. High blood sugar inhibits leukocyte function.

III. BLOODSTREAM INFECTION (BSI)

Central venous catheters (CVCs) are the predominant cause of nosocomial bacteremia and fungemia.

A. Signs and Symptoms are typically nonspecific (mental status change, hemodynamic instability, altered tolerance for nutrition, malaise), with no obvious candidate source other than an indwelling catheter. A sudden change in a patient's condition should alert the clinician to the possibility of a BSI.

B. Diagnosis. Catheter-associated BSIs are defined as bacteremia/fungemia in a patient with an intravascular catheter and at least one positive blood culture obtained from a peripheral vein, clinical manifestations of infection, and no apparent source for the BSI except the catheter. The diagnosis is more compelling if, when a catheter is removed, the same organisms that grew from blood grows from the catheter tip. **Table 19-4** lists some pathogens associated with BSI.

345

TABLE 19-4	Most Common Pathogens Associated with Bloodstream Infections
Coagulase-negative staphylococci (37%)	
Staphylococcus aureus (13%)	
Enterococcus (13%)	
Gram-negative bacilli (14%)	
• *Escherichia coli* (2%)	
• *Enterobacter* species (5%)	
• *Pseudomonas aeruginosa* (4%)	
• *Klebsiella penumoniae* (3%)	
Candida species (8%)	

C. Treatment. The best treatment is prevention. The source of the infection, usually a central venous catheter, should be removed and broad-spectrum empirical antimicrobial therapy should be initiated pending the results of the cultures, at which point therapy should be appropriately targeted.

D. Anesthesia Management

   1. Preoperative Management. Many CVCs are placed by anesthesiologists who are unaware of BSIs that occur days later. The subclavian and internal jugular routes carry less risk of infection than the femoral route. Hand washing, use of full-barrier precautions during central venous catheter insertion, cleaning the skin with chlorhexidine, avoiding the femoral site if possible, and removing unnecessary catheters all are effective in reducing catheter-related BSIs. Sterility must be maintained when accessing catheter ports. CVCs that are coated or impregnated with antimicrobial or antiseptic agents have been associated with lower rates of BSIs.

   2. Intraoperative Management. Blood transfusions are associated with immunosuppression, and transmission of infectious agents (hepatitis, human immunodeficiency [HIV]).

   a. Immunosuppression from blood transfusion may be decreased by leukodepletion of blood products.

   b. Transmission of Infectious Agents. During early viral infection with HIV and hepatitis C virus, there is a "window period" during which circulating antibodies are not yet present but there is a significant viral count. Bacterial contamination of blood products is about 1 in 1000 to 3000 platelet units (coagulase-negative staphylococci, *S. aureus, Bacillus cereus, Serratia marcescens,* streptococci, and *Pseudomonas aeruginosa*). Only organisms that grow at cold temperature, such as *Yersinia enterocolitica,* are able to grow in refrigerated blood. Transmission of variant Creutzfeldt-Jakob disease by blood transfusion has now been demonstrated. The best way to avoid the infectious complications of transfusion is to avoid transfusion.

   3. Postoperative Management. Remove central lines and pulmonary artery catheters as soon as they are no longer needed. Avoid unnecessary parenteral nutrition and even dextrose-containing fluids because these may be associated with increased risk of BSI.

IV. SEPSIS

Sepsis is a spectrum of disorders, with localized inflammation at one end and a severe generalized inflammatory response with multiorgan failure at the other (**Fig. 19-1**). Surgery and anesthesia should be postponed until sepsis is at least partially treated. However, sometimes the underlying cause of sepsis (abscess, endocarditis, bowel perforation, necrotizing fasciitis) requires urgent surgical intervention.

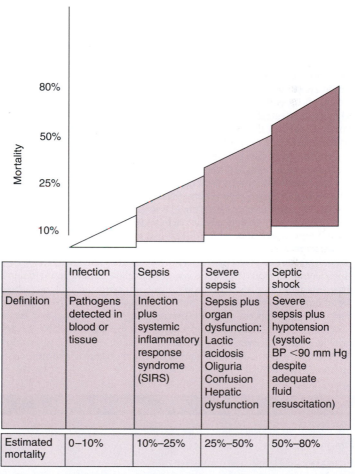

	Infection	Sepsis	Severe sepsis	Septic shock
Definition	Pathogens detected in blood or tissue	Infection plus systemic inflammatory response syndrome (SIRS)	Sepsis plus organ dysfunction: Lactic acidosis Oliguria Confusion Hepatic dysfunction	Severe sepsis plus hypotension (systolic BP <90 mm Hg despite adequate fluid resuscitation)
Estimated mortality	0–10%	10%–25%	25%–50%	50%–80%

Figure 19-1 • Continuum of sepsis with definitions and approximate mortality rates. (Adapted from Bone RC: Toward an epidemiology and natural history of systemic inflammatory response syndrome. JAMA 1992;268:3452–3455.)

A. Signs and Symptoms of sepsis are often nonspecific. The systemic inflammatory response syndrome (**Table 19-5**) is an important component of sepsis. Sepsis may result in multiple organ system failure. Classically, there is hypotension, bounding pulses, and wide pulse pressure.

B. Diagnosis is surmised from history, signs, and symptoms. Confirmation is based on the isolation of specific causative pathogens from blood, urine, sputum, cerebrospinal fluid (CSF), or tissue samples.

C. Treatment (Fig. 19-2)

    1. Rapid Initiation of Broad Antimicrobial Coverage is the initial treatment. Therapy should be tailored to the specific organism and its sensitivities. In addition to their antimicrobial spectrum, antibiotics should be chosen by their ability to penetrate various tissues, including bone, cerebrospinal fluid, lung tissue, and abscess cavities.

    2. Supportive Treatment relating to organ system dysfunction is essential (**Table 19-6**). Support should be directed at optimizing oxygen delivery and cardiac output. Mixed venous or central venous saturation may be useful guides for therapeutic end points. Early fluid resuscitation is usually indicated. Appropriate use of inotropes and vasoconstrictors may be important. (**Fig. 19-2**).

D. Prognosis depends on the virulence of the infecting pathogen(s), the stage at which appropriate treatment is initiated, the inflammatory response of the patient, the immune status of the patient, and the extent of organ system dysfunction.

E. Management of Anesthesia

    1. Preoperative. The most important questions are whether the surgery may be postponed pending treatment of sepsis and whether, if surgery is urgent, the patient's condition may be improved prior to surgery. Preoperative resuscitation should aim to achieve mean arterial pressure greater than 65 mm Hg, central venous pressure of 8 to 12 mm Hg, adequate urine output, a normal pH without a metabolic (lactic) acidosis, and mixed venous or central venous saturation above 70%.

    2. Intraoperative. Invasive monitoring, (arterial blood pressure, central venous pressure or pulmonary artery pressure), is usually indicated. Sufficient intravenous (IV) access is needed to allow volume resuscitation and transfusion of blood and blood components. Prophylactic antibiotics should be administered within the 30 minutes prior to skin incision. Normothermia and normoglycemia are a priority. Inotropes (e.g., epinephrine) and vasoconstrictors (e.g., norepinephrine and vasopressin) should be available. IV steroids may be indicated for refractory shock.

    3. Postoperative. Continued hemodynamic monitoring and support as needed (**Fig. 19-2**).

TABLE 19-5 Systemic Inflammatory Response Syndrome
Two or more of the following:
• White blood count >11,000 or <4,000 × 10^9/L or >10% immature forms
• Heart rate >90 bpm
• Temperature >38° C or <36° C
• Respiratory rate >20 breaths per minute or PaCO$_2$ <32 mm Hg

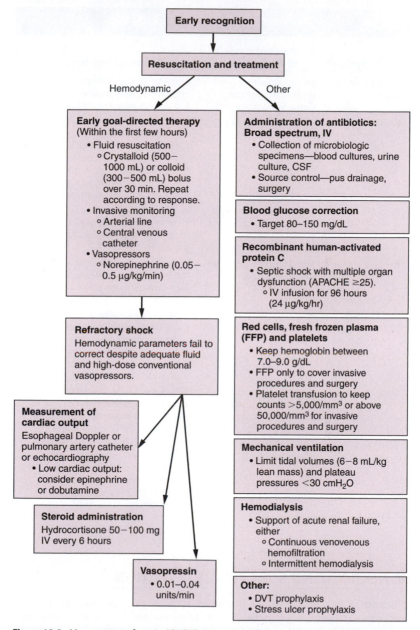

Figure 19-2 • Management of sepsis. APACHE, Acute Physiology and Chronic Health Evaluation II; DVT, deep vein thrombosis; FFP, fresh frozen plasma.

	TABLE 19-6 Organ System Dysfunction in Sepsis	
Organ System	Manifestations of Dysfunction	Treatment and Support
Central nervous system	Encephalopathy, decreased Glasgow Coma Scale score	Consider airway protection (e.g., intubation), daily interruption of sedation to assess neurologic status
Cardiovascular	Vasodilatory shock, myocardial depression	Maintain mean arterial pressure >65 mm Hg, central venous pressure of 8–12 cm H_2O, and central or mixed venous saturation >70%; fluid resuscitation, vasoconstrictors (e.g., norepinephrine, vasopressin); inotropes (e.g., epinephrine)
Respiratory	Impaired oxygenation (decreased PaO_2/FiO_2), acute respiratory distress syndrome	Assisted ventilation with low tidal volumes (6–8 mL/kg ideal body mass) and target mean airway pressures <30 cm H_2O
Renal	Renal failure (elevated creatinine)	Attempt to maintain urine output >0.5 mL/kg/hr; venovenous hemofiltration or hemodialysis if needed
Hematologic	Thrombocytopenia or disseminated intravascular coagulopathy	Treatment is controversial; consider heparin or recombinant activated protein C; anticoagulants are contraindicated at the time of surgery; platelet transfusion may be indicated for surgery
Gastrointestinal	Hepatic dysfunction (elevated bilirubin)	Treatment is supportive; fresh frozen plasma or vitamin K may be required to correct an abnormal prothrombin time (PT) at the time of surgery
Endocrine	Hyperglycemia, adrenal insufficiency	Insulin infusion to achieve blood glucose of 80–150 mg/dL; check random and stimulated adrenal function; consider hydrocortisone (50–100 mg intravenously for refractory hypotension)

V. NECROTIZING SOFT-TISSUE INFECTION

Necrotizing infection includes diagnoses such as gas gangrene, toxic shock syndrome, Fournier's gangrene, severe cellulitis, and flesh-eating infection. Severity may be underappreciated at the time of presentation. The organisms responsible are highly virulent, the clinical course is rampant, and mortality is high (up to 75%).

A. Signs and Symptoms include general features of infection, including malaise, fever, sweating, and altered mental status. Pain is always present and may be out of proportion to physical signs. Because the infection begins in deep tissue planes, cutaneous signs are often surprisingly mild and are not reflective of the extent of tissue necrosis or the severity of the disease. Hypotension is an ominous sign.

B. Diagnosis. Patients with a history of alcohol abuse, malnutrition, obesity, trauma, cancer, burns, older age, vascular disease, diabetes, and immunocompromise are more susceptible. There may be a high white blood cell count, thrombocytopenia, coagulopathy, electrolyte abnormalities, acidosis, hyperglycemia, elevated markers of inflammation such as C reactive protein, and radiographic evidence of extensive necrotic inflammation with subcutaneous air. Computed tomography or magnetic resonance imaging may delineate the extent of necrotic tissue. Blood, urine, and tissue samples should be sent to the laboratory for culture.

C. Treatment is extensive surgical debridement of necrotic tissue coupled with appropriate antimicrobial therapy, which typically includes coverage of gram-positive, gram-negative, and anaerobic organisms. Other therapies include topical unprocessed honey (to digest necrotic tissue) and hyperbaric treatment.

D. Prognosis. Mortality rate is high, and if patients survive the initial insult, they may remain vulnerable to secondary infection.

E. Management of Anesthesia

1. Preoperative. The anesthesiologist should treat such patients as having severe sepsis and try to resuscitate preoperatively. However, surgical debridement should not be postponed because delay is associated with increased mortality.

2. Intraoperative. Concern has been raised about the use of etomidate when patients have septic shock because they may already have adrenal insufficiency, and this may theoretically be worsened by even a single dose of etomidate. Major fluid shifts, blood loss, and release of cytokines may occur intraoperatively. Good IV access is essential, and invasive arterial and central venous monitoring may be useful. Blood should be cross-matched and readily available. Patients are at risk of developing both hypovolemic and septic shock.

3. Postoperative. As with sepsis, patients are at risk of developing multiorgan failure. Postoperative admission to an intensive care unit (ICU) is advisable. Antibiotic therapy should be continued in the postoperative period and should be targeted to the organisms that grow from tissue specimens.

VI. TETANUS

The neurotoxin tetanospasmin produced by vegetative forms of *Clostridium tetani* organisms causes the clinical manifestations of tetanus. Tetanospasmin suppresses inhibitory internuncial neurons in the spinal cord, resulting in generalized skeletal muscle contractions (spasms). In the brain, the fourth ventricle is believed to have selective permeability for tetanospasmin, resulting in early manifestations of trismus and neck rigidity. Sympathetic nervous system hyperactivity may develop.

A. Signs and Symptoms (Table 19-7)

B. Treatment

1. Control of Skeletal Muscle Spasms is achieved by use of diazepam, muscle relaxants, and mechanical ventilation.

2. Prevention of Sympathetic Nervous System Hyperactivity is possible with use of beta-blockers.

3. Ventilatory Support includes tracheal intubation to control secretions and prevention of airway obstruction caused by laryngospasm.

4. Neutralize Circulating Exotoxin with intramuscular administration of human hyperimmunoglobulin.

5. Surgical Debridement can eliminate the source of the exotoxin.

6. Antibiotic treatment (penicillin) destroys the exotoxin-producing vegetative forms of *C. tetani.*

C. Management of Anesthesia. General anesthesia with volatile agents (to decrease sympathetic nervous system activity) and tracheal intubation (due to increased potential for laryngospasm) is the usual approach. Surgical debridement is delayed for several hours after the patient has received antitoxin because tetanospasmin will be mobilized into the systemic circulation during surgical resection. Invasive blood pressure and central venous pressure monitoring is often indicated. Drugs such as lidocaine, esmolol, metoprolol, magnesium, nicardipine, and nitroprusside should be readily available.

VII. PNEUMONIA

Community-acquired pneumonia is one of the 10 leading causes of death in the United States. *Streptococcus pneumoniae* is the most common cause of bacterial pneumonia in adults (typical pneumonia). Other common organisms include

TABLE 19-7 Symptoms and Signs of Tetanus
• Trismus (75%)
• Laryngospasm
• Facial muscle rigidity ("risus sardonicus")
• Dysphagia
• Abdominal and lumbar muscle rigidity (opisthotonic posture)
• Excruciating skeletal muscle spasms, precipitated by external stimulation, such as sudden exposure to light, unexpected noise, or tracheal suction
• Increased body temperature due to increased skeletal muscle work and increased oxygen consumption
• Hypotension (myocarditis) or transient hypertension
• Tachydysrhythmias
• Peripheral vasoconstriction
• Diaphoresis
• Inappropriate antidiuretic hormone secretion with hyponatremia and decreased plasma osmolality

Haemophilus influenzae, Mycoplasma pneumoniae, S. aureus, Legionella pneumophilia, Klebsiella pneumoniae, and *Chlamydia pneumoniae* and Influenza virus (atypical pneumonias).

A. Diagnosis. An initial chill, followed by abrupt onset of fever, chest pain, dyspnea, fatigue, rigors, cough, and copious sputum production characterizes bacterial pneumonia. Nonproductive cough is a feature of atypical pneumonias. Patient history may suggest possible causative organisms, such as exposure to hotels and whirlpools (*L. pneumophila*), cave exploration (*Histoplasma capsulatum*), diving (*Scedosporium angiospermum*), contact with birds (*Chlamydia psittaci*), contact with sheep (*Coxiella burnetti*), alcoholism (*K. pneumoniae*), and immunocompromise such as in AIDS (*Pneumocystis jirovecii* pneumonia [PCP]). Chest radiograph, microscopic examination of sputum and cultures, urine testing for the presence of *L. pneumophila* antigen, blood antibody titers for *M. pneumoniae,* sputum polymerase chain reaction for *Chlamydia* and serum testing for HIV infection can be helpful.

B. Treatment for severe pneumonia is empirical therapy (typically a combination such as a cephalosporin plus a macrolide antibiotic such as azithromycin or clarithromycin). Therapy should be narrowed and targeted when the pathogen is identified.

C. Prognosis (Table 19-8)

D. Aspiration Pneumonia. Risks include depressed consciousness (alcohol abuse, drug abuse, head trauma, seizures and other neurologic disorders, administration of sedatives), abnormalities of deglutition or esophageal motility resulting from placement of nasogastric tubes, esophageal cancer, bowel obstruction, repeated vomiting, poor oral hygiene and periodontal disease, and induction and recovery from anesthesia. Clinical manifestations depend on the nature and volume of aspirated material and can include

TABLE 19-8	Pneumonia: Factors Associated with Worse Outcomes
Temperature >40°C or <35°C	
Respiratory rate >30/min	
Altered mental status	
Systolic blood pressure <90 mm Hg	
Heart rate >125/min	
Hypoxia (PO_2 <60 mm Hg or saturation <90% on room air)	
Pleural effusion	
Anemia (hematocrit <30%)	
BUN >64 mg/dL	
Glucose >250 mg/dL	
Acidosis (pH <7.35)	
Sodium <130 mmol/L	

BUN, blood urea nitrogen.

fulminating arterial hypoxemia, airway obstruction, atelectasis, and pneumonia.

E. Management of Anesthesia. Anesthesia and surgery should ideally be deferred with acute pneumonia. Fluid management is challenging; fluid overload may worsen hypoxia. During general anesthesia, ventilation should generally be with tidal volumes of 6 to 8 mL/kg ideal body mass and mean airway pressures less than 30 cm H_2O.

F. Postoperative Pneumonia occurs in approximately 20% of patients undergoing major thoracic, esophageal, or upper abdominal surgery but is rare in other procedures in previously fit patients.

G. Lung Abscesses may develop after bacterial pneumonia. The finding of an air-fluid level on the chest radiograph signifies rupture of the abscess into the bronchial tree, and foul-smelling sputum is characteristic. Surgery is indicated only when complications such as empyema occur.

VIII. VENTILATOR-ASSOCIATED PNEUMONIA

Ventilator-associated pneumonia (VAP) is the most common nosocomial infection in the ICU and makes up one third of all nosocomial infections. Mortality is 15% to 50%. Several simple interventions may decrease the occurrence of VAP, including meticulous hand hygiene, oral care, limiting patient sedation, positioning patients semiupright, suctioning subglottic secretions, limiting intubation time, and considering the appropriateness of noninvasive ventilation support.

A. Diagnosis (Table 19-9). The National Nosocomial Infections Surveillance System uses a standardized diagnostic algorithm for VAP and a clinical pulmonary infection score to promote diagnostic consistency among clinicians and investigators. A clinical pulmonary infection score greater than 6 is consistent with a diagnosis of VAP. Both the NNIS and the clinical pulmonary infection score are relatively sensitive for VAP (>80%) but nonspecific.

B. Treatment (Fig. 19-3)

C. Management of Anesthesia. Patients with VAP often require anesthesia for tracheostomy. Major surgery should be deferred until the pneumonia has resolved and respiratory function has improved. Patients with respiratory failure may be positive end-expiratory pressure (PEEP) dependent. Ideally, the same ventilator settings that were used in the ICU should be used in the operating room, including mode of ventilation and PEEP. The lowest inspired oxygen necessary to achieve adequate oxygen saturation (SpO_2 >95%) should be administered.

IX. SEVERE ACUTE RESPIRATORY SYNDROME AND INFLUENZA

Influenza A and SARS-associated viruses are examples of viruses that have rampant courses, high virulence, and high mortality.

A. Signs and Symptoms include nonspecific complaints (cough, sore throat, headache, diarrhea, arthralgia, muscle pain). In more severe cases, patients may present with respiratory distress, confusion (encephalitis), and hemoptysis. Other signs include fever, tachycardia, sweating, conjunctivitis, rash, tachypnea,

TABLE 19-9 Clinical Pulmonary Infection Score Calculation

Parameter	Options	Score
Temperature (°C)	≥36.5 and ≤38.4	0
	≥38.5 and ≤38.9	1
	≥39 or ≤36	2
Blood leukocytes (mm³)	≥4000 and ≤11,000	0
	<4000 or >11000	1
	+ band forms ≥50%	Add 1
Tracheal secretions	Absence of tracheal secretions	0
	Presence of nonpurulent tracheal secretions	1
	Presence of purulent tracheal secretions	2
Oxygenation: PaO_2/FiO_2 (mm Hg)	>240 or ARDS	0
	≤240 and no ARDS	2
Pulmonary radiography	No infiltrate	0
	Diffuse (or patchy) infiltrate	1
	Localized infiltrate	2
Progression of pulmonary infiltrate	No radiographic progression	0
	Radiographic progression (after cardiac failure and ARDS excluded)	2
Culture of tracheal aspirate	Pathogenic bacteria cultured in rare or light quantity	0
	Pathogenic bacteria cultured in moderate or heavy quantity	1
	Same pathogenic bacteria seen on Gram stain	Add 1

ARDS, acute respiratory distress syndrome.
Reproduced from Luyt CE, Chastre J, Fagon JY: Value of the clinical pulmonary infection score for the identification and management of ventilator-associated pneumonia. Intensive Care Med 2004;30:844–852; with permission.

use of accessory respiratory muscles, cyanosis, and pulmonary features of pneumonia, pleural effusion, or pneumothorax. A chest radiograph may be helpful.

B. Diagnosis. In the context of an outbreak, history, symptoms, and presentation are usually sufficient to suggest a diagnosis. The incubation period for SARS-Coronavirus (CoV) and H5N1 influenza A, "bird flu," is about 1 week. For influenza, the range is 2 to 17 days. Serologic testing is not usually helpful because it may take 2 to 3 weeks for seroconversion after infection. Polymerase chain reaction tests can be useful for diagnosing SARS-CoV and H5N1 influenza A.

C. Treatment. Vaccine development is key in prevention of widespread infection and reduction of morbidity and mortality. No vaccine currently exists for the SARS-CoV or for the H5N1 influenza A virus. In the case of influenza, neuraminidase inhibitors (zanamivir, oseltamivir) may decrease the severity of infection. Amantadine and rimantadine may also be used. These drugs are only of

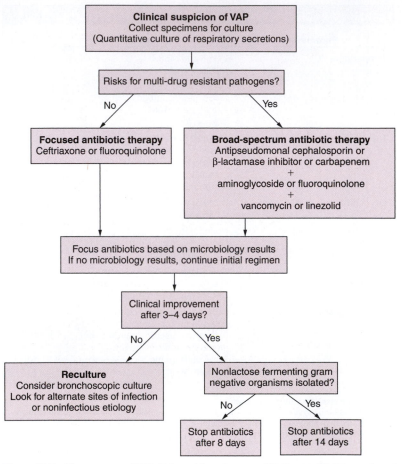

Figure 19-3 • Management of VAP. (Adapted from Porzecanski I, Bowton DL: Diagnosis and treatment of ventilator-associated pneumonia. Chest 2006;130:597–604.)

modest benefit and are helpful only if administered within the first 48 hours of symptoms. The mainstay of treatment for influenza and SARS is supportive care.
D. Prognosis depends on the pathogenicity of the infecting virus as well as the susceptibility of the infected person.
E. Management of Anesthesia
   1. Preoperative. Barrier precautions should be used with patients infected with SARS-CoV and newly evolved virulent influenza strains, including full-body disposable oversuits, double gloves, goggles, and powered air-purifying respirators with high-efficiency particulate air filters. If these are not available, N95 masks (block 95% of particles) should be used rather than regular surgical masks. Filters should be

placed in both limbs of breathing circuits to protect ventilators and anesthesia machines from contamination. All surfaces should be sterilized with alcohol, and ideally rooms should not be used for other patients (if practical) for up to 48 hours after a person with SARS-CoV or H5N1 influenza A has been in the room.

2. Intraoperative. Fears about contagion should not blind anesthesiologists to the high level of care required for these vulnerable patients. When appropriate precautions are taken, spread of infection may be prevented. If mechanical ventilation is required, protective ventilation as for acute respiratory distress syndrome is indicated. Tidal volumes should be limited to 6 to 8 mL/kg lean body mass and mean airway pressure should be less than 30 cm H_2O.

3. Postoperative. Precautions to prevent spread of infection should be ongoing.

X. ACQUIRED IMMUNODEFICIENCY SYNDROME

It is estimated that more than 40 million people worldwide are infected with HIV, which is thought to have caused more than 25 million deaths to date. The predominant mode of HIV transmission is heterosexual sex. There is a variable period during which the patient remains healthy but is viremic.

A. Pathogenesis. Acute seroconversion illness occurs with a high viral load soon after infection. After several months, there is a decrease in the viremia as the immune response occurs. Gradual involution of lymph nodes occurs, with a concomitant decrease in T-helper lymphocytes (CD4 T cells) and an increase in viral load as the inexorable onset of AIDS occurs. Pneumcystis pneumonia does not usually occur until the CD4 count is less than 200 cells/mL.

B. Signs and Symptoms (Table 19-10)

C. Diagnosis is via an enzyme-linked immunosorbent assay (ELISA), which usually becomes positive when the antibodies to HIV increase 4 to 8 weeks after infection. During this period, patients are more infectious. Infection may be confirmed with a Western blot test or by measurement of HIV viral load in the blood.

D. Treatment. Five major classes of antiretroviral agents are currently in use:

1. Nucleoside Analogue Reverse-Transcriptase Inhibitors (NRTIs) bind to the evolving viral DNA and prevent completion of reverse transcription.

2. Non-nucleoside Analogue Reverse-Transcriptase Inhibitors (NNRTIs) interfere with the transcriptional activity of this enzyme by binding to it directly, downstream of the active catalytic site.

3. Protease Inhibitors (PIs) inhibit the HIV protease, which cleaves the polyprotein precursors that ultimately make up the core proteins of mature virions. PIs bind specifically to the active cleavage site.

4. Integrase Inhibitors act on the integrase enzyme, inhibiting HIV, which the virus needs for incorporation of its DNA into the infected cell's DNA.

5. Chemokine Receptor 5 (CCR5) Antagonists (e.g., maraviroc) prevent the binding of HIV to one of the co-receptors it uses to enter target cells.

A typical antiretroviral regimen consists of three agents: a PI or NNRTI combined with two NRTIs. Numerous side effects (hypersensitivity reactions, severe myopathy, respiratory muscle dysfunction) and drug interactions complicate treatment and decrease compliance (**Table 19-11**). Of particular importance to anesthesiologists is the fact that patients are

TABLE 19-10   Signs and Symptoms of AIDS

Constitutional	Night sweats, weight loss
Respiratory	Breathlessness, abnormal chest x-ray
Lymph nodes	Diffuse adenopathy
Neurologic	Dementia
	Cerebral toxoplasmosis
	CNS lymphoma
	Progressive multifocal leukoencephalopathy
	Meningitis (*Cryptococcus,* HIV, tuberculosis)
Cardiac	Often silent involvement
	Abnormal ECG in up to 50% of patients
	Pericardial effusion in up to 25% of patients
Generalized vascular disease	Complication of antiviral therapy
Adrenal insufficiency	Hypotension
Kaposi's sarcoma	Skin and endobronchial involvement; may cause hemoptysis

CNS, central nervous system; ECG, electrocardiogram.

subject to long-term metabolic complications, including lipid abnormalities and glucose intolerance, which may result in the development of diabetes, coronary artery disease, and cerebrovascular disease.

E. Management of Anesthesia

1. Intraoperative

a. Universal Precautions require that every patient be regarded as potentially infected with a blood-borne virus. Following an accident with high-risk body fluid, such as a (hollow) needlestick injury, postexposure prophylaxis should begin as soon as possible after the injury, ideally within 1 to 2 hours, but can be considered up to 1 to 2 weeks after the injury. A recommended postexposure prophylaxis regimen for a duration of 4 weeks is zidovudine 250 mg every 12 hours, lamivudine 150 mg every 12 hours, and indinavir 800 mg every 8 hours.

b. Focal Neurologic Lesions May Increase Intracerebral Pressure precluding neuraxial anesthesia. Neurologic involvement may make the use of succinylcholine hazardous. Steroid supplementation should be considered for unexplained hypotension.

2. Postoperative.
HIV infection does not increase the risk of postprocedural complications including death up to 30 days post-procedure. Little information exists concerning the overall risk of anesthesia and surgery in the HIV-seropositive patient. In studies of HIV-seropositive parturients who were given regional anesthesia, no neurologic or infectious complications occurred related to the anesthetic or obstetric course. In the immediate postpartum period, immune function measurements remained essentially unchanged, as did the severity of the disease. The safety of epidural blood patches for treatment of postdural puncture headache has been reported in

TABLE 19-11 Antiretroviral Drugs: Administration Tips and Side Effects

Drug Name	Administration	Common Side Effects
NRTIs:		
Zidovudine	Oral/IV	Bone marrow suppression (neutropenia), GI upset, headache
Didanosine	Empty stomach, oral	Peripheral neuropathy, pancreatitis, diarrhea
Zalcitabine	Oral	Peripheral neuropathy, pancreatitis, oral ulcers
Stavudine	Oral	Peripheral neuropathy
Lamivudine	Oral	Anemia, GI upset
Abacavir	Oral	GI upset, potentially fatal acute hypersensitivity reactions
NNRTIs:		
Nevirapine	Oral	Rash, hepatitis, liver enzyme (P-450) induction
Delavirdine	Oral	Rash, liver enzyme (P-450) induction
Efavirenz	Oral	Dizziness, rash, dysphoria, liver enzyme (P-450) induction
PIs:		
Saquinavir	With fatty meal or up to 2 hr after meals	Diarrhea, increased transaminases, hyperlipidemia, P-450 inhibition
Indinavir	Empty stomach; 1.5 L water in 24 hr	Nephrolithiasis, hyperbilirubinemia, hyperlipidemia, lipodystrophy, P-450 inhibition
Ritonavir	Refrigerate tablets With food	GI upset, circumoral paresthesia, hyperlipidemia, lipodystrophy, P-450 inhibition
Nelfinavir		Diarrhea, hyperlipidemia, lipodystrophy, P-450 inhibition

GI, gastrointestinal; NNRTIs, non-nucleoside reverse transcriptase inhibitors; NRTIs, nucleoside reverse transcriptase inhibitors; PIs, protease inhibitors.

HIV-seropositive patients, but, given the theoretical risk of introducing virus into the central nervous system, other treatment strategies should be tried first.

XI. TUBERCULOSIS

Mycobacterium tuberculosis is an obligate aerobe responsible for TB, which survives most successfully in tissues with high oxygen concentrations. At present, most cases of TB in the United States occur in racial and ethnic minorities, foreign-born individuals from areas where TB is endemic (Asia and Africa), IV drug abusers, and those with HIV infection or AIDS. Any patient with TB should be tested for HIV. The appearance of multidrug-resistant strains of *M. tuberculosis* has contributed to the resurgence of TB worldwide.

A. **Diagnosis** of TB is based on the presence of clinical symptoms (persistent nonproductive cough, anorexia, weight loss, chest pain, hemoptysis, night sweats), the epidemiologic likelihood of infection, and results of diagnostic tests. The most common test for TB is the tuberculin skin (Mantoux) test. This test may be positive if people have received a bacille Calmette-Guérin (BCG) vaccine or if they have been exposed to TB, even if there are no viable mycobacteria present at the time of the skin test. Chest radiographs show apical or subapical infiltrates, or bilateral upper lobe infiltration with the presence of cavitation. Patients with AIDS may demonstrate a less classic picture on chest radiography. Tuberculous vertebral osteomyelitis (Pott's disease) is a common manifestation of extrapulmonary TB. Sputum smears may show presence of acid-fast bacilli.

B. Anesthesiologists Are at Increased Risk of nosocomial TB and should participate in annual tuberculin screening so that those who develop a positive skin test may be offered chemotherapy.

C. Treatment is chemotherapy with isoniazid. Other drugs include pyrazinamide, rifampicin, and ethambutol. In order to be curative, treatment for pulmonary TB is recommended for 6 months. Extrapulmonary TB usually requires a longer course.

D. Management of Anesthesia

1. Preoperative Assessment includes a detailed history, including the presence of a persistent cough and the tuberculin status. Elective surgical procedures should be postponed until patients are no longer infectious (i.e., they have received antituberculous chemotherapy, are improving clinically, and have had three consecutive negative sputum smears). If surgery cannot be delayed, limit the number of involved personnel. High-risk procedures (bronchoscopy, tracheal intubation, tracheal suctioning) should be performed in a negative-pressure environment. Patients should be transported wearing a tight-fitting N-95 face mask and staff should also wear N-95 masks.

2. Intraoperative. Special precautions should be taken not to injure the spine during airway manipulation in patients with TB of the spine. A high-efficiency particulate air (HEPA) filter should be placed between the Y connector and the mask, laryngeal mask airway, or tracheal tube. Bacterial filters should be placed on the exhalation limb of the anesthesia delivery circuit to decrease the discharge of tubercle bacilli into the ambient air. Use of a dedicated anesthesia machine and ventilator is recommended.

3. Postoperative care should take place in an isolation room, preferably with negative pressure.

XII. CLOSTRIDIUM DIFFICILE

C. difficile is an anaerobic, gram-positive, spore-forming bacterium that is the major identifiable cause of antibiotic-associated diarrhea and pseudomembranous colitis. *C. difficile* produces two toxins (A and B) that cause diarrhea.

A. Risk Factors (Table 19-12)

B. Signs and Symptoms are most commonly diarrhea and abdominal pain. Patients may be febrile with abdominal tenderness and distension.

C. Diagnosis. The most common confirmatory study is an enzyme immunoassay for *C. difficile* toxins A and B in the stool. The results are available in 2 to 4 hours. Specificity is high (up to 100%), but sensitivity ranges from 63% to 99%.

TABLE 19-12	Risk Factors for Developing *C. difficile*–Associated Diarrhea

Increasing age (except infants)

Severe underlying disease

Nonsurgical gastrointestinal procedures

Presence of a nasogastric tube

Receiving antiulcer medication

ICU stay

Long duration of hospital stay

Long duration of antibiotic course (risk doubles after 3 days)

Multiple antibiotic therapy

Immunosuppressive therapy

Recent surgical procedure

Sharing hospital room with a *C. difficile*–infected patient

Therefore, it is advisable to send stool for *C. difficile* toxin detection over 3 sequential days in order to exclude the diagnosis of *C. difficile* associated diarrhea.
D. Treatment is fluid and electrolyte replacement, withdrawal of current antibiotic therapy if possible, and targeted antibiotic treatment to eradicate *C. difficile* (oral metronidazole 400 mg 3 times daily, or oral vancomycin 125 mg 4 times daily). Treatment is typically for at least 10 days but should be continued until symptoms and diarrhea resolve.

E. Management of Anesthesia

   1. Preoperative. Generally the sickest patients with *C. difficile* colitis, including those who do not improve with conventional therapy, present for surgery, such as subtotal colectomy and ileostomy. Surgery carries a high mortality.

   2. Intraoperative. Hemodynamic instability is likely, and invasive monitoring may guide fluid administration and the use of inotropes and vasopressors. Dehydration, acid-base, and electrolyte abnormalities may occur following episodes of diarrhea. Opiates decrease intestinal motility, which may exacerbate toxin-mediated disease.

   3. Postoperative. One of the most important considerations is prevention of the spread of *C. difficile*; therefore contact and isolation precautions are essential, and routine use of disposable gloves and gowns is important. Vigorous hand washing with soap and water may remove spores.

CHAPTER 20

Cancer

ancer is the second most common cause of death in the United States, exceeded only by heart disease.

I. MECHANISM

Cancer results from an accumulation of mutations in genes that regulate cellular proliferation (oncogenes). An example of a critical gene is tumor suppressor p53. This gene is critical in monitoring damage to DNA and essential for cell viability. Inactivation of p53 is an early step in the development of many types of cancer. Stimulation of oncogene formation by carcinogens (tobacco, alcohol, sunlight) is estimated to be responsible for 80% of cancers in the United States. Evidence of a protective role of the immune system in fighting cancer is the increased incidence of cancer in immunosuppressed patients, such as those with acquired immunodeficiency syndrome and those receiving organ transplants.

II. DIAGNOSIS (Table 20-1)

Cancer often becomes evident when tumor bulk compromises the function of vital organs. The initial diagnosis is often by aspiration cytology or biopsy (needle, incisional, excisional). Monoclonal antibodies against specific cancers (prostate, lung, breast, ovary) may aid in the diagnosis. A commonly used staging system for solid tumors is the TNM system based on tumor size (T), lymph node involvement (N), and distant metastasis (M). This system further groups patients into stages from I to IV. Stage I has the best prognosis and stage IV the worst. Imaging techniques, including computed tomography and magnetic resonance imaging, are used for further delineation of tumor presence and spread.

III. TREATMENT

Treatment of cancer includes chemotherapy, radiation, and surgery. Surgery is often necessary for the initial diagnosis of cancer (biopsy) and subsequent definitive treatment. Palliative and rehabilitative therapy may require surgery. Adequate relief of acute and chronic pain associated with cancer is a mandatory part of treatment.

A. Chemotherapy administered for cancer chemotherapy may produce significant side effects (see **Table 20-1**) that may have important implications for anesthesia management.

B. Surgery is often needed in the initial diagnosis of cancer (biopsy), as well as definitive treatment, and may be required for tumor palliation.

C. Angiogenesis Inhibitors (e.g., endostatin) interfere with the ability of cancer cells to secrete proteins that facilitate angiogenesis and tissue invasion, such as vascular endothelial growth factor, fibroblast growth factors, and matrix metalloproteinases.

D. Treatment of Acute and Chronic Pain, which can result from pathologic fractures, tumor invasion, surgery, radiation, and chemotherapy, is an essential part of cancer management.

   1. Pathophysiology of cancer pain may be subdivided into nociceptive and neuropathic pain.

      a. Nociceptive Pain includes somatic and visceral pain and refers to pain caused by the stimulation of nociceptors in somatic (bones, muscle) or visceral structures. It typically responds to both nonopioids and opioids.

      b. Neuropathic Pain involves peripheral or central afferent neural pathways, is commonly described as burning or lancinating, and responds poorly to opioids.

      c. Trauma Associated with Surgery for removal of cancerous tissue may cause both acute and chronic pain. Multimodal analgesia with local anesthetics and gabapentin may be used for treatment. Gabapentin has been shown to reduce analgesic requirements for acute postoperative pain but does not significantly affect the development of chronic pain.

TABLE 20-1 Principal Toxicities of Commonly Used Cancer Chemotherapeutic Drugs	
Drug	**Effect**
Bleomycin (Blenoxane)	Interstitial pneumonitis/pulmonary fibrosis
Busulfan (Myleran)	Interstitial pneumonitis/pulmonary fibrosis
Cisplatin (Platinol)	Ototoxicity, peripheral neuropathy, renal failure
Cyclophosphamide (Cytoxan)	Plasma cholinesterase inhibition, hemorrhagic cystitis
Doxorubicin (Adriamycin)	Dose-dependent cardiomyopathy
L-Asparaginase (Elspar)	Hypersensitivity reactions/anaphylaxis, pancreatitis
Melphalan (Alkeran)	Development of secondary leukemias, sterility
Mitomycin	Hemolytic uremic syndrome
Paclitaxel (Taxol)	Hypersensitivity reactions, peripheral neuropathy
Vincristine (Oncovin)	Peripheral neuropathy, autonomic neuropathy

2. Drug therapy

   a. Nonsteroidal Anti-Inflammatory Drugs (NSAIDs) and acetaminophen are often initial therapy. NSAIDs are especially effective for managing bone pain, the most common cause of cancer pain.

   b. Codeine or one of its analogues is often the next step in management
   of moderate to severe pain.

   c. Opioids often used include morphine (routes of administration include
   oral, intravenous, subcutaneous, epidural, intrathecal, transmucosal, transdermal) and fentanyl (transdermal, transmucosal). There is no maximum
   safe dose of morphine and other μ-agonist opioids. Tolerance to these
   drugs occurs, but addiction is rare when these drugs are used correctly.

   d. Tricyclic Antidepressant Drugs are recommended for depression and
   appear to have direct analgesic effects that potentiate those of opioids.

   e. Anticonvulsants are useful for management of chronic neuropathic pain.

   f. Corticosteroids can decrease pain perception, have a sparing effect
   on opioid requirements, improve mood, increase appetite, and lead to
   weight gain.

3. Neuraxial Analgesia provides effective pain control after cancer surgery.
Neuraxial analgesia with local anesthetics provides immediate pain relief in
patients whose pain cannot be relieved with oral or intravenous analgesics.
Morphine may be administered intrathecally or epidurally. Spinal opioids
may be delivered for weeks to months via a long-term, subcutaneously
tunneled, exteriorized catheter or an implanted intrathecal or epidural
drug delivery system. Some patients require an additional low concentration
of neuraxial local anesthetic to achieve adequate pain control.

4. Neurolytic Procedures intended to destroy sensory components of
nerves may help control pain but also destroy motor and autonomic nervous
system fibers. Constant pain is more amenable to destructive nerve blocks
than is intermittent pain. Neurolytic celiac plexus block (alcohol, phenol) has
been used to treat pain originating from abdominal viscera—for example,
resulting from pancreatic cancer—and may last as long as 6 months.

5. Neurosurgical Procedures (neuroablative or neurostimulatory) are
reserved for patients unresponsive to other less invasive procedures.
Cordotomy (interruption of the spinothalamic tract in the spinal cord)
is considered for unilateral pain involving the lower extremity, thorax, or
upper extremity. Dorsal rhizotomy (interruption of sensory nerve roots) is
used when pain is localized to specific dermatomal levels. Dorsal column
stimulators or deep brain stimulators may be used in selected patients.

IV. IMMUNOLOGY OF CANCER CELLS

Tumor cells are antigenically different from normal cells and may therefore elicit
immune reactions similar to those that cause rejection of allografts. Antigens present in cancer cells but not in normal cells are designated tumor-specific antigens.
Tumor-associated antigens (α-fetoprotein, prostate-specific antigen [PSA],
carcinoembryonic antigen [CEA]) are present in both cancer cells and normal
cells, but concentrations are higher in tumor cells. Antibodies to tumor-associated
antigens can be used for the immunodiagnosis of cancer. Most spontaneously
occurring tumors appear to be weakly antigenic.

V. PARANEOPLASTIC SYNDROMES

Paraneoplastic syndromes manifest as pathophysiologic disturbances that may accompany cancer (**Table 20-2**).

A. Fever may reflect tumor necrosis, inflammation, the release of toxic products by cancer cells, or the production of endogenous pyrogens.

B. Neuromuscular Abnormalities occur in 5% to 10% of patients. The most common is the skeletal muscle weakness (myasthenic syndrome) associated with lung cancer.

C. Ectopic Hormone Production. Active hormones are produced by a number of tumors, resulting in predictable physiologic effects (**Table 20-3**).

D. Hypercalcemia in hospitalized patients is most often caused by cancer, reflecting local osteolytic activity from bone metastases (especially breast cancer) or the ectopic parathyroid hormonal activity associated with tumors of the kidneys, lungs, pancreas, or ovaries. Hypercalcemia occurring in patients with cancer may manifest as lethargy and coma, polyuria, and/or dehydration.

E. Tumor Lysis Syndrome is caused by sudden destruction of tumor cells by chemotherapy, with release of uric acid, potassium, and phosphate. This syndrome can result in acute renal failure (caused by hyperuricemia), cardiac dysrhythmias (caused by hyperkalemia), and hypocalcemia (caused by hyperphosphatemia).

TABLE 20-2	Pathophysiologic Manifestations of Paraneoplastic Syndromes
Fever	
Anorexia	
Weight loss	
Anemia	
Thrombocytopenia	
Coagulopathy	
Neuromuscular abnormalities	
Ectopic hormone production	
Hypercalcemia	
Hyperuricemia	
Tumor lysis syndrome	
Adrenal insufficiency	
Nephrotic syndrome	
Ureteral obstruction	
Pulmonary hypertrophic osteoarthropathy and digital clubbing	
Pericardial effusion	
Pericardial tamponade	
Superior vena cava obstruction	
Spinal cord compression	

TABLE 20-3	Ectopic Hormone Production	
Hormone	**Associated Cancer**	**Manifestations**
Corticotropin	Lung (small cell), thyroid (medullary), thymoma, carcinoid islet, cell tumor	Cushing's syndrome
Antidiuretic hormone	Lung (small cell), pancreas, lymphoma	Water intoxication
Gonadotropin	Lung (large cell), ovary, adrenal	Gynecomastia, precocious puberty
Parathyroid hormone	Lung, kidney, pancreas, ovary	Hyperpigmentation, hyperparathyroidism
Thyrotropin	Choriocarcinoma, testicular (embryonal)	Hyperthyroidism
Thyrocalcitonin	Thyroid (medullary)	Hypocalcemia
Insulin	Retroperitoneal tumors	Hypoglycemia

F. Adrenal Insufficiency is usually relative insufficiency caused by partial replacement of the adrenal cortex by tumor or suppression of adrenal cortical function by prolonged treatment with corticosteroids. It is most often seen in patients with metastatic disease caused by melanoma, retroperitoneal tumors, lung cancer, or breast cancer. Clinical manifestations include fatigue, dehydration, oliguria, and cardiovascular collapse, and treatment is administration of cortisol either intravenously or (if possible) orally.

G. Acute Respiratory Complications. The acute onset of dyspnea may reflect extension of the tumor or the effects of chemotherapy. Bleomycin-induced interstitial pneumonitis and fibrosis are the most commonly encountered pulmonary complications of chemotherapy. Pulmonary toxicity rarely occurs when the total dose is less than 150 mg/m². The most common symptoms of interstitial pneumonitis are the insidious onset of nonproductive cough, dyspnea, tachypnea, and occasionally fever 4 to 10 weeks after initiation of bleomycin therapy. Once interstitial and alveolar fibrosis have occurred, they are irreversible.

H. Acute Cardiac Complications. Malignant invasion of the pericardium can cause pericardial effusion (possibly with pericardial tamponade) and atrial fibrillation or flutter. Cardiac toxicity can accompany doxorubicin or daunorubicin chemotherapy. Cardiomyopathy can result from radiation therapy, particularly in patients receiving radiation to the mediastinum or who are on concurrent cyclophosphamide therapy.

I. Superior Vena Cava Obstruction is caused by spread of cancer into the mediastinum or directly into the caval wall, resulting in engorgement of veins above the level of the heart, edema of the arms and face, and sometimes dyspnea, hoarseness, and airway obstruction. Increased intracranial pressure caused by increased cerebral venous pressure may cause nausea, seizures, and decreased levels of consciousness. Treatment is prompt radiation or chemotherapy to decrease the size of the tumor and relieve venous and airway obstruction. Bronchoscopy and/or mediastinoscopy to obtain a tissue diagnosis may be very hazardous in the presence of co-existing airway obstruction and increased pressure in the mediastinal veins.

J. Spinal Cord Compression caused by the presence of metastatic lesions in the epidural space may cause pain, skeletal muscle weakness, sensory loss, and autonomic nervous system dysfunction. Radiation therapy is a useful treatment when neurologic deficits are only partial or are in development. Once total paralysis has developed, the results of surgical laminectomy or of radiation to decompress the spinal cord are poor.

K. Increased Intracranial Pressure can manifest as mental deterioration, focal neurologic deficits, or seizures. Treatment includes corticosteroids, diuretics, and mannitol. Radiation or surgery may be indicated to treat intracranial tumor. Intrathecal chemotherapy may be necessary if tumor involves the meninges.

VI. MANAGEMENT OF ANESTHESIA

Preoperative evaluation of patients with cancer includes consideration of the pathophysiologic effects of the disease (see **Tables 20-2** and **20-3**) and recognition of the potential adverse effects of cancer chemotherapeutic drugs (see **Table 20-1**). Preoperative tests to detect side effects of chemotherapy are listed in **Table 20-4**.

A. Side Effects of Chemotherapy

1. Pulmonary and Cardiac Toxicity. A history of drug-induced pulmonary fibrosis (dyspnea, nonproductive cough) or congestive heart failure will influence anesthesia management. Bleomycin-treated patients are vulnerable to the development of interstitial pulmonary edema because of impaired lymphatic drainage from the pulmonary fibrosis. Bleomycin therapy may increase the risk of oxygen toxicity in the presence of high inspired oxygen concentrations, and it is prudent to use the minimum oxygen concentration that provides the desired SpO_2. The myocardial depressant effects of anesthetic drugs may be enhanced in patients with drug-induced cardiac toxicity.

TABLE 20-4 Preoperative Tests in Patients with Cancer
Hematocrit
Platelet count
White blood cell count
Prothrombin time
Electrolytes
Liver function tests
Renal function tests
Blood glucose concentrations
Arterial blood gases
Chest radiography
Electrocardiography

2. Neurotoxicity

a. Peripheral Neuropathy

1.) *Vinca Alkaloids* (e.g., vincristine) cause sensorimotor peripheral neuropathy. Virtually all patients treated with vincristine develop reversible paresthesias in their digits.

2.) *Cisplatin* causes dose-dependent large-fiber neuropathy and loss of proprioception by damaging dorsal root ganglia. Subclinical neurotoxicity is present in a large percentage of patients and may extend several months beyond discontinuation of treatment. Administration of regional anesthesia containing local anesthetics and epinephrine to such patients might cause clinically significant injury.

b. Encephalopathy

1.) *Cyclophosphamide* may be associated with acute delirium.

2.) *Cytarabine* may cause acute delirium or cerebellar degeneration, both of which are usually reversible.

3.) *Methotrexate* can cause acute reversible encephalopathy, and prolonged administration of methotrexate, especially in conjunction with radiation therapy, can lead to progressive irreversible dementia.

3. Paclitaxel causes dose-dependent ataxia that may be accompanied by paresthesias in the hands and feet and proximal skeletal muscle weakness.

4. Corticosteroids (prednisone or its equivalent at 60 to 100 mg/day) may cause myopathy and neuromuscular toxicity, which are usually reversible.

B. Preoperative Preparation. Correction of nutrient deficiencies, anemia, coagulopathy, and electrolyte abnormalities may be necessary. The presence of hepatic or renal dysfunction may influence the choice of anesthetic drugs and muscle relaxants. Attention to aseptic technique is critical because immunosuppression occurs with most chemotherapeutic agents. Cancer patients may have life-threatening airway difficulties and upper airway obstruction with head, neck, and chest tumors.

C. Postoperative mechanical ventilation may be required, particularly following invasive or prolonged operations and in patients with drug-induced pulmonary fibrosis. Patients with drug-induced cardiac toxicity are more likely to experience postoperative cardiac complications.

VII. COMMON CANCERS ENCOUNTERED IN CLINICAL PRACTICE

A. Lung Cancer is the leading cause of adult cancer deaths and accounts for nearly one third of all cancer deaths in the United States. It is largely a preventable disease, because more than 90% of lung cancer deaths are related to cigarette smoking.

1. Etiology. In addition to cigarette smoking, lung cancer is associated with marijuana smoking, ionizing radiation, asbestos exposure, and exposure to radon gas.

2. Signs and Symptoms usually reflect features related to the extent of the disease, including local and regional manifestations, signs and symptoms of metastatic disease, and various paraneoplastic syndromes related indirectly to the cancer (see **Table 20-2**).

3. Histologic Subtypes (Table 20-5)

4. Diagnosis. Cytologic analysis of sputum is often sufficient for the diagnosis. Flexible fiber-optic bronchoscopy with biopsy, brushings, or washings may be used in initial evaluation. Peripheral lung lesions can be diagnosed by percutaneous fine-needle aspiration guided by fluoroscopy, ultrasonography, or computed tomography. Video-assisted thoracoscopic surgery is useful for diagnosing peripheral lung lesions and pleura-based tumors. Mediastinoscopy and video-assisted thoracoscopy are employed to biopsy lymph nodes and stage the tumor.

5. Treatment. Surgical resection (lobectomy, pneumonectomy) is the most effective treatment. Surgery has little effect on survival when the disease has spread to unilateral mediastinal lymph nodes. The 5-year survival is unaffected by radiation, chemotherapy, immunotherapy, and combinations of these treatments. Radiotherapy is effective in palliating symptoms from tumor invasion in most patients.

6. Management of Anesthesia in patients with lung cancer includes preoperative consideration of tumor-induced effects such as malnutrition, pneumonia, pain, and ectopic endocrine effects, including hyponatremia (see **Table 20-3**). When resection of lung tissue is planned, it is important to evaluate underlying pulmonary and cardiac function, especially for the presence of pulmonary hypertension.

> *a. Mediastinoscopy.* Hemorrhage and pneumothorax are the most commonly encountered complications of mediastinoscopy. The mediastinoscope can exert pressure on the right innominate artery, with loss of the distal pulse and an erroneous diagnosis of cardiac arrest. Compression of the right innominate artery of which the right carotid artery is a branch may manifest as a postoperative neurologic deficit. Bradycardia can occur because of stretching of the vagus nerve or tracheal compression by the mediastinoscope.

TABLE 20-5	Clinical and Pathologic Features of Lung Cancer			
Histologic Subtype	**Incidence (%)**	**5-Year Survival (%)**		**Associated Symptoms**
		All Cases	**Resectable Cases**	
Squamous cell	25–40	11	40	Hypercalcemia
Adenocarcinoma	30–50	5	30	Hypercoagulability, osteoarthropathy
Large cell	10	4	30	Gynecomastia, galactorrhea
Small cell	15–24	2	5–10	Inappropriate antidiuretic hormone secretion, ectopic corticotropin secretion, Eaton-Lambert syndrome

Adapted from Skarin AT: Lung cancer. Sci Am Med 1997;1–20.

B. Colorectal Cancer. Colon cancer is second only to lung cancer as a cause of cancer death in the United States.

1. Etiology. Most colorectal cancers arise from premalignant adenomatous polyps. Colorectal cancer appears to be increased by high intake of animal fat. Familial history of colon cancer, history of inflammatory bowel disease, and cigarette smoking all increase the risk of colon cancer.

2. Diagnosis. Early detection and removal of localized superficial tumors and precancerous lesions in asymptomatic individuals increases the cure rate. Screening programs (digital rectal examination, examination of the stool for occult blood, colonoscopy) are particularly useful for persons with a family history of colon cancer.

3. Signs and Symptoms of colorectal cancer reflect the anatomic location of the cancer, ranging from anemia and fatigue (ascending colon) to obstruction (descending colon). Colorectal cancers initially spread to regional lymph nodes and then through the portal venous circulation to the liver, which represents the most common visceral site of metastases.

4. Treatment. Radical surgical resection, including the blood vessels and lymph nodes draining the involved bowel, offers the best potential for cure. Radiation therapy is a consideration in patients with rectal tumors because the risk of recurrence following surgery is significant.

5. Management of Anesthesia for surgical resection of colorectal cancers may be influenced by anemia and the effects of metastatic lesions in liver, lung, bone, or brain. Blood transfusion during surgical resection of colorectal cancers appears to be associated with a decrease in the length of patient survival, possibly because of immunosuppression produced by transfused blood. For this reason, careful review of the risks and benefits of blood transfusions in these patients is prudent.

C. Prostate Cancer. Prostate cancer is the second leading cause of cancer death among men.

1. Diagnosis. Increased serum PSA concentration (particularly levels >10 ng/mL) may indicate the presence of prostate cancer in asymptomatic men and prompt a digital rectal examination. Rectal examination can evaluate only the posterior and lateral aspects of the prostate. If the rectal examination indicates the possible presence of cancer, transrectal ultrasonography and biopsy are needed regardless of the PSA concentration.

2. Treatment. Focal, well-differentiated prostate cancers are usually cured by transurethral resection. If lymph nodes are involved, radical prostatectomy or definitive radiation therapy may be recommended. Radiation therapy can be delivered either by an external beam or by implantation of radioactive seeds. Hormone therapy is indicated for management of metastatic prostate cancer because these tumors are under the trophic influence of androgens.

When advanced prostate cancers become resistant to hormone therapy, incapacitating bone pain often develops. Systemic chemotherapy with mitoxantrone plus corticosteroids or estramustine plus a taxane may be effective in palliating pain. In the terminal phases of the disease, high doses of prednisone for short periods may produce subjective improvement.

D. Breast Cancer. Women in the United States have a 12.6% lifetime risk of developing breast cancer.

1. Risk Factors. The principal risk factors for development of breast cancer are increasing age and family history. Other risk factors are early menarche, late menopause, late first pregnancy, and nulliparity. Two breast cancer susceptibility genes (BRCA1, BRCA2) are mutations that are inherited as autosomal dominant traits.

2. Screening Strategies for breast cancer include the triad of breast self-examination, clinical breast examination by a professional, and screening mammography.

3. Prognosis. Axillary lymph node invasion and tumor size are the two most important determinants of outcome in patients with early breast cancer. The absence of estrogen and progesterone receptor expression in the tumor is associated with a poorer prognosis.

4. Treatment

a. Surgery. Breast conservation therapy (lumpectomy with radiation therapy), simple mastectomy, and modified radical mastectomy provide similar survival rates. Distant micrometastastic disease is correlated with the number of lymph nodes containing tumor invasion. Morbidity associated with breast cancer surgery is largely related to side effects of lymph node dissection (lymphedema, restricted arm motion).

b. Radiation is an important component of breast conservation therapy because lumpectomy alone is associated with a high incidence of recurrence. High-dose radiation therapy may be associated with brachial plexopathy or nerve damage, pneumonitis, pulmonary fibrosis, and cardiac injury.

c. Systemic Treatment. Many women with early-stage breast cancer already have distant micrometastases at the time of diagnosis. Tamoxifen therapy, chemotherapy, and ovarian ablation are intended to prevent or delay recurrence of the disease. The most serious late sequelae of chemotherapy are leukemia and doxorubicin-induced cardiac impairment.

d. Supportive Treatment in advanced breast cancer includes administration of bisphosphonates (pamidronate, clodronate) in addition to hormone therapy or chemotherapy to decrease bone pain. Erythropoietin may be useful for diminishing symptoms of chemotherapy-related bone marrow suppression. Adequate pain control is usually achieved with sustained-release oral and/or transdermal opioid preparations.

5. Management of Anesthesia. Preoperative evaluation includes a review of potential side effects related to chemotherapy. Placement of intravenous catheters in the arm at risk of lymphedema is avoided because of exacerbation of lymphedema and susceptibility to infection. The arm should also be protected from compression (as with a blood pressure cuff) and heat exposure. The presence of bone pain and pathologic fractures is noted when considering regional anesthesia and when positioning patients. If isosulfan blue dye is injected during the surgical procedure, pulse oximetry may demonstrate a transient spurious decrease in the measured SpO_2 value.

VIII. LESS COMMON CANCERS ENCOUNTERED IN CLINICAL PRACTICE

A. Cardiac Tumors may be primary or secondary, benign or malignant. Metastatic cardiac involvement, usually from adjacent lung cancer, occurs 20 to 40 times more often than a primary malignant cardiac tumor.

    1. Cardiac Myxomas account for most benign cardiac tumors that occur in adults.

        a. Signs and Symptoms reflect interference with filling and emptying of the involved cardiac chamber (heart failure, syncope, arrhythmias, pulmonary hypertension) and release of emboli composed of myxomatous material or thrombi that have formed on the tumor.

        b. Diagnosis. Echocardiography can determine the location, size, shape, attachment, and mobility of cardiac myxomas.

        c. Treatment. Surgical resection of cardiac myxomas is usually curative.

        d. Management of Anesthesia considers the possibility of low cardiac output and arterial hypoxemia caused by obstruction at the mitral or tricuspid valve. Symptoms of obstruction may be exacerbated by changes in body position. The presence of a right atrial myxoma prohibits placement of right atrial or pulmonary artery catheters.

B. Head and Neck Cancers account for approximately 5% of all cancers in the United States, with a predominance in men older than 50 years of age. Most patients have a history of excessive alcohol use and cigarette smoking. The most common sites of metastases are lung, liver, and bone. Preoperative nutritional therapy may be indicated before surgical resection of the tumor.

C. Thyroid Cancer. Papillary and follicular thyroid cancers are among the most curable cancers. Medullary thyroid cancers may be associated with pheochromocytomas in an autosomal dominant disorder known as multiple endocrine neoplasia type 2. Subtotal and total thyroidectomies are the primary treatment, and external beam radiation can be used for palliative treatment of obstruction and bony metastases.

D. Esophageal Cancer. Excessive alcohol consumption and cigarette smoking are risk factors for development of squamous cell carcinoma of the esophagus, while Barrett's esophagus, a complication of gastroesophageal reflux disease, is the primary risk factor for adenocarcinoma. The results of primary radiation therapy resemble those of radical surgery. The likelihood of underlying alcohol-induced liver disease, chronic obstructive pulmonary disease from cigarette smoking, and cross-tolerance with anesthetic drugs in alcohol abusers are considerations during anesthetic management of patients with esophageal cancer.

E. Gastric Cancer. Achlorhydria (loss of gastric acidity), pernicious anemia, chronic gastritis, and *Helicobacter* infection contribute to the development of gastric cancer. Gastric cancer is usually far advanced when signs such as weight loss, palpable epigastric mass, jaundice, or ascites appear. Complete surgical resection is the only treatment that may be curative.

F. Liver Cancer occurs most often in men with liver disease caused by hepatitis B or hepatitis C virus, alcohol consumption, and hemochromatosis. Radical surgical resection or liver transplantation offers the only hope for survival, but most patients with liver cancer are not surgical candidates because of extensive cirrhosis, impaired liver function, and the presence of extrahepatic disease.

G. Pancreatic Cancer. Abdominal pain, anorexia, and weight loss are the usual initial symptoms. Pain suggests retroperitoneal invasion and jaundice reflects biliary obstruction in patients with tumor in the head of the pancreas. Complete surgical resection (total pancreatectomy and pancreaticoduodenectomy or Whipple procedure) is the only effective treatment of ductal pancreatic cancer. The median survival for patients with unresectable tumors is 5 months. Celiac plexus block with alcohol or phenol is the most effective intervention for treating the pain associated with pancreatic cancer.

H. Renal Cell Cancer most often manifests itself as hematuria, mild anemia, and flank pain. Risk factors include a family history of renal cancer and cigarette smoking. Paraneoplastic syndromes especially hypercalcemia due to ectopic parathyroid hormone secretion and erythrocytosis due to ectopic erythropoietin production are common.

I. Bladder Cancer is associated with cigarette smoking and chronic exposure to chemicals used in the dye, leather, and rubber industries. The most common presenting feature is hematuria. Treatment of noninvasive bladder cancer includes endoscopic resection and intravesical chemotherapy.

J. Testicular Cancer is the most common cancer in young men and represents a tumor that can be cured even when distant metastases are present. Testicular cancer usually presents as a painless testicular mass and is diagnosed at the time of orchiectomy.

K. Uterine Cervix Cancer is the most common gynecologic cancer in females 15 to 34 years old. Human papillomavirus infection of the uterine cervix is the principal cause. Carcinoma in situ as detected by a Papanicolaou smear is treated with a cone biopsy, whereas more extensive local disease or disease that has metastasized is treated with some combination of surgery, radiation therapy, and chemotherapy.

L. Uterine Cancer most often presents as postmenopausal or irregular bleeding. Initial evaluation is usually fractional dilation and curettage. In the absence of metastatic disease, a total abdominal hysterectomy and bilateral salpingo-oophorectomy with or without radiation is the treatment.

M. Ovarian Cancer. Advanced disease is usually present by the time the cancer is discovered. Aggressive surgical tumor debulking, even if all cancer cannot be removed, improves the length and quality of survival. Intraperitoneal chemotherapy is indicated postoperatively in most women and is usually well tolerated.

N. Cutaneous Melanoma. The initial treatment of a suspected lesion is wide and deep excisional biopsy, often with sentinel node mapping. Melanoma can metastasize to virtually any organ. Treatment of metastatic melanoma is directed at palliation and can include resection of a solitary metastasis, simple or combination chemotherapy, and immunotherapy.

O. Bone Cancer

    1. Multiple Myeloma (plasma cell myeloma, myelomatosis) is characterized by poorly controlled growth of a single clone of plasma cells that produce a monoclonal immunoglobulin.

        a. Signs and Symptoms are bone pain (often from vertebral collapse), anemia, thrombocytopenia, neutropenia, hypercalcemia (from bone destruction), renal failure (from deposition of Bence-Jones protein in renal tubules or renal amyloidosis), and recurrent bacterial infection (due to bone marrow invasion by tumor cells and decreased cell-mediated immunity).

b. Treatment includes autologous stem cell transplantation and chemotherapy. Palliative radiation is limited to patients who have disabling pain and a well-defined focal process that has not responded to chemotherapy. Hypercalcemia requires prompt treatment with intravenous saline infusion and administration of furosemide.

c. Management of Anesthesia. The presence of compression fractures requires caution when positioning these patients. Pathologic fractures of the ribs may impair ventilation and predispose to development of pneumonia.

2. Osteosarcoma occurs most often in adolescents and typically involves the distal femur and proximal tibia. Treatment consists of combination chemotherapy followed by surgical excision/amputation.

3. Ewing's Tumor or sarcoma usually occurs in children and young adults and most often involves the pelvis, femur, and tibia. Ewing's sarcoma is highly malignant, and metastatic disease is often present at the time of diagnosis. Treatment consists of surgery, local radiation, and combination chemotherapy.

4. Chondrosarcoma usually involves the pelvis, ribs, or upper end of the femur or humerus in young or middle-aged adults. This tumor is treated by radical surgical excision of larger lesions and radiation of smaller lesions.

IX. LYMPHOMAS AND LEUKEMIAS

A. Hodgkin's Disease is a lymphoma that appears to have infective (Epstein-Barr virus), genetic, and environmental associations. Impaired immunity as seen in patients after organ transplantation or in patients who are HIV positive appears to predispose to lymphoma.

1. Signs and Symptoms include lymphadenopathy, night sweats, and unexplained weight loss. Moderately severe anemia is often present. Peripheral neuropathy and spinal cord compression may occur as a direct result of tumor growth.

2. Treatment. Radiation therapy is curative for localized early-stage Hodgkin's disease. Bulkier or more advanced Hodgkin's disease is treated by combination chemotherapy.

B. Leukemia is the uncontrolled production of leukocytes due to cancerous mutation of lymphogenous cells or myelogenous cells. Lymphocytic leukemias begin in lymph nodes, whereas myeloid leukemia begins in myelogenous cells in bone marrow with spread to extramedullary organs. Bone marrow failure is the cause of fatal infections or hemorrhage due to thrombocytopenia. Leukemia cells may also infiltrate the liver, spleen, lymph nodes, and meninges, producing organ dysfunction.

1. Acute Lymphoblastic Leukemia accounts for approximately 15% of all leukemias in adults. Central nervous system dysfunction is common.

2. Chronic Lymphocytic Leukemia rarely occurs in children and accounts for approximately 25% of all leukemias. Signs and symptoms are highly variable, with the extent of bone marrow infiltration often determining the clinical course.

3. Acute Myeloid Leukemia is characterized by an increase in the number of myeloid cells in bone marrow and arrest of their maturation, resulting in hematopoietic insufficiency (granulocytopenia, thrombocytopenia, anemia). Many patients present with life-threatening infections. Other presenting signs include fatigue, bleeding gums or nose bleeds, pallor, and headache. Hyperleukocytosis (more than 100,000 cells/mm^3) can result in signs of leukostasis with ocular and cerebrovascular dysfunction or bleeding. Chemotherapy and bone marrow transplantation are usual treatments.

4. Chronic Myeloid Leukemia presents as myeloid leukocytosis with splenomegaly. Cytoreduction therapy with hydroxyurea, chemotherapy, leukopheresis, and splenectomy may be necessary. Bone marrow transplantation may be considered.

C. Treatment of Leukemia

1. Chemotherapy is intended to decrease the number of tumor cells so organomegaly regresses and function of the bone marrow improves. Drugs used for chemotherapy are principally those that depress bone marrow activity. Therefore, hemorrhage and infection will determine the maximum doses of the chemotherapeutic drugs. Destruction of tumor cells by chemotherapy produces a uric acid load that may result in urate nephropathy and/or gouty arthritis.

2. Bone Marrow Transplantation offers a potential cure of several otherwise fatal diseases. Autologous bone marrow transplantation entails collection of the patient's own bone marrow for subsequent reinfusion, and allogeneic transplantation uses bone marrow or peripheral blood elements from an immunocompatible donor. Recipients undergo a combination of total body radiation and chemotherapy to achieve bone marrow ablation.

a. Anesthesia for Bone Marrow Transplantation. General or regional anesthesia is required during aspiration of bone marrow from the iliac crests. Nitrous oxide might be avoided in the donor because of potential bone marrow depression associated with this drug. However, there is no evidence that nitrous oxide administered during bone marrow harvesting adversely affects marrow engraftment and subsequent function. Blood replacement may be necessary, either with autologous blood transfusion or by reinfusion of separated erythrocytes obtained during the harvest.

b. Complications of Bone Marrow Transplantation

  1.) Graft-versus-Host Disease (Table 20-6) is a life-threatening complication of bone marrow transplantation in which the donor cells attack antigens on the recipient's cells. It manifests as organ system dysfunction, most often involving the skin (rash, desquamation), liver (jaundice), and gastrointestinal tract (diarrhea).

  2.) Graft Rejection occurs when immunologically competent cells of host origin destroy the cells of donor origin.

TABLE 20-6	Manifestations of Graft-Versus-Host Disease

Pancytopenia and immunodeficiency

Maculopapular rash, erythroderma, desquamation

Oral ulceration and mucositis

Esophageal ulceration

Diarrhea

Hepatitis with coagulopathy

Bronchiolitis obliterans

Interstitial pneumonitis

Pulmonary fibrosis

Renal failure

3.) Pulmonary Complications include infection, adult respiratory distress syndrome, chemotherapy-induced lung damage, and interstitial pneumonia (often cytomegalovirus or fungal infection).

4.) Veno-Occlusive Disease of the Liver may present as jaundice, tender hepatomegaly, ascites, and weight gain. Progressive hepatic failure and multiorgan failure can develop, and mortality is high.

CHAPTER 21

Diseases Related to Immune System Dysfunction

T he immune system can be divided into innate immunity (rapid response consisting of neutrophils, macrophages, monocytes, killer cells, the complement system, acute-phase proteins, and contact activation pathways) that has no specific memory, and adaptive or acquired immunity (delayed response, mediated by B cells, antibodies, and cellular response via T cells), which has memory for previous exposures. Defects specific to each of these immune systems generally predispose to infection with a characteristic subset of pathogenic organisms (**Table 21-1**). Both innate and acquired immunity exhibit defects that can be divided into three injury categories: those caused by (1) an inadequate immune response, (2) an excessive immune response, and (3) misdirection of the immune response.

I. INADEQUATE INNATE IMMUNITY

A. Neutropenia is defined as an absolute granulocyte count less than $2000/\mu L$ in whites or $1500/\mu L$ in African Americans. Infectious risk increases when the granulocyte count is less than $500/\mu L$ and increases dramatically if the count decreases to less than $100/\mu L$ (**Table 21-2**).
B. Abnormalities of Phagocytosis include chronic granulomatous disease (high rate of staphylococcal infection), neutrophil glucose 6-phosphate dehydrogenase deficiency (infections with catalase-positive bacteria), Chediak-Higashi syndrome (partial albinism, frequent bacterial infections, mild bleeding disorder, neuropathy, cranial nerve defects), specific granule deficiency syndrome (impaired neutrophil chemotaxis and bactericidal activity—recurrent abscesses and fungal infections).

TABLE 21-1 Pathogens Associated with Specific Immune Defects

Organism	Phagocyte Defect	Complement Defect	B-Cell Defect and Antibody Deficiency	T-Cell Defect or Deficiency	Combined B- and T-Cell Deficiency
Bacteria	Staphylococci, *Pseudomonas*, enteric flora	*Neisseria*, pyogenic bacteria	Streptococci, staphylococci, *Haemophilus*, *Neisseria* meningitidis	Bacterial sepsis, especially *Salmonella typhi*	Similar to antibody deficiency, especially *N. meningitides*
Viruses			Enteroviruses	Cytomegalovirus, Epstein-Barr virus, varicella, chronic respiratory and intestinal viruses	All
Mycobacterium	Nontuberculous mycobacteria			Nontuberculous mycobacteria	
Fungi	*Candida, Nocardia, Aspergillus*		Severe intestinal giardiasis	*Candida, Pneumocystis, Histoplasma, Aspergillus*	Similar to T-cell defect, especially *Pneumocystis* and *Toxoplasma*
Special features			Recurrent sinopulmonary infections, sepsis, chronic meningitis	Aggressive disease with opportunistic pathogens, failure to clear infections	

TABLE 21-2	Causes of Neutropenia
Pediatric Patients	Neonatal sepsis
	Transient neonatal neutropenia (caused by maternal disease or drugs)
	Cyclic neutropenia (autosomal dominant genetic disorder)
	Kostmann's syndrome (autosomal recessive disorder of neutrophil maturation)
Adult Patients	Acquired neutropenia (chemotherapy)
	Other drug side effects (gold salts, chloramphenicol, antithyroid mediations, analgesics, tricyclic antidepressants, phenothiazines)
	Autoimmune-related neutropenia (lupus, rheumatoid arthritis, Felty's syndrome)
	Lymphoma, other myeloproliferative diseases
	Severe liver disease with portal hypertension
	Sepsis
	Alcoholism
	HIV infection
	Idiopathic

HIV, human immunodeficiency virus.

C. Management of Patients with Neutropenia or Abnormal Phagocytosis is antibiotic therapy and recombinant granulocyte colony stimulating factor (G-CSF), which reduces the duration of absolute neutropenia in patients receiving chemotherapy.

D. Deficiencies in Components of the Complement System (Table 21-3)

II. EXCESSIVE INNATE IMMUNITY

A. Neutrophilia is defined as an absolute granulocyte count higher than 7000 segmented granulocytes plus bands per microliter. Major causes of neutrophilia are listed in **Table 21-4**. Granulocyte counts higher than 100,000 are associated with splenic infarction, and leukostasis in the lungs that is associated with

TABLE 21-3	Deficiencies of Complement System Components
Early components of the classic pathway: C1q, C1r, C2, C4	Autoimmune inflammatory disorders resembling lupus
Common pathway component C3	Usually fatal in utero
Terminal components C5–C8	Recurrent infection and rheumatic disease
C9 and components of the alternate pathway	Neisserial infection
Factor H deficiency	Familial relapsing hemolytic uremic syndrome
C1 inhibitor deficiency	Hereditary angioedema

TABLE 21-4	Clinical Conditions Associated with Neutrophilia	
Disorder	**Mechanism**	
Infection/inflammation	Increased neutrophil production and marrow release of neutrophils	
Stress/metabolic disorders (preeclampsia, diabetic ketoacidosis)	Increased neutrophil production	
Steroid treatment	Demargination of neutrophils	
Myeloproliferative disease	Increased marrow neutrophil release and demargination of neutrophils	
Splenectomy	Decrease in splenic trapping of neutrophils	

decreased oxygen diffusion capacity. Moderate granulocytosis is associated with infection, malignant disease myeloproliferative disorders, and glucocorticoid therapy.

B. Asthma. Triggers for bronchospasm that are unrelated to the immune system such as exposure to cold, exercise, stress, or inhaled irritants are considered part of innate immunity. Treatment consists of administration of β-agonists, anticholinergic drugs, corticosteroids, and leukotriene inhibitors.

III. MISDIRECTED INNATE IMMUNITY

A. Angioedema (episodic edema of the skin and mucous membranes) may be hereditary or acquired.

1. Hereditary Angioedema most commonly results from an autosomal dominant deficiency or dysfunction of C1 esterase inhibitor, which leads to a release of vasoactive mediators that increase vascular permeability and produce edema.

2. Acquired Angioedema occurs in some lymphoproliferative disorders because of antibodies to C1 inhibitor. Angiotensin-converting enzyme inhibitors can also precipitate angioedema in 0.1% to 0.7% of patients.

3. Prophylaxis. Patients experiencing recurrent angioedema, whether hereditary or acquired, require prophylaxis with danazol or stanozolol before a stimulating procedure such as endotracheal intubation. Acute attacks can be treated with C1 inhibitor concentrate (25 U/kg) or fresh frozen plasma (2–4 units) to replace the deficient enzyme.

4. Management of Anesthesia. Pretreatment of patients with hereditary angioedema should be considered prior to elective surgery in which airway manipulation, including LMA placement, is anticipated. C1 inhibitor concentrates should be readily available.

5. Emergency Airway Management during an acute attack includes administration of supplemental oxygen and endotracheal intubation, with standby personnel and equipment for emergency tracheostomy.

IV. INADEQUATE ADAPTIVE IMMUNITY (TABLE 21-5)

V. EXCESSIVE ADAPTIVE IMMUNITY

A. Allergic Reactions are classified according to their mechanism. Type I allergic reactions (e.g., anaphylaxis) are IgE mediated and involve mast cells and basophils. Type II reactions mediate cytotoxicity with IgG, IgM, and complement. Type III reactions produce tissue damage via immune complex formation or deposition. Type IV reactions exhibit T lymphocyte-mediated delayed hypersensitivity. Anaphylactoid reactions appear to be caused by mediator release from mast cells and basophils through a nonimmune mechanism.

    1. Anaphylaxis is a life-threatening manifestation of antigen-antibody interaction in which previous exposure to antigens has evoked production of antigen-specific IgE antibodies. Vasoactive mediators released by degranulation of mast cells and basophils are responsible for the clinical manifestations of anaphylaxis (**Table 21-6**).

    a. Diagnosis of anaphylaxis can be suggested by the often dramatic nature of the clinical manifestations in close temporal relationship to exposure to a particular antigen (may mimic pulmonary embolism, acute myocardial infarction, aspiration, or vasovagal reaction).

        1.) Hypotension and Cardiovascular Collapse may be the only manifestations of anaphylaxis in patients under general anesthesia.

        2.) Proof of Anaphylaxis is an increased plasma tryptase concentration within 1 to 2 hours of the suspected reaction. Plasma histamine concentration returns to baseline within 30 to 60 minutes of an anaphylactic reaction.

TABLE 21-5   **Diseases of Inadequate Adaptive Immunity**

1) Antibody production defect
   - X-linked agammaglobulinemia   • B-cell maturation defect. Therapy is with intravenous immunoglobulin every 3–4 months
2) Combined immunodeficiency syndromes
   - X-linked combined immunodeficiency   • Normal B-cell numbers, low immunoglobulin levels. Treatment is bone marrow transplant
   - Adenosine deaminase deficiency   • T cell death and lymphopenia. Treatment is bone marrow transplant
   - Ataxia-telangiectasia   • Cerebellar ataxia, oculocutaneous telangiectasias, sinopulmonary disease, immunodeficiency. Dysfunctional lymphocytes. Supportive therapy and immunoglobulins are treatment of choice.
3) T-lymphocyte defects
   - DiGeorge syndrome   • Absent or diminished thymic development and no T cells. T-cell infusions and thymus transplantation are treatments

TABLE 21-6	Vasoactive Mediators Released During Anaphylaxis
Mediator	**Physiologic Effect**
Histamine	Increased capillary permeability, peripheral vasodilation, bronchoconstriction
Leukotrienes	Increased capillary permeability, intense bronchoconstriction, negative inotropy, coronary artery vasoconstriction
Prostaglandins	Bronchoconstriction
Eosinophil chemotactic factor	Attraction of eosinophils
Neutrophil chemotactic factor	Attraction of neutrophils
Platelet-activating factor	Platelet aggregation and release of vasoactive amines

3.) *Identification of the Offending Antigen* can be provided by a positive intradermal test (wheal and flare response), which confirms the presence of specific IgE antibodies.

b. Treatment. The immediate goals of treatment of anaphylaxis are reversal of hypotension and hypoxemia, replacement of intravascular volume and inhibition of further cellular degranulation and release of vasoactive mediators (i.e., intravenous fluids, vasopressors such as epinephrine 10–100 μg intravenously doubled every 1-2 minutes until blood pressure increases, antihistamines, bronchodilators, corticosteroids, and support of oxygenation and ventilation).

2. Drug Allergy has been implicated in 3.4% to 4.3% of anesthesia-related deaths. Regardless of the mechanism responsible for life-threatening allergic drug reactions, the manifestations and treatment are identical to that for anaphylaxis. Allergic drug reactions must be distinguished from drug intolerance, idiosyncratic reactions, and drug toxicity (**Table 21-7**).

a. The Perioperative Period. Allergic drug reactions have been reported with most drugs that may be administered during anesthesia (**Table 21-8**), except possibly ketamine and benzodiazepines.

1.) *Cardiovascular Collapse* is the predominant manifestation of a life-threatening allergic drug reaction in an anesthetized patient. Bronchospasm is present in fewer patients.

2.) *Latex Allergy* should be considered. It is estimated that as many as 15% of allergic reactions during anesthesia are caused by latex.

3.) *Most Drug-Induced Allergic Reactions* manifest within 5 to 10 minutes of exposure to the offending drug. An important exception is the allergic response to latex, which is typically delayed for as long as 30 minutes. An allergic reaction should be considered whenever there is an abrupt decrease in blood pressure.

TABLE 21-7	Characteristics of Drug Allergy Versus Drug Toxicity	
Parameter	**Drug Allergy**	**Drug Toxicity**
Mechanism	Antigen-antibody interaction	Dependent on chemical properties of drug
Manifestations	Hypotension Bronchospasm Urticaria	Variable
Predictability	Poor	Good
Previous exposure	Required	Not required
Dose related	No	Yes
Onset	Usually within 5–10 min	Usually delayed
Incidence	Low	High if dose is sufficient

b. Local Anesthetic-Induced Allergic Reactions are rare. Ester-type local anesthetics are metabolized to the highly antigenic compound para-aminobenzoic acid and are more likely than amide-type local anesthetics that are not metabolized to this compound to evoke an allergic reaction. Anaphylaxis may also actually be caused by stimulation of antibody production by the preservative and not by the local anesthetic. It is acceptable to administer amide-based local anesthetics to patients with a history of allergy to ester-based local anesthetics and vice versa.
c. Protamine. Anaphylactic reactions following administration of protamine are more likely to occur in patients who are allergic to seafood (protamine is derived from salmon sperm) and in patients with diabetes mellitus who are being treated with protamine-containing insulin preparations.

TABLE 21-8	Intraoperative Allergic Drug Reactions		
Drug	**Incidence (%)**	**Anaphylactic**	**Anaphylactoid**	**Nonspecific Mast Cell/Basophil Degranulation**
Muscle relaxants	60	X		X
Latex	15	X		
Antibiotics	5–10	X		
Hypnotics	<5	X		
Opioids	<5	X		X
Radiocontrast media	<5		X	
Protamine	<5	X	X	

d. Antibiotics. The incidence of life-threatening allergic reactions following administration of cephalosporins is low (0.02%) and is only minimally increased in patients with a history of penicillin allergy.

e. Blood and Plasma Volume Expanders. Allergic reactions to properly cross-matched blood occur in approximately 1% to 3% of patients. Synthetic colloid solutions have been implicated in anaphylactic and anaphylactoid reactions. Dextran may also activate the complement system.

f. Radiocontrast Media evokes allergic reactions in approximately 5% of patients. Many of the allergic reactions to contrast media seem to be anaphylactoid and can be modified by pretreatment with corticosteroids and histamine antagonists and limitation of the iodine dose.

g. Latex. Cardiovascular collapse during anesthesia and surgery may be caused by latex allergy. Onset is typically more than 30 minutes after exposure. Skin testing can confirm latex hypersensitivity. Questions about itching, conjunctivitis, rhinitis, rash, or wheezing after inflating toy balloons or wearing latex gloves or following dental or gynecologic examinations involving latex gloves may be helpful in identifying sensitized patients. Operating room personnel and patients with spina bifida have an increased incidence of latex allergy.

> 1.) *Intraoperative Management* consists of maintaining a latex-free environment. Intravenous and bladder catheters, drains, anesthesia delivery tubing, ventilator bellows, endotracheal tubes, laryngeal mask airways, nasogastric tubes, blood pressure cuffs, pulse oximeter probes, electrocardiogram pads, and syringes must be latex free.

3. Eosinophilia is defined as a sustained absolute eosinophil count of greater than 1000 to 1500/μL, often seen with parasitic infections, systemic allergic disorders, collagen vascular disease, dermatitis, drug reactions, and tumors (Hodgkin's lymphoma). Hypereosinophilia (an eosinophil count >5000/μL) is associated with restrictive cardiomyopathy due to endomyocardial fibrosis. Hypereosinophilic patients need aggressive treatment with both corticosteroids and hydroxyurea. Leukopheresis may be helpful.

VI. MISDIRECTED ADAPTIVE IMMUNITY

A. Autoimmune Disorders (Table 21-9)

1. Anesthetic Implications of autoimmune disorders relate to the organ pathology specific to the particular autoimmune disorder, the consequences of therapy, and the risk of accelerated atherosclerosis and associated cardiovascular complications such as heart disease and stroke (cardiovascular morbidity and mortality may be increased approximately 8-fold by autoimmune diseases alone and 50-fold by autoimmune diseases treated with corticosteroids).

VII. ANESTHESIA AND IMMUNOCOMPETENCE

A. Resistance to Infection. Anesthesia-induced depression of the immune system may increase the risk of perioperative infection. Local and inhaled anesthetics (nitrous oxide) may produce dose-dependent inhibition of

TABLE 21-9	Examples of Autoimmune Diseases

Rheumatic
Rheumatoid arthritis
Scleroderma
Sjögren syndrome
Mixed connective tissue disease
Systemic lupus erythematosus
Gastrointestinal
Chronic active hepatitis
Ulcerative colitis
Crohn's disease
Endocrine
Type I diabetes mellitus
Hashimoto's thyroiditis
Graves' disease
Neurologic
Myasthenia gravis
Multiple sclerosis
Hematologic
Idiopathic thrombocytopenic purpura
Renal
Goodpasture syndrome

mobilization and migration of polymorphonuclear leukocytes. Mild perioperative hypothermia (<36°C) has been associated with an increased risk of postoperative infection.

B. Resistance to Cancer. There is no evidence that the short-term effects of anesthetic drugs are of any significance in the resistance of a host to cancer.

CHAPTER

Psychiatric Disease/ Substance Abuse/ Drug Overdose

MOOD DISORDERS

I. DEPRESSION

Depression is the most common psychiatric disorder, affecting 2% to 4% of the population. It is distinguished from normal sadness and grief by the severity and duration of the mood disturbances. Pathophysiologic causes of major depression are unknown, although abnormalities of amine neurotransmitter pathways are the most likely etiologic factors.

A. Diagnosis is based on the persistent presence of at least five of the symptoms noted in **Table 22-1**. Alcoholism and major depression often co-exist. Depression and dementia may be difficult to distinguish in elderly patients. All patients with depression should be evaluated for the potential to commit suicide. Physicians have significantly higher suicide rates than the general population.

B. Treatment is with antidepressant medications, psychotherapy, and/or electroconvulsive therapy (ECT). An estimated 70% to 80% of patients respond to pharmacologic therapy, and 50% or more who do not respond to antidepressant drugs respond favorably to ECT.

    1. Antidepressant Drugs almost all affect catecholamine and/or serotonin availability in the central nervous system (**Table 22-2**).

        a. Selective Serotonin Reuptake Inhibitors (SSRIs) block reuptake of serotonin at presynaptic membranes with relatively little effect on adrenergic, cholinergic, histaminergic, or other neurochemical systems. As a result, they are associated with few side effects.

            1.) Serotonin Syndrome is a potentially life-threatening adverse drug reaction that may occur with therapeutic drug use, overdose, or

TABLE 22-1 Characteristics of Severe Depression

Depressed mood

Markedly diminished interest or pleasure in almost all activities

Fluctuations in body weight and appetite

Insomnia or hypersomnia

Restlessness

Fatigue

Feelings of worthlessness or guilt

Decreased ability to concentrate

Suicidal ideation

TABLE 22-2 Commonly Used Antidepressant Medications

Drug Class	Generic Name	Trade Name
SSRI	Fluoxetine	Prozac
	Paroxetine	Paxil
	Sertraline	Zoloft
	Fluvoxamine	Luvox
	Citalopram	Celexa
Tricyclics	Amitriptyline	Elavil
	Imipramine	Tofranil
	Protriptyline	Vivactil
	Doxepin	Sinequan
MAOI	Phenelzine	Nardil
	Tranylcypromine	Parnate
Atypical	Bupropion	Wellbutrin
	Trazodone	Desyrel
	Nefazodone	Serzone
	Venlafaxine	Effexor

MAOI, monoamine oxidase inhibitor; SSRI, selective serotonin reuptake inhibitor.

interaction between serotoninergic drugs. A large number of drugs have been associated with the serotonin syndrome (**Table 22-3**). Symptoms include agitation, delirium, autonomic hyperactivity, hyperreflexia, clonus, and hyperthermia. Additional syndromes to consider in the differential diagnosis of serotonin syndrome are listed in **Table 22-4**. Treatment includes supportive measures and control of autonomic instability, excess muscle

TABLE 22-3	Drug and Drug Interactions Associated with Serotonin Syndrome
Drugs Associated with Serotonin Syndrome	
SSRIs	
Atypical and cyclic antidepressants	
Monoamine oxidase inhibitors	
Anticonvulsant drugs: valproate	
Analgesics: meperidine, fentanyl, tramadol, pentazocine	
Antiemetic drugs: ondansetron, granisetron, metoclopramide	
Antimigraine drugs: sumatriptan	
Bariatric medications: sibutramine	
Antibiotics: linezolide, ritonavir	
Over-the-counter cough medicine: dextromethorphan	
Drugs of abuse: ecstasy, LSD, foxy methoxy, Syrian rue	
Dietary supplements: St. John's wort, ginseng	
Other: lithium	
Drug Interactions Associated with Severe Serotonin Syndrome	
Phenylzine and meperidine	
Tranylcypromine and imipramine	
Phenylzine and SSRIs	
Paroxetine and buspirone	
Linezolide and citalopram	
Modobemide and SSRIs	
Tramadol, venlafaxine, and mirtazapine	

Modified from Boyer EW, Shannon M: The serotonin syndrome. N Engl J Med 2005;352:1112–1120. Copyright 2005 Massachusetts Medical Society. All rights reserved.

activity, and hyperthermia. Cyproheptadine, an oral $5-HT_{2A}$ antagonist, can be used to bind serotonin receptors.

b. Tricyclic Antidepressants inhibit synaptic reuptake of norepinephrine and serotonin and affect other neurochemical systems, including histaminergic and cholinergic systems. They have a large range of side effects (postural hypotension, cardiac dysrhythmias, urinary retention). Tachydysrhythmias have been observed following administration of pancuronium to patients who were also receiving imipramine. Ketamine, meperidine, and epinephrine-containing local anesthetic solutions might produce similar adverse responses and are best avoided.

c. Monoamine Oxidase Inhibitors (MAOIs) change the concentration of neurotransmitters by preventing breakdown of catecholamines and serotonin. Significant systemic hypertension can occur if patients ingest foods containing tyramine (cheeses, wines) or receive sympathomimetic

TABLE 22-4	Drug-Induced Hyperthermic Syndromes			
Syndrome	**Time to Onset**	**Causative Drugs**	**Outstanding Features**	**Treatment**
Malignant hyperthermia	Within minutes	Succinylcholine, inhalation anesthetics	Muscle rigidity, severe hypercarbia	Dantrolene, supportive care
Neuroleptic malignant syndrome	24–72 hr	Dopamine antagonist antipsychotic drugs	Muscle rigidity, stupor/coma, bradykinesia	Bromocriptine or dantrolene, supportive care
Serotonin syndrome	Up to 12 hr	Serotoninergic drugs including SSRIs, MAOIs, and atypical antidepressants	Clonus, hyperreflexia, agitation; may have muscle rigidity	Cyproheptadine, supportive care
Sympathomimetic syndrome	Up to 30 min	Cocaine, amphetamines	Agitation, hallucinations, myocardial ischemia, dysrhythmias, no rigidity	Vasodilators, α- and β-blockers, supportive care
Anticholinergic poisoning	Up to 12 hr	Atropine, belladonna	Toxidrome of hot, red, dry skin, dilated pupils, delirium, no rigidity	Physostigmine, supportive care
Cyclic antidepressant overdose	Up to 6 hr	Cyclic antidepressants	Hypotension, stupor/coma, wide-complex dysrhythmias, no rigidity	Serum alkalinization, magnesium

drugs, because tyramine and sympathomimetic drugs are potent stimuli for norepinephrine release. Orthostatic hypotension is the most common side effect of MAOI therapy.

  1.) Management of Anesthesia in Patients on MAOIs (Table 22-5)
1. Electroconvulsive Therapy. The mechanism of the therapeutic effect of ECT remains unknown. ECT is indicated for treating patients who are unresponsive to drug therapy or who are acutely suicidal.

  a. Adverse Effects (Table 22-6). ECT produces significant cardiovascular and central nervous system effects that may be undesirable in patients with ischemic heart disease. Because of marked increases in cerebral blood flow and intracranial pressure, ECT is contraindicated in patients with known space-occupying lesions, cerebral aneurysms, or head injury.

  b. Management of Anesthesia (Table 22-7)

TABLE 22-5	Anesthesia Considerations in Patients Treated with MAOIs
Preoperative	• Anesthesia can be managed safely without discontinuing MAOIs. • Benzodiazepine premedication is acceptable.
Intraoperative	• Anesthetic requirements may be increased. • Most intravenous induction agents are safe. • Fentanyl appears to be safe. • Ketamine should probably be avoided. • Succinylcholine dose should be reduced. • Provide maintenance anesthesia with volatile agents and nitrous oxide. • Pancuronium should probably be avoided. • Regional anesthesia is acceptable but may have higher incidence of hypotension. • Avoid epinephrine in local anesthetic solutions. • Avoid light anesthesia, topical cocaine, and indirect-acting vasopressors (ephedrine). • Treat hypotension with direct-acting vasopressors (phenylephrine) in decreased doses.
Postoperative	• Avoid meperidine (severe serotonin syndrome). • Consider alternatives to opioid analgesics.

II. BIPOLAR DISORDER

Bipolar disorder is characterized by marked mood swings from depressive episodes to manic episodes with normal behavior often seen in between these episodes (**Table 22-8**). The evaluation of mania must exclude the effects of substance abuse drugs, medications, and concomitant medical conditions.

TABLE 22-6	Side Effects of Electroconvulsive Therapy
Parasympathetic nervous system stimulation	
Bradycardia	
Hypotension	
Sympathetic nervous system stimulation	
Tachycardia	
Hypertension	
Dysrhythmias	
Increased cerebral blood flow	
Increased intracranial pressure	
Increased intraocular pressure	
Increased intragastric pressure	

TABLE 22-7	Management of Anesthesia for ECT Therapy
Preoperative	• Patient should be NPO. • Preanesthesia sedation should be omitted to avoid prolonged emergence. • Anticholinergic drugs (atropine, glycopyrrolate) decrease secretions and reduce the likelihood of bradycardia. • Esmolol 1 mg/kg IV just prior to induction attenuates tachycardia and hypertension (nitroglycerin is an alternative treatment of hypertension). • Pacer devices are usually shielded, but an external magnet should be available. • Implantable defibrillators *must* be turned off prior to treatment and reactivated afterward.
Intraoperative	• Induction is usually with methohexital 0.5–1.0 mg/kg. • Propofol can be used, but may shorten duration of seizure and reduce efficacy of ECT. • Succinylcholine 0.3–0.5 mg/kg attenuates skeletal muscle contractions and risk of bone fractures from seizure activity. • EEG is best monitor of seizure activity. • A tourniquet placed on a limb and inflated to arterial pressure prior to administration of succinylcholine permits evaluation of tonic-clonic movement in that limb to signal seizure activity.
Postoperative	• Support of ventilation and supplemental oxygen until recovered.

NPO, nothing by mouth.

A. Treatment. Lithium remains a mainstay of treatment, but antiepileptic drugs such as carbamazepine and valproate are often used. Olanzapine is another treatment option.

1. Lithium. Because of its narrow therapeutic index, monitoring serum lithium concentration is necessary to prevent toxicity.

   a. Toxicity (Table 22-9) occurs at serum lithium concentrations above 2 mEq/L. Thiazide diuretics trigger lithium reabsorption in the kidneys and should be avoided (loop diuretics are safe).

TABLE 22-8	Manifestations of Mania
Expansive, euphoric mood	
Inflated self-esteem	
Decreased need for sleep	
Flight of ideas	
More talkative than usual	
Distractibility	
Psychomotor agitation	

TABLE 22-9	Signs of Lithium Toxicity
Skeletal muscle weakness	
Ataxia	
Sedation	
Widening of the QRS complex	
Heart block	
Hypotension	
Seizures	

b. Management of Anesthesia. The patient should be evaluated for lithium toxicity, including recent serum lithium concentrations. Thiazide diuretics should be avoided. The ECG should be monitored for evidence of lithium-induced conduction problems or dysrhythmias. The duration of all muscle relaxants may be prolonged in the presence of lithium.

III. SCHIZOPHRENIA

Schizophrenia is the major psychotic mental disorder and is characterized by abnormal reality testing or thought processes. Symptoms include delusions, hallucinations, flattened affect, apathy, social, or occupational dysfunction including withdrawal, and changes in appearance and hygiene.

  A. Treatment. Schizophrenia is likely the result of neurotransmitter dysfunction, specifically of the neurotransmitters dopamine and serotonin. Drugs that block dopamine receptors, especially D_2 and D_4 receptors, improve a variety of psychotic symptoms, especially delusions and hallucinations. Troubling side effects include tardive dyskinesia (choreoathetoid movements), akathisia (restlessness), acute dystonia (contraction of skeletal muscles of the neck, mouth and tongue), and parkinsonism. Newer "atypical" antipsychotic drugs have variable effects on dopamine receptor subtypes and on serotonin receptors, especially the $5\text{-}HT_{2A}$ receptor and appear to be effective in relieving the symptoms of schizophrenia, and with fewer extrapyramidal side effects than the classic drugs (**Table 22-10**).

   1. Anesthesia Considerations. Important effects of antipsychotic medications include α-adrenergic blockade causing postural hypotension, prolongation of the QT interval potentially producing torsade de pointes, seizures, hepatic enzyme elevations, abnormal temperature regulation, and sedation. Drug-induced sedation may decrease anesthetic requirements.

  B. Neuroleptic Malignant Syndrome is a rare, potentially fatal complication of antipsychotic drug therapy. Clinical manifestations include hyperpyrexia, severe skeletal muscle rigidity, rhabdomyolysis, autonomic hyperactivity (tachycardia, hypertension, cardiac dysrhythmias), altered consciousness, and acidosis. Skeletal muscle spasm may be so severe that mechanical ventilation becomes necessary. Renal failure may occur due to myoglobinuria and dehydration.

TABLE 22-10	Commonly Used Antipsychotic Medications			
Class	Generic Name	Trade Name	EPSEs	Special Side Effects
Phenothiaziness	Chlorpromazine	Thorazine	Common	
	Perphenazine	Trilafon		
	Fluphenazine	Prolixin		
	Trifluoperazine	Stelazine		
	Thioridazine	Mellaril		
Butyrophenones	Haloperidol	Haldol	Common	Retinal pigmentation
Thioxanthines	Thiothixene	Navane	Common	
Atypical Drugs	Risperidone	Risperdal	Uncommon	Agranulocytosis,
	Clozapine	Clozaril	Rare	Cataracts,
	Quetiapine	Seroquel	Uncommon	Neutropenia,
	Olanzapine	Zyprexa	Uncommon	Prolonged
	Ziprasidone	Geodon	Uncommon	QT interval

EPSEs, extrapyramidal side effects.

1. Treatment is immediate cessation of antipsychotic drug therapy and supportive therapy (ventilation, hydration, cooling). Bromocriptine (5 mg PO every 6 hours) or dantrolene (up to 6 mg/kg daily as a continuous infusion) may decrease skeletal muscle rigidity Mortality rates approach 20% in untreated patients. At the present time there is no evidence of a pathophysiologic link between neuroleptic malignant syndrome and malignant hyperthermia.

IV. ANXIETY DISORDERS

Anxiety disorders are associated with distressing symptoms such as nervousness, sleeplessness, hypochondriasis, and somatic complaints. There are two patterns: (1) chronic generalized anxiety and (2) episodic, often situation-dependent, anxiety. Anxiety resulting from identifiable stresses is usually self-limited and rarely requires pharmacologic treatment. Benzodiazepines can be helpful. β-blockers are useful for performance anxiety ("stage fright"). Cognitive behavioral therapy, relaxation techniques, hypnosis, and psychotherapy may be useful. Panic disorders are qualitatively different from generalized anxiety and involve discrete periods of unprovoked intense fear, apprehension, and a sense of impending doom. SSRIs, benzodiazepines, cyclic antidepressants, and MAOIs are effective treatments.

SUBSTANCE ABUSE

Psychoactive drug dependence is diagnosed when patients manifest at least three of nine characteristic symptoms, with some of the symptoms having persisted for at least 1 month or occurred repeatedly (**Table 22-11**). Substance abuse is often first during the medical management of other conditions (hepatitis, acquired immunodeficiency syndrome [AIDS], pregnancy). Sociopathic characteristics (school dropout, criminal record, multiple drug abuse) seem to predispose to,

TABLE 22-11	Characteristic Symptoms of Psychoactive Drug Dependence

Drug taken in higher doses or for longer periods than intended

Unsuccessful attempts to reduce use of the drug

Increased time spent obtaining the drug

Frequent intoxication or withdrawal symptoms

Restricted social or work activities because of drug use

Continued drug use despite social or physical problems related to drug use

Evidence of tolerance to the effects of the drug

Characteristic withdrawal symptoms

Drug use to avoid withdrawal symptoms

rather than result from, drug addiction. Drug overdose is the leading cause of unconsciousness in patients presenting to the emergency room.

A. Alcoholism is defined as a primary chronic disease with genetic, psychosocial, and environmental factors that influence its development and manifestations. Up to one third of adult patients have medical problems related to alcohol (**Table 22-12**).

   1. Treatment of alcoholism mandates total abstinence from alcohol. Disulfiram, which produces unpleasant symptoms when alcohol is ingested (flushing, vertigo, diaphoresis, nausea, vomiting) may be administered as an adjunctive drug along with psychiatric counseling.

   2. Overdose. In nonalcoholic patients, blood alcohol levels of 25 mg/dL are associated with impaired cognition and coordination. At blood alcohol concentrations greater than 100 mg/dL, signs of vestibular and cerebellar dysfunction (nystagmus, dysarthria, ataxia) increase. Intoxication with alcohol is defined as a blood alcohol concentrations above 80 to 100 mg/dL. Levels greater than 500 mg/dL are usually fatal. Treatment of life-threatening overdose is support of ventilation and treatment of hypoglycemia if needed.

   3. Alcohol Withdrawal Syndrome (Table 22-13)

   4. Wernicke-Korsakoff Syndrome may accompany alcoholism and reflects a loss of neurons in the cerebellum (Wernicke's encephalopathy) and a loss of memory (Korsakoff's psychosis) caused by the lack of thiamine (vitamin B_1), which is required for the intermediary metabolism of carbohydrates. Signs include global confusion, drowsiness, nystagmus, orthostatic hypotension, and peripheral neuropathy. Treatment consists of intravenous thiamine, then oral intake when possible.

   5. Alcohol and Pregnancy. Alcohol crosses the placenta and may result in decreased birth weight. High blood concentrations of alcohol (>150 mg/dL) may result in the fetal alcohol syndrome (craniofacial dysmorphology, growth retardation, mental retardation). There is increased risk of cardiac malformations (patent ductus arteriosus, septal defects).

   6. Management of Anesthesia. The presence of disulfiram-induced sedation and hepatotoxicity should be suspected in alcoholic patients being treated with this drug. Acute, unexplained hypotension during general

397

TABLE 22-12	Medical Problems Related to Alcoholism
Central Nervous System Effects	
Psychiatric disorders (depression, antisocial behavior)	
Nutritional disorders (Wernicke-Korsakoff)	
Withdrawal syndrome	
Cerebellar degeneration	
Cerebral atrophy	
Cardiovascular Effects	
Cardiomyopathy	
Cardiac dysrhythmias	
Hypertension	
Gastrointestinal and Hepatobiliary Effects	
Esophagitis	
Gastritis	
Pancreatitis	
Hepatic cirrhosis	
Portal hypertension	
Skin and Musculoskeletal Effects	
Spider angiomata	
Myopathy	
Osteoporosis	
Endocrine and Metabolic Effects	
Decreased serum testosterone concentrations (impotence)	
Decreased gluconeogenesis (hypoglycemia)	
Ketoacidosis	
Hypoalbuminemia	
Hypomagnesemia	
Hematologic Effects	
Thrombocytopenia	
Leukopenia	
Anemia	

anesthesia could reflect inadequate stores of norepinephrine caused by disulfiram-induced inhibition of dopamine β-hydroxylase. Direct-acting sympathomimetics (phenylephrine) produce a more predictable response than indirect agents (ephedrine). Use of regional anesthesia may be influenced by the presence of disulfiram-induced polyneuropathy. Alcohol-containing solutions, as used for skin cleansing, probably should be avoided in disulfiram-treated patients.

TABLE 22-13	Alcohol Withdrawal Syndrome
Early signs (6–8 hr after decreased alcohol levels, most pronounced in 24–36 hr)	• Tremors • Nightmares, hallucinations, insomnia, confusion • Autonomic nervous system hyperreactivity (tachycardia, hypertension, cardiac dysrhythmias) • Nausea, vomiting • May be treated with benzodiazepines, β-receptor antagonists or $α_2$-agonists.
Delirium tremens (2–4 days after alcohol cessation) *Life threatening!*	• Hallucinations, combativeness • Hyperthermia, tachycardia • Hypertension or hypotension • Seizures
	Treatment of delirium tremens
	o Diazepam 5–10 mg IV every 5 min until patient is calm o β-adrenergic antagonists IV (propranolol, esmolol) until heart rate <100 bpm o Correction of fluid and electrolyte disturbances o Lidocaine for cardiac dysrhythmias o Airway protection if consciousness is affected o Physical restraint if necessary to prevent injury to self or others

B. Cocaine produces sympathetic nervous system stimulation by blocking the presynaptic uptake of norepinephrine and dopamine, thereby increasing the postsynaptic concentrations of these neurotransmitters. Dopamine is present in high concentrations in synapses, producing the characteristic "cocaine high."

1. Side Effects of acute cocaine administration include hypertension, tachycardia, coronary vasospasm, myocardial ischemia, myocardial infarction, and ventricular cardiac dysrhythmias, including ventricular fibrillation. Lung damage and pulmonary edema can occur in patients who smoke cocaine. Cocaine-abusing parturients are at higher risk of spontaneous abortion, abruptio placenta, and fetal malformations. Long-term abuse is associated with nasal septal atrophy, agitated behavior, paranoid thinking, and heightened reflexes. Symptoms associated with cocaine withdrawal include fatigue, depression, and increased appetite.

2. Treatment of cocaine overdose includes nitroglycerin to manage myocardial ischemia and α-adrenergic blockade to treat coronary vasoconstriction. Intravenous benzodiazepines such as diazepam are effective in controlling seizures. Active cooling may be necessary for hyperthermia.

3. Management of Anesthesia in patients acutely intoxicated with cocaine must consider the vulnerability of these patients to myocardial ischemia and cardiac dysrhythmias. Nitroglycerin should be readily available.

Thrombocytopenia associated with cocaine abuse may influence the selection of regional anesthesia. In the absence of acute intoxication long-term abuse of cocaine has not been shown to be predictably associated with adverse anesthetic interactions.

C. Opioids. Numerous medical problems are encountered in opioid addicts, especially intravenous abusers (Table 22-14). Dependence rarely develops in the setting of opioid use to treat postoperative pain.

1. Overdose. The most obvious sign of opioid overdose (usually heroin) is a slow breathing rate with a normal to increased tidal volume. Pupils are usually miotic. Central nervous system manifestations range from dysphoria to unconsciousness; seizures are unlikely. Pulmonary edema occurs in a large proportion of patients with heroin overdose. Naloxone is the specific opioid antagonist administered to maintain an acceptable respiratory rate, usually 12 breaths or more per minute.

2. Withdrawal Syndrome from opioids is rarely life threatening. The time course is summarized in Table 22-15. Clonidine may also attenuate opioid withdrawal symptoms (diaphoresis, mydriasis, hypertension, tachycardia). Other symptoms include insomnia, abdominal cramps, diarrhea, hyperthermia, skeletal muscle spasms, and jerking of the legs. Rapid detoxification using high doses of an opioid antagonist (nalmefene) administered during general anesthesia followed by naltrexone maintenance has been proposed as a cost-effective alternative to conventional detoxification approaches.

3. Management of Anesthesia. Opioid addicts should have opioids or methadone maintained during the perioperative period. Opioid addicts often seem to experience exaggerated degrees of postoperative pain. For reasons that are not clear, satisfactory postoperative analgesia may be achieved when average doses of meperidine are administered in addition to the usual daily maintenance dose of methadone or other opioids. Alternative methods of postoperative pain relief include continuous

TABLE 22-14	Medical Problems Associated with Chronic Opioid Abuse
Hepatitis	
Cellulitis	
Superficial skin abscesses	
Septic thrombophlebitis	
Endocarditis	
Systemic septic emboli	
Acquired immunodeficiency syndrome	
Aspiration pneumonitis	
Malnutrition	
Tetanus	
Transverse myelitis	

TABLE 22-15	Time Course of Opioid Withdrawal Syndrome		
Drug	**Onset**	**Peak Intensity**	**Duration**
Meperidine Oxycodone Codeine	2–6 hours	8–12 hours	4–5 days
Morphine Heroin	6–18 hours	36–72 hours	7–10 days
Methadone	24–48 hours	3–21 days	6–7 weeks

regional anesthesia with local anesthetics, neuraxial opioids, and transcutaneous electrical nerve stimulation.

D. Barbiturates

1. Overdose. Central nervous system depression is the principal manifestation of barbiturate overdose. Treatment is supportive: maintenance of a patent airway, protection from aspiration, and support of ventilation using a cuffed endotracheal tube if necessary. Hypotension, hypothermia, acute renal failure, and rhabdomyolysis may occur. Forced diuresis and alkalinization of the urine promote elimination of phenobarbital but are of lesser value with many of the other barbiturates.

2. Withdrawal Syndrome (Table 22-16). The abrupt cessation of excessive barbiturate ingestion is associated with delayed but potentially life-threatening responses. Barbiturate withdrawal symptoms include anxiety, skeletal muscle tremors, hyperreflexia, diaphoresis, tachycardia, orthostatic hypotension, grand mal seizures, and cardiovascular collapse. Pentobarbital may be administered if evidence of barbiturate withdrawal manifests. Phenobarbital and diazepam may also be useful for suppressing evidence of barbiturate withdrawal.

3. Management of Anesthesia. There are no reports of increased anesthetic requirements (MAC) in chronic barbiturate abusers. Venous access is a likely problem in intravenous barbiturate abusers, as the alkalinity of the self-injected solutions is likely to sclerose veins.

E. Substance Abuse as an Occupational Hazard in Anesthesiology.

Anesthesiologists are represented in addictive treatment programs at a rate three times higher than any other physician group.

TABLE 22-16	Time Course of Barbiturate Withdrawal Syndrome		
Drug	**Onset (hr)**	**Peak Intensity (days)**	**Duration (days)**
Pentobarbital	12–24	2–3	7–10
Secobarbital	12–24	2–3	7–10
Phenobarbital	48–72	6–10	10+

1. Characteristics/Demographics of the Addicted Anesthesiologist:
- 50% are younger than 35 years old.
- Residents are overrepresented.
- 67% to 88% are male, and 75% to 96% are white.
- 76% to 90% use opiates as the drug of choice.
- 33% to 50% are polydrug users.
- 33% have a family history of addictive disease, most commonly alcohol.
- 65% of anesthesiologists with a history of addiction are associated with academic departments.

2. Most Commonly Abused Drugs. Fentanyl and sufentanil are the most commonly abused drugs, followed by meperidine and morphine. Alcohol abuse occurs more often in anesthesia practitioners who have been out of residency for more than 5 years. Sevoflurane has been reported as the drug of choice among inhalational agents.

3. Signs and Symptoms of Addictive Behavior. Any unusual and persistent changes in behavior should be cause for alarm. Classically, these behaviors include wide mood swings, such as periods of depression, anger, and irritability alternating with periods of euphoria.
- Denial is universal.
- Symptoms at work are the last to appear (symptoms appear first in the community and then at home).
- Detected addicts are often found comatose.
- *Untreated addicts are often found dead!*
- The most commonly overlooked symptoms of addictive behavior are:
  - The desire to work alone
  - Refusing lunch relief or breaks
  - Frequently relieving others
  - Volunteering for extra cases or call
  - Patient pain needs in the postanesthetic care unit that are out of proportion to the narcotics recorded as given
  - Weight loss
  - Frequent bathroom breaks

4. Associated Risks of Physician Drug Addiction
a. Physician. The relapse rate for anesthesiologists is the highest of all physicians and is greatest in the first 5 years. Death is the primary presenting sign of relapse.
b. Patient. Impaired physicians (those who are actively abusing drugs) are at increased risk of malpractice suits.

5. What to Do When Substance Abuse is Suspected
a. Reporting and Intervention. Admission to an alcohol or drug addiction treatment program is not a reportable event to state or national agencies. After an individual has been confronted and is awaiting final disposition, he or she should not be left alone because newly identified addictive physicians are at increased risk of suicide.
b. Treatment. There is no cure for addiction, and recovery is a lifelong process. The most effective treatment programs are multidisciplinary in composition and can provide long-term follow-up for the impaired physician.

F. Benzodiazepines. Addiction requires ingestion of large doses of drug. Symptoms of withdrawal generally occur later than with barbiturates and are less severe owing to the prolonged elimination half-lives of most benzodiazepines and the fact that many of these drugs are metabolized to pharmacologically active metabolites that also have prolonged elimination half-lives. Anesthetic considerations in chronic benzodiazepine abusers are similar to those described for chronic barbiturate abusers.

1. Acute Benzodiazepine Overdose. Supportive treatment and flumazenil, a specific benzodiazepine antagonist, are used for severe or life-threatening overdose.

G. Amphetamines stimulate the release of catecholamines, resulting in increased cortical alertness, appetite suppression, and decreased need for sleep. Approved medical uses of amphetamines are treatment of narcolepsy, attention-deficit disorders, and hyperactivity associated with minimal brain dysfunction in children.

1. Overdose causes anxiety, a psychotic state, progressive central nervous system irritability (hyperactivity, hyperreflexia, seizures), cardiovascular stimulation (hypertension, tachycardia, dysrhythmias), decreased gastrointestinal motility, mydriasis, diaphoresis, and hyperthermia.

a. Treatment is induced emesis or gastric lavage and administration of activated charcoal and a cathartic. Phenothiazine and diazepam may be useful. Acidification of the urine promotes elimination of amphetamines.

2. Withdrawal Syndrome. Abrupt cessation of excessive amphetamine use is accompanied by extreme lethargy, depression that may be suicidal, increased appetite, and weight gain.

3. Management of Anesthesia. Amphetamines administered chronically for medically indicated uses (narcolepsy, attention-deficit disorder) need not be discontinued before elective surgery. In the acutely intoxicated patient undergoing emergency surgery, effects from amphetamines may include hypertension, tachycardia, hyperthermia, and increased requirements for volatile anesthetics, intracranial hypertension and cardiac arrest. Direct-acting vasopressors, including phenylephrine and epinephrine, should be available to treat hypotension because the response to indirect-acting vasopressors such as ephedrine may be attenuated by the amphetamine-induced catecholamine depletion.

H. Hallucinogens, such as LSD and phencyclidine, are usually ingested orally. There is no evidence of physical dependence or withdrawal symptoms. The effects of these drugs consist of visual, auditory, and tactile hallucinations and distortions of the surroundings and body image. Evidence of sympathetic nervous system stimulation includes mydriasis, increased body temperature, hypertension, and tachycardia.

1. Overdose is usually not life threatening. Patients should be placed in a calm, quiet environment with minimal external stimuli. Benzodiazepines may be useful. Supportive care (airway management, mechanical ventilation, treatment of seizures, control of the manifestations of sympathetic nervous system hyperactivity) is warranted. Forced diuresis and acidification of the urine promotes elimination of phencyclidine but increases the risk of fluid overload and electrolyte abnormalities, especially hypokalemia.

2. Management of Anesthesia may be complicated by acute panic episodes and exaggerated responses to sympathomimetic drugs. Diazepam is likely to be useful.

I. Marijuana abuse is associated with lethargy, sedation, tachycardia, orthostatic hypotension, and bronchitis (related to smoke ingestion).

1. Management of Anesthesia includes consideration of the known effects of THC on the heart, lungs, and central nervous system. Barbiturate and ketamine sleep times are prolonged in THC-treated animals, and opioid-induced respiratory depression may be potentiated.

J. Tricyclic Antidepressant Overdose is a common cause of drug ingestion death. Signs are intense anticholinergic effects (delirium, fever, tachycardia, mydriasis, flushed dry skin, ileus, urinary retention, cardiovascular toxicity (tachycardia, prolonged PR interval, QRS and QTc, ventricular dysrhythmias, myocardial depression), and seizures. The risk of life-threatening cardiac dysrhythmias may persist for several days.

1. Treatment of cyclic antidepressant overdose in the presence of preserved upper airway reflexes includes gastric lavage and activated charcoal. Emesis should not be induced because of the risk of pulmonary aspiration. Serum alkalinization is the principal treatment and results in an increase of protein-bound drug, less free drug, and thereby less toxicity. Intravenous administration of sodium bicarbonate or hyperventilation to a pH between 7.45 and 7.55 should be accomplished to a clinical end point such as narrowing of the QRS or cessation of dysrhythmias. Lidocaine may be an additional treatment for cardiac dysrhythmias. If torsade de pointes is present, magnesium should be administered. Vasopressor or inotropic support may be needed. Diazepam is useful for seizure control. Hemodialysis is ineffective in removing cyclic antidepressants.

K. Salicylic Acid Overdose. Symptoms and signs include tinnitus, nausea and vomiting, fever, seizures, obtundation, hypoglycemia, low cerebrospinal fluid glucose concentration, coagulopathy, hepatic dysfunction, and direct stimulation of the respiratory center. Noncardiogenic pulmonary edema often occurs during the first 24 hours after aspirin overdose.

1. Initial Treatment includes gastric lavage and activated charcoal, administration of dextrose to prevent low cerebrospinal fluid glucose concentrations, administration of sodium bicarbonate to increase arterial pH to 7.45 to 7.55 (alkalinizes the urine and dramatically increases renal clearance of salicylate), and hemodialysis for potentially lethal concentrations of salicylic acid (>100 mg/dL), refractory acidosis, coma, seizures, volume overload, or renal failure.

L. Acetaminophen Overdose

1. Treatment is administration of activated charcoal to impede drug absorption. Four hours after drug ingestion, a plasma acetaminophen concentration is measured and plotted on the Rumack-Matthew nomogram, which stratifies the patient's risk of hepatotoxicity. All patients with possible or probable risk and anyone in whom the time of ingestion is not known are treated with N-acetylcysteine, which repletes glutathione, combines directly with N-acetylbenzoquinonimine, and enhances sulfate conjugation of acetaminophen. N-acetylcysteine is virtually 100% effective in preventing hepatotoxicity when administered within 8 hours of drug ingestion.

POISONING

I. METHYL ALCOHOL

Methyl alcohol is found in paint remover, gas-line antifreeze, windshield washing fluid, and camper fuel. It is metabolized by alcohol dehydrogenase to formaldehyde and formic acid, resulting in an anion-gap metabolic acidosis. Toxicity occurs in the retina, the optic nerve, and the central nervous system.

A. Treatment includes supportive care and a secure airway. Intravenous administration of ethyl alcohol will decrease the metabolism of methanol. Alternatively, the activity of alcohol dehydrogenase may be specifically inhibited by administration of fomepizole. Hemodialysis may be indicated for refractory acidosis or visual impairment.

II. ETHYLENE GLYCOL

Ethylene glycol is found in antifreeze, de-icers, and industrial solvents.

A. Treatment is similar to that described for methyl alcohol ingestion. Inhibition of formation of toxic metabolites can be accomplished by administration of ethyl alcohol or fomepizole. Thiamine, pyridoxine, and sufficient calcium to reverse hypocalcemia are also given. Urgent hemodialysis may be necessary.

III. ORGANOPHOSPHATE PESTICIDES, CARBAMATE PESTICIDES, AND ORGANOPHOSPHORUS COMPOUNDS

Organophosphate pesticides, carbamate pesticides, and organophosphorus compounds ("nerve agents") were developed for chemical warfare. All inhibit acetylcholinesterase, resulting in cholinergic overstimulation. The manifestations of pesticide and nerve agent poisoning are influenced by the route of absorption, with the most severe effects occurring after inhalation (**Table 22-17**).

A. Treatment involves three strategies: an anticholinergic drug to counteract the acute cholinergic crisis, an oxime drug to reactivate inhibited acetylcholinesterase, and an anticonvulsant drug to prevent or treat seizures (**Table 22-18**).

IV. CARBON MONOXIDE (CO) POISONING

A. Pathophysiology. CO competes with oxygen for binding to hemoglobin, shifting the oxygen-hemoglobin dissociation curve to the left, with impaired release of oxygen to tissues (**Fig. 22-1**). CO also disrupts oxidative metabolism, increases nitric oxide concentrations, causes brain lipid peroxidation, generates oxygen free radicals, and produces other metabolic changes that may result in neurologic and cardiac toxicity. CO binds more tightly to fetal hemoglobin than adult hemoglobin, making infants particularly vulnerable to its effects.

B. Signs and Symptoms include headache, nausea, vomiting, weakness, difficulty concentrating, confusion, syncope, and seizures. Angina pectoris,

405

TABLE 22-17	Signs of Organophosphate Poisoning
Muscarinic Effects	
Copious secretions	
Salivation	
Tearing	
Diaphoresis	
Bronchorrhea	
Rhinorrhea	
Bronchospasm	
Miosis	
Hyperperistalsis	
Bradycardia	
Nicotinic Effects	
Skeletal muscle fasciculations	
Skeletal muscle weakness	
Skeletal muscle paralysis	
Central Nervous System Effects	
Seizures	
Coma	
Central apnea	

dysrhythmias, and pulmonary edema may result from the increased cardiac output necessitated by the hypoxemia. Persistent or delayed neurologic effects may be seen (cognitive dysfunction, memory loss, seizures, personality changes, parkinsonism, dementia, mutism, blindness, psychosis) following apparent recovery from the acute phase of CO intoxication.

C. Diagnosis. Serum carboxyhemoglobin concentrations should be obtained from patients suspected of CO exposure. SpO_2 values may be misleading.

TABLE 22-18	Goals of Treatment in Organophosphate Poisoning
Reverse the acute cholinergic crisis created by the poison	
Atropine 2 mg IV every 5–10 min as needed until ventilation improves	
Reactivate the function of acetylcholinesterase	
Pralidoxime 600 mg IV	
Prevent/treat seizures	
Diazepam or midazolam as needed	
Supportive care	

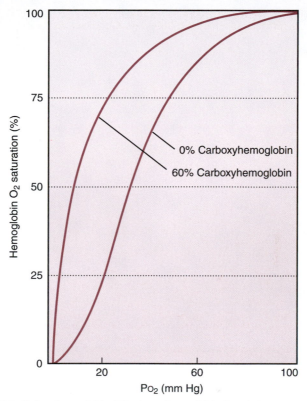

Figure 22-1 • Carboxyhemoglobin shifts the oxyhemoglobin dissociation curve to the left and changes it to a more hyperbolic shape. This results in decreased oxygen-carrying capacity and impaired release of oxygen at the tissue level. (Adapted from Ernst A, Zibrak JD: Carbon monoxide poisoning. N Engl J Med 1998;339:1603–1608. Copyright 1998 Massachusetts Medical Society. All rights reserved.)

D. Treatment consists of removing the individual from the source of the CO production, immediate administration of supplemental oxygen, and aggressive supportive care: airway management, blood pressure support, and cardiovascular stabilization. Oxygen therapy shortens the elimination half-time of CO by competing at the binding sites for hemoglobin and improves tissue oxygenation. Hyperbaric oxygen therapy accelerates the elimination of CO and may be indicated in selected patients who are comatose or neurologically abnormal at presentation, who have carboxyhemoglobin concentrations greater than 40%, and who are pregnant and have carboxyhemoglobin concentrations above 15%.

CHAPTER 23

Pregnancy-Associated Diseases

I. PHYSIOLOGIC CHANGES ASSOCIATED WITH PREGNANCY

A. **General Physiologic Changes (Table 23-1)**

B. **Specific Concerns**

　　1. Obstruction of the Inferior Vena Cava by the gravid uterus when the pregnant woman is in the supine position results in supine hypotension syndrome in about 10% of parturients. It can be minimized by positioning the patient in the lateral position or mechanically displacing the uterus to the left.

　　2. Capillary Engorgement of the Respiratory Mucosa results in swelling of the nasal and oral pharynx, larynx, and trachea. Manipulation of the airway may cause bleeding and further edema.

　　3. Lower Esophageal Sphincter Tone is decreased as a result of upward displacement of the stomach and muscle relaxation resulting from the effects of progestins.

　　4. Insulin Resistance is caused by placental lactogen secretion.

　　5. Hypercoagulability. Pregnancy is a state of both increased platelet turnover and clotting.

C. **Anesthetic Considerations**

　　1. Induction and Emergence from anesthesia are more rapid than in the nonpregnant state because of increased minute ventilation, decreased functional residual capacity, and the decreased MAC of volatile agents.

　　2. Teratogenicity. Few, if any, studies support teratogenic effects of anesthetic or sedative medications in the doses used for anesthesia care in humans.

　　　　a. Diazepam. Some studies have suggested a connections between high-dose diazepam in the first trimester and cleft palate; medicinal doses of benzodiazepine are safe when needed to treat perioperative anxiety.

　　　　b. Nitrous Oxide. Teratogenesis has been seen only in animals under extreme conditions and is not likely to be reproduced in clinical care.

TABLE 23-1	Physiologic Changes Accompanying Pregnancy
Parameter	**Average Change from Nonpregnant Value (%)**
Intravascular fluid volume	+35
Plasma volume	+45
Erythrocyte volume	+20
Cardiac output	+40
Stroke volume	+30
Heart rate	+15
Peripheral circulation	
Systolic blood pressure	No change
Systemic vascular resistance	−15
Diastolic blood pressure	−15
Central venous pressure	No change
Femoral venous pressure	+15
Minute ventilation	+50
Tidal volume	+40
Breathing rate	+10
PaO_2	+10 mm Hg
$PaCO_2$	−10 mm Hg
pHa	No change
Total lung capacity	No change
Vital capacity	No change
Functional residual capacity	−20
Expiratory reserve volume	−20
Residual volume	−20
Airway resistance	−35
Oxygen consumption	+20
Renal blood flow and glomerular filtration rate	−50
Serum cholinesterase activity	−25

3. Avoid Intrauterine Fetal Asphyxia by maintaining maternal PaO_2, $PaCO_2$ (maternal alkalosis can cause uterine vasoconstriction and shift the oxyhemoglobin dissociation curve to the left, releasing less oxygen to the fetus), and uterine blood flow (avoid hypotension, alkalosis, uterine irritability).

4. Preterm Labor can occur during the intraoperative and postoperative periods. For monitoring, at least preoperative and postoperative fetal heart rate and uterine activity must be assessed.

D. Obstetric Anesthesia Care

a. Regional Analgesic Techniques during Labor and Delivery. During the first stage of labor, pain is visceral and supplied by spinal cord segments T10–L1. During the second stage of labor, pain is somatic from S2–4 spinal cord segments via the pudendal nerves. Neuraxial analgesia in early labor does not increase the incidence of cesarean delivery and may shorten labor when compared with systemic analgesia.

b. Lumbar Epidural Analgesia. (See **Table 23-2** for analgesic choices.) It is important to confirm the absence of intravascular or subarachnoid placement of the epidural catheter. This is usually done by administering a test dose of a solution containing local anesthetic and epinephrine (15 μg) through the catheter. Tachycardia and/or hypertension alert the anesthesiologist to the possibility of an intravascular catheter. Rapid onset of analgesia suggests subarachnoid placement. Hypotension may require administration of small doses of ephedrine (5 to 10 mg intravenously [IV]) or phenylephrine (20 to 100 μg IV).

c. Combined Spinal-Epidural Analgesia (CSE). Analgesia via CSE in labor is an alternative to epidural analgesia. Advantages include rapid onset of analgesia, increased reliability, effectiveness when instituted in a rapidly progressing labor, and minimal motor block. Subarachnoid administration of low doses of opioids (fentanyl 12.5 to 25 μg, sufentanil 5 to 10 μg) results in rapid (5 minutes), nearly complete pain relief during the first stage of labor. Disadvantages of CSE include increased technical complexity and the possible risk of postdural puncture headache.

d. Anesthesia for Cesarean Delivery. Epidural analgesia for labor can be converted to a surgical anesthetic by changing the drug dose and concentration administered. Spinal anesthesia with hyperbaric bupivacaine solution provides reliable anesthesia, often with the addition of morphine or meperidine for postoperative analgesia. General anesthesia is reserved for the most emergent cases or when maternal condition contraindicates regional anesthesia.

TABLE 23-2	Epidural Labor Analgesia	
	Infusion	
Bolus (10 mL)	**Local Anesthetic +**	**Opioid**
Bupivacaine 0.125% with hydromorphine 10 μg/mL	Bupivacaine 0.0625%–0.125%	Hydromorphine 3 μg/mL
Bupivacaine 0.125% with fentanyl 5 μg/mL	Bupivacaine 0.0625%–0.125%	Fentanyl 2 μg/mL
Bupivacaine 0.125% with sufentanil 1 μg/mL	Bupivacaine 0.0625%–0.125%	Sufentanil 2 μg/mL
(Ropivacaine 0.075% may be used with opioid as above)	(Ropivacaine 0.075%–0.125% may be used)	(Any of the above)

1.) *Availability.* The American College of Obstetricians and Gynecologists/American Society of Anesthesiologists consensus is that hospitals should have the capability to begin a cesarean delivery within 30 minutes of the decision to operate, although not all indications for cesarean delivery require that 30-minute response time.

2.) *Maternal Risks for Anesthesia (Table 23-3).* Pulmonary aspiration and failed intubation account for three fourths of all maternal deaths related to anesthesia care. Prevention includes premedication with H_2-blockers, the use of a nonparticulate antacid, and/or metoclopramide and/or famotidine. General anesthesia should be avoided whenever possible; cricoid pressure and an endotracheal tube should be used if general anesthesia is required. The incidence of failed intubation in the obstetric population is 10 times that in the general surgical population.

II. PREGNANCY-INDUCED HYPERTENSION (PIH)

PIH encompasses a range of disorders collectively and formerly known as toxemia of pregnancy, which includes gestational hypertension (nonproteinuric hypertension), preeclampsia (proteinuric hypertension), and eclampsia.

A. Gestational Hypertension is characterized by the onset of systemic hypertension, without proteinuria or edema, during the last few weeks of gestation or during the immediate postpartum period.

B. Preeclampsia, a syndrome exhibited after 20 weeks of gestation, manifests as systemic hypertension, proteinuria, and generalized edema (**Table 23-4**). Systemic blood pressures higher than 140/90 mm Hg with daily urine protein losses of more than 2 g are sufficient for the diagnosis of preeclampsia. Severe preeclampsia is present if systemic blood pressure is higher than 160/110 mm Hg with daily urine protein losses of more than 5 g (**Table 23-5**).

   1. Etiology (see Fig. 23-1). Preeclampsia is a syndrome that affects virtually all organ systems. It is associated with placental ischemia resulting from

TABLE 23-3	Factors That Increase Anesthetic Risk
Obesity	
Facial and neck edema	
Extremely short stature	
Difficulty opening mouth	
Arthritis of neck/short neck/small mandible	
Abnormalities of face, mouth, or teeth	
Large thyroid	
Pulmonary disease	
Cardiac disease	

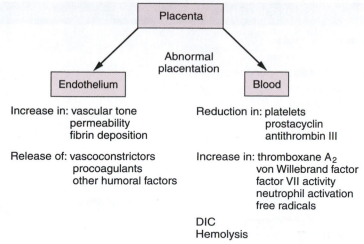

Figure 23-1 • Primary initiating change for the development of pregnancy-induced hypertension (preeclampsia) may be placental ischemia. DIC, disseminated intravascular coagulation. (Adapted from Mushambi MC, Halligan AW, Williamson K: Recent developments in the pathophysiology of pre-eclampsia. Br J Anaesth 1996;76:133–148. © The Board of Management and Trustees of the British Journal of Anaesthesia.)

an abnormal placenta that releases factors that produce generalized vascular endothelial cell damage and lead to multiple organ system dysfunction.

2. Signs include hypertension, decreased intravascular volume, heart failure, pulmonary edema, visual disturbances, headache, seizures, oliguria, thrombocytopenia, and impaired placental circulation. Abnormal liver function tests are seen alone and in conjunction with HELLP syndrome (see "HELLP Syndrome").

3. Treatment. The definitive treatment is delivery. If the preeclampsia is mild and the patient remote from term, conservative management with bed rest and monitoring until 37 weeks of gestation or until the status of the mother or fetus deteriorates are recommended. Management includes administration of magnesium sulfate to prevent seizures, antihypertensive therapy (hydralazine, labetolol, nifedipine), and fluid resuscitation (**Table 23-6**). Arterial and central venous pressure monitoring may be necessary.

4. Prognosis

a. Maternal. Cerebral hemorrhage is a major cause of maternal death that results from preeclampsia and eclampsia. Patients may develop seizures or pulmonary edema within 24 to 48 hours of delivery; anticonvulsant therapy and antihypertensive therapy should continue for 48 hours or longer postpartum.

b. Neonatal. Babies are at greater risk of prematurity, of being small for gestational age, and of drug-related respiratory depression at the time of delivery.

TABLE 23-4	Manifestations and Complications of Preeclampsia
Systemic hypertension	
Congestive heart failure	
Decreased colloid osmotic pressure	
Pulmonary edema	
Arterial hypoxemia	
Laryngeal edema	
Cerebral edema (headaches, visual disturbances, changes in levels of consciousness)	
Grand mal seizures	
Cerebral hemorrhage	
Hypovolemia	
HELLP Syndrome (*h*emolysis, *e*levated *l*iver enzymes, *l*ow *p*latelets)	
Disseminated intravascular coagulation	
Proteinuria	
Oliguria	
Acute tubular necrosis	
Epigastric pain	
Decreased uterine blood flow	
Intrauterine growth retardation	
Premature labor and delivery	
Abruptio placentae	

TABLE 23-5	Diagnostic Features of Severe Preeclampsia
≥5 g proteinuria over 24 hr	
Oliguria	
Pulmonary edema	
Abnormal liver function	
Right upper quadrant pain	
Cerebral disturbances	
Thrombocytopenia	

5. Management of Anesthesia

a. Preanesthetic Assessment

1.) *Airway Assessment.* Facial edema or stridor may indicate airway edema and thus a difficult intubation.

2.) *Volume Assessment.* Preeclamptic patients are hypovolemic and prone to hypotension with the institution of neuraxial anesthesia, but they are also at risk of pulmonary edema. A 500 to 1000 mL crystalloid preload is appropriate before initiating neuroaxial

TABLE 23-6	Treatment of Preeclampsia

Maintain diastolic blood pressure <110 mm Hg

Hydralazine 5–10 mg IV every 20–30 min

Hydralazine 5–20 mg/hr IV as a continuous infusion following administration of 5 mg IV

Labetalol 50 mg IV or 100 mg PO

Labetalol 20–160 mg/hr IV as a continuous infusion

Nitroglycerin 10 μg/min IV, titrated to response

Nitroprusside 0.25 μg/kg/min IV, titrated to response

Fenoldopam 0.1 μg/kg/min IV, increase by 0.05–0.2 μg/kg/min until desired response reached; average dose 0.25–0.5 μg/kg/min

Seizure prophylaxis

Magnesium 4–6 g IV followed by concentrations continuous infusion of 1–2 g/hr (goal is to maintain serum magnesium concentration of 2.0–3.5 mEq/L)

Monitor for magnesium toxicity

4.0–6.5 mEq/L associated with nausea, vomiting, diplopia, somnolence, loss of patellar reflex

6.5–7.5 mEq/L associated with skeletal muscle paralysis, apnea

$\geq$10 mEq/L associated with cardiac arrest

PO, by mouth.

analgesia. Invasive monitoring may be indicated if the patient develops either pulmonary edema or oliguria unresponsive to a fluid challenge. Intra-arterial blood pressure monitoring is indicated for refractory hypertension, especially if an antihypertensive infusion is needed.

3.) *Laboratory Assessment* should include a complete blood cell count. An elevated hematocrit suggests hypovolemia. A platelet count of less than 70,000/mm³ indicates an increased risk of epidural hematoma. A test of platelet function is useful in evaluating the patient's eligibility for regional anesthesia if the platelet count is in the range of 70,000 to 100,000/mm³. Liver function tests, blood urea nitrogen, and creatinine are essential in determining the severity of the preeclampsia or in identifying the presence of HELLP syndrome.

b. Labor Analgesia. Vaginal delivery in the presence of PIH and in the absence of fetal distress is acceptable. Epidural analgesia is the preferred technique for labor analgesia, if not contraindicated (reduces maternal catecholamine levels and facilitates blood pressure control). Because of the hypersensitivity of the maternal vasculature to catecholamines, use of local anesthetic solutions without the addition of epinephrine should be considered.

415

c. Anesthetic for Cesarean Delivery

1.) *General Anesthesia* is indicated for preeclamptic patients undergoing cesarean section who refuse regional anesthesia or who are coagulopathic or septic. Risks include potentially difficult tracheal intubation, risk of aspiration, increased sensitivity to nondepolarizing muscle relaxants, exaggerated pressor responses to direct laryngoscopy and tracheal intubation, and impaired placental blood flow. Before induction of anesthesia, it is essential to restore intravascular fluid volume and control blood pressure. Hydralazine (5 to 10 mg IV 10 to 15 minutes before induction of anesthesia), labetalol (10 to 20 mg IV 5 to 10 minutes before induction of anesthesia), or nitroglycerin (1 to 2 μg/kg IV just prior to induction) may attenuate hypertensive responses to direct laryngoscopy.

2.) *Spinal Anesthesia.* Although spinal anesthesia has traditionally been discouraged in parturients with preeclampsia because of the theoretical risk of severe hypotension, the magnitude of maternal blood pressure decreases are similar following the administration of either spinal or epidural anesthesia for cesarean section in preeclamptic patients. As with epidural anesthesia, institution of intravenous hydration before performing spinal anesthesia is essential.

C. HELLP Syndrome, a severe form of preeclampsia, is characterized by hemolysis (H), elevated liver transaminase enzymes (EL), and low platelet counts (LP). In addition to other signs of preeclampsia, HELLP syndrome patients may present with epigastric pain, upper abdominal tenderness, and jaundice. Disseminated intravascular coagulation (DIC) is a risk, and maternal and perinatal mortality is increased.

1. Treatment. Definitive treatment of HELLP syndrome is the delivery of the fetus, often by cesarean section.

2. Management of Anesthesia. Regional techniques must often be avoided because of coagulation defects. The precise selection of drugs will be influenced by the presence of renal and hepatic dysfunction that could alter drug clearance, metabolism, and elimination.

D. Eclampsia is present when seizures are superimposed on preeclampsia. It is associated with a maternal mortality of approximately 10%. The obstetric and anesthetic management of the eclamptic patient is directed at controlling the seizures (airway support, oxygenation, antiseizure treatment with thiopental, a benzodiazepine, or magnesium) and protecting the patient from aspiration pneumonitis. Lateralizing neurologic signs following a seizure may be the first sign of intracranial hemorrhage.

III. OBSTETRIC COMPLICATIONS

Obstetric complications include hemorrhagic complications, amniotic fluid embolism, uterine rupture, vaginal birth after cesarean delivery (VBAC), abnormal presentations, and multiple births.

A. Obstetric Hemorrhage (Table 23-7)

1. Placenta Previa is classified as complete when the entire cervical os is covered by placental tissue, partial when the internal cervical os is covered

TABLE 23-7	Differential Diagnosis of Third-Trimester Bleeding		
Parameter	Placenta Previa	Abruptio Placentae	Uterine Rupture
Signs and symptoms	Painless vaginal bleeding	Abdominal pain Bleeding partially or wholly concealed Uterine irritability Shock Acute renal failure Fetal distress	Abdominal pain Vaginal pain Recession of presenting part Disappearance of fetal heart tones/fetal bradycardia Hemodynamic instability
Predisposing conditions	Advanced age	Advanced parity Advanced age, Cigarette smoker Cocaine abuse Trauma	Previous uterine incision
	Multiple parity	Uterine anomalies Compression of the inferior vena cava Chronic systemic hypertension	Rapid spontaneous delivery Excessive uterine stimulation Cephalopelvic disproportion Multiple parity Polyhydramnios

by placental tissue when closed but not when fully dilated, and marginal when placental tissue encroaches on or extends to the margin of the internal cervical os. Parturients with a total or partial previa will deliver by cesarean section. Large-bore intravenous access should be established, and cross-matched blood should be immediately available.

2. Placenta Accreta occurs when the placenta is abnormally adherent to the myometrium. Massive hemorrhage may occur when removal of the placenta is attempted after delivery. The majority of cases require cesarean hysterectomy. Large-bore intravenous catheters should be placed, and blood should be immediately available.

3. Abruptio Placentae (separation of the placenta from the uterus) can cause severe blood loss, fetal distress or demise, clotting abnormalities, and acute renal failure. Definitive treatment is delivery of the fetus and placenta, often by cesarean section. Anesthetic management is similar to that employed with placenta previa. Blood and blood products should be readily available because of the risk of bleeding and DIC.

4. Postpartum Hemorrhage

 a. Uterine Atony. Treatment is with intravenous oxytocin resulting in contraction of the uterus. Intravenous or intramuscular methylergonovine or intrauterine carboprost tromethamine (misoprostol) may also be used. Rarely, it may be necessary to perform an emergency hysterectomy.

417

5. Retained Placenta. Manual removal of the retained placenta may be attempted under epidural or spinal anesthesia. Low doses (40-µg boluses, as needed) of intravenous nitroglycerin are used to relax the uterus for placental removal when indicated.

B. Amniotic Fluid Embolism is a rare catastrophic and life-threatening complication of pregnancy heralded by abrupt onset of dyspnea, arterial hypoxemia, cyanosis, seizures, loss of consciousness, and hypotension disproportionate to blood loss. Fetal distress is present at the same time. Coagulopathy resembling DIC with associated bleeding may be the only presenting symptom. Treatment includes tracheal intubation, mechanical ventilation with 100% oxygen, inotropic support, and correction of coagulopathy. Even with aggressive treatment, mortality from amniotic fluid embolism is greater than 80%.

C. Uterine Rupture may present with severe abdominal pain (often referred to the shoulder), maternal hypotension, and disappearance of fetal heart tones. Treatment is immediate laparotomy, delivery, and surgical repair of the uterus or hysterectomy.

D. Vaginal Birth after Cesarean Section. The risk of uterine rupture increases with the number of previous uterine incisions. Both the American College of Obstetricians and Gynecologists and the American Society of Anesthesiologists recommend that personnel, including the obstetrician, anesthetist, and operating room personnel, be immediately available at all times to perform an emergency cesarean delivery when VBAC is being attempted.

    1. Anesthetic Management. Epidural analgesia is an ideal technique for pain control in parturients attempting a VBAC. Approximately 60% to 80% of patients undergoing a trial for VBAC ultimately have a cesarean delivery, and epidural analgesia can be quickly converted to surgical anesthesia in these patients.

E. Abnormal Presentations and Multiple Births

    1. Breech Presentation. Breech vaginal deliveries result in increased maternal morbidity (cervical lacerations, perineal injury, retained placenta, shock caused by hemorrhage) and neonatal morbidity and mortality. Preferred delivery is by elective cesarean section. Dense perineal anesthesia is needed if vaginal instrumentation is anticipated and must be administered rapidly (3% 2-chloroprocaine epidurally or by the induction of general anesthesia).

    2. Multiple Gestations. All triplet and higher-order gestations are delivered by cesarean section. For twin gestations, presentation of the twins is considered when determining mode of delivery. If both are vertex, vaginal delivery is appropriate. If twin A is breech, cesarean delivery is recommended.

        a. Anesthetic Concerns include worsened functional residual capacity, worsened supine hypotension syndrome, and increased risk of postpartum hemorrhage.

IV. CO-EXISTING MEDICAL DISEASES

A. Heart Disease

    1. Circulatory Changes and Co-existing Heart Disease. Pregnancy and labor may lead to cardiovascular decompensation of an already diseased cardiovascular system because of pregnancy-induced and labor-induced increases in cardiac output. Relief of aortocaval obstruction at delivery may further increase cardiac output. Approximately 50% of patients with symptoms of heart disease during minimal activity or at rest in the non-pregnant state develop congestive heart failure during pregnancy. Epidural analgesia can minimize the adverse effects of increased cardiac output caused by pain or anxiety during labor and delivery. Invasive monitoring is usually not necessary in the absence of cardiac symptoms. Exceptions are parturients with pulmonary hypertension, right-to-left intracardiac shunts, or coarctation of the aorta. Hemodynamic changes during labor and delivery can persist into the postpartum period, and invasive cardiac monitoring should be continued for 48 hours after delivery in these patients.

2. Mitral Stenosis is associated with increased incidence of pulmonary edema, atrial fibrillation, and paroxysmal atrial tachycardia. Epidural analgesia minimizes the undesirable effects of pain on maternal heart rate and cardiac output. Perineal analgesia prevents the parturient's urge to push and eliminates the deleterious effects of the Valsalva maneuver on venous return. General or regional anesthesia can be used for cesarean section.

3. Mitral Regurgitation. These patients usually tolerate pregnancy well. Epidural analgesia is recommended for labor and vaginal delivery, as it decreases the peripheral vasoconstriction associated with pain and thus helps to maintain forward left ventricular stroke volume.

4. Aortic Regurgitation. These patients usually have an uneventful pregnancy, although congestive heart failure may develop in severe cases. As with mitral regurgitation, epidural analgesia is recommended for analgesia during labor and vaginal delivery. General anesthesia is acceptable when cesarean section is planned.

5. Aortic Stenosis. Asymptomatic parturients are not at increased risk during labor and delivery. These patients are vulnerable to decreased stroke volume and hypotension if systemic vascular resistance is abruptly decreased. If regional anesthesia is used, a gradual onset of analgesia/anesthesia with epidural anesthesia is preferred. General anesthesia is acceptable when cesarean section is planned.

6. Tetralogy of Fallot. Pregnancy increases the morbidity and mortality associated with tetralogy of Fallot. Regional anesthesia must be used with caution because of the hazards of decreased systemic blood pressure due to peripheral sympathetic nervous system blockade. General anesthesia is the preferred anesthetic technique for cesarean section. Invasive monitoring, including continuous measurement of arterial and cardiac filling pressures, is helpful.

7. Eisenmenger Syndrome consists of obliterative pulmonary vascular disease with resultant pulmonary hypertension, right-to-left intracardiac shunts, and arterial hypoxemia. If these anomalies are not well-compensated or completely corrected, then pregnancy is not well tolerated and maternal mortality approaches 30%.

   a. Anesthesia Concerns

      1.) Labor Analgesia. Events that decrease systemic vascular resistance (hypotension, vasodilation) and those that increase pulmonary vascular resistance (hypercarbia, increased arterial hypoxemia) are both detrimental. Infusion of air through the intravenous line tubing must be avoided because of the risk of paradoxical air embolism. If epidural analgesia is used, it is crucial that decreases in systemic vascular resistance be minimized. Epinephrine probably should not be added to local anesthetic solutions, but intrathecal opioid in early labor is useful.

2.) *Delivery by Cesarean Section* is most often accomplished under general anesthesia. Antibiotics are indicated for protection against infective endocarditis. Arm-to-brain circulation times are rapid because of right-to-left intracardiac shunts, and intravenous drugs therefore have a rapid onset of action. Nitrous oxide may increase pulmonary vascular resistance and should be avoided. Positive-pressure ventilation can decrease venous return. Invasive monitoring of arterial and cardiac filling pressures is indicated. The right ventricle is at greater risk of dysfunction than the left ventricle so monitoring of right atrial pressure is particularly useful.

8. Coarctation of the Aorta. During labor, acute left ventricular failure can occur. The increased heart rate and myocardial contractility that accompany labor may predispose to aortic dissection. General anesthesia is recommended for cesarean section. In all cases, invasive monitoring of arterial and cardiac filling pressures is helpful.

9. Primary Pulmonary Hypertension. Pain during labor and vaginal delivery may increase pulmonary vascular resistance and decrease venous return. Epidural analgesia is useful for preventing pain-induced increases in pulmonary vascular resistance. Diluting local anesthetic solutions with the addition of opioids will minimize the decrease in systemic vascular resistance. Spinal anesthesia is not recommended because of potentially sudden decreases in systemic vascular resistance. Supplemental oxygen and isoproterenol may help decrease pulmonary vascular resistance. Invasive hemodynamic monitoring is indicated. Maternal mortality is greater than 50%, usually because of heart failure during labor and the early postpartum period.

10. Cardiomyopathy of Pregnancy is left ventricular failure late in the course of pregnancy or during the first 6 weeks postpartum. The precise etiology remains unknown. Medical treatment of peripartum cardiomyopathy is similar to that for other dilated cardiomyopathies, except that angiotensin-converting enzyme inhibitors, which are routinely used for afterload reduction in nonpregnant patients, are contraindicated during pregnancy. Nitroglycerin or nitroprusside can be used for afterload reduction.

a. Anesthetic Management. Invasive hemodynamic monitoring is usually needed. Cardiac decompensation during labor can be treated with intravenous nitroglycerin or nitroprusside (preload, afterload reduction) and dopamine or dobutamine (inotropic support). Early epidural labor analgesia minimizes the cardiac stress associated with the pain of labor. If cesarean delivery is required, epidural or spinal anesthetic may be used with fluid management guided by the use of the invasive monitors. If general anesthesia is required, a high-dose opioid technique is often preferred; neonatal depression from the opioid is expected, and personnel for neonatal resuscitation must be available.

B. Diabetes Mellitus. Pregnancy is a state of progressive insulin resistance. Women who cannot produce enough insulin to compensate for this develop gestational diabetes. Patients with diabetes prior to pregnancy have increased insulin requirements in pregnancy. Diabetic ketoacidosis occurs at lower glucose levels in pregnancy.

1. Diagnosis. If the routine 1-hour glucose tolerance test is abnormal, a 3-hour glucose tolerance test is administered and, if abnormal, establishes the diagnosis of gestational diabetes (**Table 23-8**).

2. Treatment. Glycemic control (blood sugar 50 to 120 mg/dL) is the goal. Management of diabetic ketoacidosis is similar to that for nonpregnant patients. In patients with gestational diabetes, diet control is used initially. If glycemic control cannot be achieved, insulin therapy is initiated.

3. Antenatal Surveillance begins in the third trimester using twice-weekly nonstress tests, beginning at 28 weeks. A nonreactive nonstress test leads to a biophysical profile to determine timing and route of delivery. Elective induction of labor is commonly chosen to avoid neonatal risks associated with maternal diabetes.

4. Fetal Effects of Diabetes include a greater risk of fetal anomalies, intrauterine fetal death including stillbirth, macrosomia, greater incidence of cesarean delivery, shoulder dystocia, and birth trauma. Neonates are at risk for hypoglycemia and respiratory distress.

5. Anesthetic Management. Patients with autonomic dysfunction are especially prone to hypotension with epidural analgesia, and thus hypervigilance and rapid treatment are indicated. Epidural analgesia is preferred to CSE as the catheter should be known to be functioning to minimize the need for general anesthesia in the event of a cesarean section.

C. Myasthenia Gravis. Anticholinesterase drugs should be continued during pregnancy and labor. Epidural analgesia is acceptable for labor and vaginal

TABLE 23-8	White's Classification of Diabetes During Pregnancy
Class	**Definition**
A_1	Diet-controlled gestational DM
A_2	Gestational DM requiring insulin
B	Preexisting DM, without complications (duration <10 yr or age at onset >20 yr)
C	Preexisting DM without complications (duration 10–19 yr or age at onset 10–19 yr)
D	Preexisting DM (duration >20 yr or age at onset <10 yr)
F	Preexisting DM with nephropathy
R	Preexisting DM with retinopathy
T	Preexisting DM S/P renal transplant
H	Preexisting DM with heart disease

DM, diabetes mellitus; S/P, postoperative status.

delivery. Regional anesthesia can be used safely for cesarean section, but co-existing skeletal muscle weakness may lead to hypoventilation during anesthesia. Neonatal myasthenia gravis occurs transiently in 20% to 30% of babies born to mothers with myasthenia. Anticholinesterase therapy is usually necessary in neonates for approximately 21 days after birth.

D. Obesity is associated with increased risk of hypertensive disorders, including chronic hypertension and preeclampsia, gestational diabetes, thromboembolic disease, abnormal labor, cesarean delivery, dystocia, maternal death, infection, and anesthesia-associated airway difficulties. Perinatal risks include increased incidence of macrosomia, birth trauma, shoulder dystocia, meconium aspiration, neural tube defects, and other congenital abnormalities.

    1. Anesthetic Management. Epidural analgesia is a reasonable choice for labor analgesia and surgical anesthesia. The sitting, rather than the lateral, position may facilitate successful identification of the epidural space. Cesarean delivery is complicated by longer surgical duration and increased blood loss in obese patients. Regional anesthesia is preferred whenever possible for the obese parturient but may be associated with exaggerated spread of local anesthetic in the obese parturient (high spinal).

E. Advanced Maternal Age (>35 years) is independently associated with higher rates of maternal morbidities, including gestational diabetes, preeclampsia, placental abruption, and cesarean delivery. Advanced maternal age is also independently associated with an increased likelihood of cesarean delivery because of co-morbidities and an increased rate of requested cesarean delivery. Anesthesia considerations are directed toward management of co-morbidities.

F. Substance Abuse

    1. Alcohol Abuse. Fetal alcohol syndrome (neurobehavioral deficit, intrauterine growth retardation, congenital abnormalities) occurs in approximately one third of infants born to mothers who drink more than 3 ounces of alcohol per day during pregnancy. Anesthetic care of the pregnant alcohol abuser is the same as in the nonpregnant patient.

    2. Tobacco Abuse is strongly associated with low birth rate, abruptio placentae, impaired respiratory function in newborns, and sudden infant death syndrome. Anesthetic considerations for care of the tobacco-abusing parturient are similar to those considerations in the nonpregnant patient.

    3. Opioid Abuse. Complications include human immunodeficiency virus (HIV) infection, hepatitis, abscesses, endocarditis, and thrombophlebitis. A pregnant patient admitted on chronic opioid therapy should be maintained on that therapy during her pregnancy and into the postpartum period. Neonates should be observed and treated for withdrawal symptoms as necessary.

    4. Cocaine Abuse among parturients is associated with maternal cardiovascular, respiratory, neurologic, and hematologic complications similar to those seen in the nonpregnant patient. An increased incidence of significant obstetric complications (spontaneous abortion, stillbirth, preterm labor, abruptio placentae) occurs in parturients who abuse cocaine during pregnancy (**Table 23-9**). Fetal complications include decreased birth weight, intrauterine growth retardation, microcephaly, and prematurity.

422

TABLE 23-9	Obstetric Complications Associated with Cocaine Abuse During Pregnancy

Spontaneous abortion

Preterm labor

Premature rupture of membranes

Abruptio placentae

Precipitous delivery

Stillbirth

Maternal hypertension

Meconium aspiration

Low Apgar scores at birth

a. Anesthetic Considerations. Cocaine-induced thrombocytopenia must be excluded prior to regional anesthesia. Phenylephrine, because of its direct actions, is a better choice for treatment of hypotension than ephedrine. Body temperature increases and sympathomimetic effects associated with cocaine toxicity may mimic malignant hyperthermia.

V. FETAL ASSESSMENT/NEONATAL PROBLEMS

A. Evaluation of the Fetus

1. Fetal Heart Rate

a. Beat-to-Beat Variability. The fetal heart rate varies 5 to 20 bpm (normal heart rate is 120 to 160 bpm). Fetal distress caused by arterial hypoxemia, acidosis, or central nervous system damage is associated with minimal to absent beat-to-beat variability. Drugs most commonly associated with loss of beat-to-beat variability are benzodiazepines, opioids, barbiturates, anticholinergics, and local anesthetics used for continuous lumbar epidural analgesia.

b. Early Decelerations are characterized by the slowing of the fetal heart rate that begins with the onset of uterine contractions (**Fig. 23-2**), is maximum at the peak of the contraction, and returns to near baseline at its termination. This fetal heart rate pattern is not associated with fetal distress.

c. Late Decelerations are characterized by slowing of the fetal heart rate that begins 10 to 30 seconds after the onset of uterine contractions and maximizes after the peak intensity of the contractions (**Fig. 23-3**). Late decelerations are associated with fetal distress, most likely reflecting myocardial hypoxia secondary to uteroplacental insufficiency. Treatment involves left uterine displacement, intravenous fluids, and, if maternal hypotension is present, ephedrine administration.

d. Variable Decelerations are the most common pattern of fetal heart changes observed during the intrapartum period. They are variable in magnitude, duration, and time of onset relative to uterine contractions (**Fig. 23-4**). Severe variable deceleration patterns that persist for 15 to

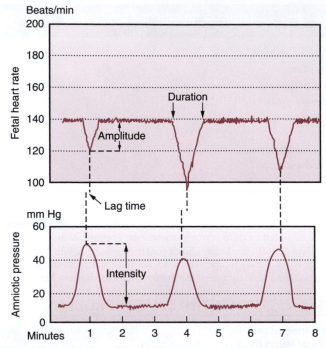

Figure 23-2 • Early decelerations of the fetal heart rate are characterized by a short lag time between the onset of uterine contractions and the beginning of fetal heart rate slowing. Maximum heart rate slowing is usually less than 20 bpm and occurs at the peak intensity of the contraction. Heart rate returns to normal by the time the contraction has ceased. The most likely explanation for this early deceleration is a vagal reflex response to compression of the fetal head. (Adapted from Shnider SM: Diagnosis of fetal distress: Fetal heart rate. In Shnider SM [ed]: Obstetrical Anesthesia: Current Concepts and Practice. Baltimore, Williams & Wilkins, 1970;197–203.)

30 minutes are associated with fetal acidosis. Variable decelerations are caused by umbilical cord compression, and delivery may become necessary if variable decelerations persist or worsen.

2. Fetal Scalp Sampling may be used to evaluate a fetus with an abnormal fetal heart rate tracing. Fetal hypoxia may be confirmed, establishing a need for urgent delivery. A pH of less than 7.20 suggests fetal compromise necessitating immediate delivery.

3. Fetal Pulse Oximetry provides continuous fetal arterial oxygen saturation readings when placed through the cervix to lie alongside the fetal cheek or temple. Normal fetal oxygen saturations range between 30% to 70%. Saturations less than 30% suggest fetal acidosis.

4. Ultrasound Examination of the fetus when the mother is in labor may be useful to determine the fetal presenting part, to confirm intrauterine fetal health or demise, and to diagnose placental abruption and placenta previa.

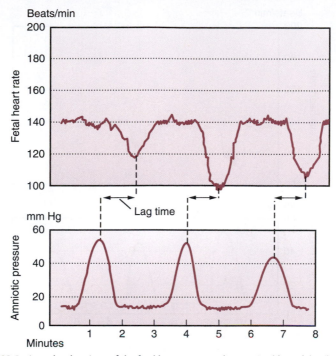

Figure 23-3 • Late decelerations of the fetal heart rate are characterized by a delay (lag time) between the onset of the uterine contraction and the beginning of fetal heart rate slowing. The fetal heart rate does not return to normal until after the contraction has ceased. A mild late deceleration pattern is present when slowing is less than 20 bpm; profound slowing is present when the fetal heart rate slows more than 40 bpm. Late fetal heart rate decelerations indicate fetal distress owing to uteroplacental insufficiency.(Adapted from Shnider SM: Diagnosis of fetal distress: Fetal heart rate. In Shnider SM [ed]: Obstetrical Anesthesia: Current Concepts and Practice. Baltimore, Williams & Wilkins, 1970;197–203.)

B. Evaluation of the Neonate

1. The Apgar Score assigns a numerical value to five vital signs measured or observed in neonates 1 minute and 5 minutes after delivery (**Table 23-10**). Apgar scores correlate well with acid-base measurements performed immediately after birth. When scores are higher than 7, neonates have either normal blood gases or mild respiratory acidosis. Infants with scores of 4 to 6 are moderately depressed; those with scores of 3 or lower have combined metabolic and respiratory acidosis. Mildly to moderately depressed infants (Apgar scores of 3 to 7) often improve in response to oxygen administered by face mask, with or without positive-pressure ventilation. Tracheal intubation and perhaps external cardiac massage are indicated when Apgar scores are less than 3.

2. Oxygenation and Ventilation. When oxygenation and ventilation are inadequate after delivery, a fetal circulation pattern persists (increased

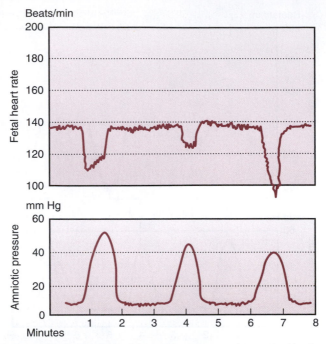

Figure 23–4 • Variable decelerations of the fetal heart rate are characterized by decreases in the heart rate of varying magnitude and duration that do not show a consistent relation to uterine contractions. This pattern of fetal heart rate slowing is associated with umbilical cord compression. (Adapted from Shnider SM: Diagnosis of fetal distress: Fetal heart rate. In Shnider SM [ed]: Obstetrical Anesthesia: Current Concepts and Practice. Baltimore, Williams & Wilkins, 1970:197–203.)

pulmonary vascular resistance and decreased pulmonary blood flow) and the ductus arteriosus and foramen ovale remain open, resulting in large right-to-left intracardiac shunts with associated arterial hypoxemia and acidosis.

3. Abnormalities Present at or Shortly after Delivery

a. Hypovolemia is likely in newborns with mean arterial pressures below 50 mm Hg at birth. Hypovolemia often follows intrauterine fetal distress, during which larger than normal portions of fetal blood are shunted to the placenta and remain there after delivery and clamping of the umbilical cord.

b. Hypoglycemia can manifest as hypotension, tremors, and seizures. Infants with intrauterine growth retardation and those born to diabetic mothers or after severe intrauterine fetal distress are vulnerable to hypoglycemia.

c. Meconium Aspiration. Meconium may be present in the major airways and is distributed to the lung periphery with the onset of spontaneous breathing. Obstruction of small airways causes ventilation-to-perfusion mismatching. In severe cases, pulmonary hypertension and right-to-left

TABLE 23-10	Evaluation of Neonates Using the Apgar Score		
Parameter	**0**	**1**	**2**
Heart rate (bpm)	Absent	<100	>100
Respiratory effort	Absent	Slow Irregular	Crying
Reflex irritability	No response	Grimace	Crying
Muscle tone	Limp	Flexion of extremities	Active
Color	Pale Cyanotic	Body pink Extremities cyanotic	Pink

shunting through the patent foramen ovale and ductus arteriosus (persistent fetal circulation) lead to severe arterial hypoxemia. Routine oropharyngeal suctioning is recommended at the time of delivery. Infants with low Apgar scores or who are clinically obstructed with meconium require active resuscitation, including tracheal intubation and attempts to remove meconium via suctioning.

d. Choanal Stenosis and Atresia. Nasal obstruction should be suspected in neonates who have good breathing efforts but become cyanotic when forced to breathe with their mouths closed. Unilateral or bilateral choanal stenosis is diagnosed based on the failure to pass a small catheter through each naris; such failure may reflect congenital (anatomic) obstruction or functional atresia caused by blood, mucus, or meconium. An oral airway may be necessary for anatomic obstruction until surgical correction can be accomplished. Functional choanal atresia is treated by nasal suctioning.

e. Diaphragmatic Hernia is characterized by severe respiratory distress at birth, associated with cyanosis and a scaphoid abdomen. Initial treatment is tracheal intubation and ventilation with oxygen.

f. Tracheoesophageal Fistula should be suspected when polyhydramnios is present (see **Chapter 24**). An initial diagnosis in the delivery room is suggested when a catheter is inserted into the esophagus but cannot be passed into the stomach. Copious amounts of oropharyngeal secretions are usually present. Chest radiographs with the catheter in place confirm the diagnosis.

g. Laryngeal Anomalies and Subglottic Stenosis are manifested at birth as stridor. Insertion of a tube into the trachea beyond the obstruction alleviates the symptoms.

CHAPTER 24

Pediatric Diseases

I. UNIQUE CONSIDERATIONS IN PEDIATRIC PATIENTS

A. Airway Anatomy. The large head and tongue, mobile epiglottis, and anterior position of the larynx characteristic of neonates makes tracheal intubation easier with the neonate's head at a neutral or slightly flexed position than with the neck hyperextended. The cricoid cartilage (as opposed to the vocal cords in adults) is the narrowest portion of the larynx and necessitates the use of tracheal tubes that minimize risks of trauma to the airway and subsequent development of subglottic edema.

B. Physiology

1. Respiratory System (Table 24-1). The single most important difference in pediatric patients is that oxygen consumption and alveolar ventilation is significantly higher (in neonates, about double that of adults per kilogram).

2. Cardiovascular System. Fetal circulation has high pulmonary vascular resistance, low systemic vascular resistance (placenta), and right-to-left shunting of blood through the foramen ovale and patent ductus arteriosus (PDA). At birth, pulmonary vascular resistance drops and pulmonary blood flow increases. The foramen ovale and PDA functionally close with increased left atrial pressure and increase arterial oxygen saturation, respectively. Neonates are highly dependent on heart rate to maintain cardiac output and systemic blood pressure.

3. Distribution of Body Water. Total body water content and extracellular fluid (ECF) volume are increased in neonates. The increased metabolic rate in neonates results in accelerated turnover of ECF and dictates meticulous attention to intraoperative fluid replacement (**Table 24-2**).

4. Renal Function. Glomerular filtration rate is greatly decreased in term neonates but increases nearly fourfold by 3 to 5 weeks.

5. Hematology. Fetal hemoglobin (FHb) has higher oxygen affinity than adult Hb, with decreased delivery of oxygen to tissues and compensatory increased Hb concentrations in neonates. At 4 to 6 months, the oxyhemoglobin dissociation curve approximates that of adults. Calculation of the estimated erythrocyte mass and the acceptable erythrocyte loss

TABLE 24-1 Mean Pulmonary Function Values

Parameter	Neonates (3 kg)	Adults (70 kg)
Oxygen consumption (mL/kg/min)	6.4	3.5
Alveolar ventilation (mL/kg/min)	130	60
Carbon dioxide production (mL/kg/min)	6	3
Tidal volume (mL/kg)	6	6
Breathing frequency (min)	35	15
Vital capacity (mL/kg)	35	70
Functional residual capacity (mL/kg)	30	35
Tracheal length (cm)	5.5	12
PaO_2 (room air, mm Hg)	65–85	85–95
$PaCO_2$ (room air, mm Hg)	30–36	36–44
pH	7.34–7.40	7.36–7.44

provides a useful guide for intraoperative blood replacement (**Table 24-3**). Routine preoperative hemoglobin determinations in children younger than 1 year of age rarely influences management of anesthesia or delays planned surgery.

6. Thermoregulation. Shivering contributes little to heat production in neonates, whose primary mechanism in heat production is nonshivering thermogenesis mediated by brown fat. "Neutral temperature" is defined as the ambient temperature that results in the least oxygen consumption. "Critical temperature" is the ambient temperature below which an unclothed, unanesthetized person cannot maintain a normal core body temperature (**Table 24-4**). Most operating rooms are below the critical temperature of a term neonate. Steps aimed at decreasing loss of body heat include transporting neonates in heated modules; increasing the ambient temperature of operating rooms; using a heating mattress, radiant warmer, and forced-air warming devices; and humidifying and warming inspired gases.

TABLE 24-2 Intraoperative Fluid Therapy for Pediatric Patients

	Normal Saline Or Lactated Ringer's Solution (mL/kg/hr)		
Procedure	Maintenance	Replacement	Total
Minor surgery (herniorrhaphy)	4	2	6
Moderate surgery (pyloromyotomy)	4	4	8
Extensive surgery (bowel resection)	4	6	10

TABLE 24-3	Estimation of Acceptable Blood Loss*	

A 3.2-kg term neonate is scheduled for intra-abdominal surgery. The preoperative hematocrit is 50%. What is the acceptable intraoperative blood loss to maintain the hematocrit at 40%?

Parameter	Calculation
Estimated blood volume	85 mL/kg × 3.2 kg = 272 mL
Estimated erythrocyte mass	272 mL × 0.5 = 136 mL
Estimated erythrocyte mass to maintain hematocrit at 40%	272 mL × 0.4 = 109 mL
Acceptable intraoperative erythrocyte loss	136 mL − 109 mL = 27 mL
Acceptable intraoperative blood loss to maintain hematocrit at 40%	27 × 2[†] = 54 mL

* These calculations are only guidelines and do not consider the potential impact of intravenous infusion of crystalloid or colloid solutions on the hematocrit.
[†] Factor to correct the original hematocrit to 50%.

7. Pharmacologic Responses

a. Anesthetic Requirements. Minimum alveolar concentration (MAC) is 25% less in neonates than in infants, and MAC in preterm infants is even lower. MAC increases until 2 to 3 months of age and steadily declines with age thereafter. The MAC of sevoflurane is unique and does not decline with advancing age in childhood. It remains constant at 2.5%.

b. Muscle Relaxants. The infant's diaphragm is paralyzed by muscle relaxants simultaneously with peripheral muscles (as opposed to later in adults). Initial doses, however, are similar on a weight basis to adult doses. Antagonism of neuromuscular blockade appears reliable in infants. Neonates and infants require more succinylcholine per kilogram than older children (probably because of increased ECF volumes and a larger volume of distribution of succinylcholine). Adverse side effects of succinylcholine (myoglobinuria, malignant hyperthermia [MH], hyperkalemia) limit the use of this drug in children (especially <age 5) to rapid securing of the airway and treatment of laryngospasm.

c. Pharmacokinetics. Uptake of inhaled anesthetics is more rapid in infants than older children or adults, and they are more sensitive to barbiturates and opioids. Neonates require higher doses of propofol than

TABLE 24-4	Neutral and Critical Temperatures	
Patient Age	Neutral Temperature (°C)	Critical Temperature (°C)
Preterm neonate	34	28
Term neonate	32	23
Adult	28	1

431

adults, and children from 5 to 15 years of age require higher doses of thiopental than do adults. Decreased hepatic and renal clearance of drugs in neonates leads to prolonged drug effects. Clearance rates increase to adult levels by 5 to 6 months of age.

d. Monitoring should include blood pressure cuff of appropriate size, temperature, and end-tidal CO_2 (because of high inspired gas flows, may be falsely low in neonates and infants). If arterial catheterization is considered, blood sampled from an artery distal to a ductus arteriosus (left radial artery, umbilical artery, posterior tibial artery) may not accurately reflect the PaO_2 delivered to the retina or brain in the presence of a PDA.

II. DISEASES OF NEONATES

Infants are "premature" if born before 37 weeks of gestation (**Table 24-5**).

A. Respiratory Distress Syndrome (RDS) or hyaline membrane disease is progressive impairment of gas exchange at the alveolar level because of deficient production and secretion of surfactant. Mature levels of surfactant are not present until 35 weeks of gestation.

1. Signs and Symptoms of RDS are usually apparent within minutes of birth (tachypnea, prominent grunting, intercostal and subcostal retractions, nasal flaring, duskiness). Apnea and irregular respirations are ominous signs.

2. Diagnosis is established by clinical course, chest radiograph (fine reticular granularity, air bronchograms) and blood gas analysis (progressive hypoxemia, hypercarbia, variable metabolic acidosis).

3. Treatment is supportive, using supplemental oxygen. Infants with severe RDS or those who develop persistent apnea or who cannot maintain an arterial oxygen tension greater than 50 mm Hg while breathing 70% to 100% oxygen require assisted mechanical ventilation. Acceptable ranges of blood gas values during mechanical ventilation are PaO_2 of 55 to 70 mm Hg, PCO_2 of 45 to 55 mm Hg, and pH of 7.25 to 7.45.

4. Prognosis. Usually gradual improvement occurs after several days, heralded by spontaneous diuresis and reduced oxygen requirements. Antenatal corticosteroid administration, postnatal surfactant use, improved modes of ventilation, and skilled supportive care have resulted in lower mortality from RDS.

TABLE 24-5 Classification of Prematurity	
Degree of Prematurity	**Gestational Age (wk)**
Borderline	36–37 wk
Moderate	31–36 wk
Severe	24–30 wk

5. Management of Anesthesia. An intra-arterial catheter is useful to assess oxygenation, avoid hyperoxia, and prevent respiratory and metabolic acidosis. Pneumothorax secondary to barotrauma should be considered if oxygenation deteriorates abruptly. Administration of albumin (1 g/kg intravenously) to premature neonates with RDS will likely increase the blood volume and glomerular filtration rate. Keeping the neonate's hematocrit near 40% optimizes tissue oxygen delivery. Excessive hydration may reopen the ductus arteriosus and should be avoided.

B. Bronchopulmonary Dysplasia (BPD) is a chronic disease of lung parenchyma and small airways that usually results from lung injury in premature infants requiring prolonged mechanical ventilation.

1. Signs and Symptoms are persistent respiratory distress characterized by increased airway reactivity and resistance, decreased pulmonary compliance, ventilation-to-perfusion mismatch, hypoxemia, hypercarbia, tachypnea, and, in severe cases, right heart failure.

2. Diagnosis. BPD is a clinical diagnosis defined as oxygen dependence at 36 weeks' postconceptual age with oxygen requirements (to maintain PaO_2 >50 mm Hg) beyond 28 days of life in infants with birth weights less than 1500 g.

3. Treatment. Maintenance of adequate oxygenation (with PaO_2 >55 mm Hg and SpO_2 >94%) is necessary to prevent cor pulmonale and to promote growth of lung tissue and remodeling of the pulmonary vascular bed. Reactive airway bronchoconstriction is treated with bronchodilators. Fluid restriction and diuretics may be needed to decrease pulmonary edema and improve gas exchange.

4. Prognosis. Pulmonary dysfunction is worst during the first year of life. Airway hyperreactivity may persist after symptoms subside.

5. Management of Anesthesia. Desaturation may be rapid during apnea. Subglottic stenosis, tracheomalacia, and bronchomalacia may be present. Increased risk of bronchospasm warrants establishing a deep level of anesthesia before instrumenting the airway. High airway pressures required during mechanical ventilation may cause pneumothorax. Fluid administration should be monitored and minimized to avoid pulmonary edema.

C. Intracranial Hemorrhage (ICH). Four types of ICH occur in neonates: subdural, primary subarachnoid, intercellular, and (the most common and significant) periventricular-intraventricular (intraventricular hemorrhage [IVH]). Incomplete autoregulation of cerebral blood flow and immaturity of neonatal cerebral capillary beds predispose vessels to rupture with abrupt or severe changes in blood flow. Newborn prematurity is the most important risk factor for ICH.

1. Signs and Symptoms range from subtle neurologic aberrations to catastrophic deterioration and rapid onset of coma.

2. Diagnosis of IVH can be made by maintaining a high index of suspicion in susceptible neonates, by clinical signs of encephalopathy, and by neuroimaging.

3. Treatment. Antenatal corticosteroids and prevention or delay of preterm delivery has reduced the incidence of ICH. Important measures in prevention of IVH are expanding intravascular volume slowly and maintaining blood pressure stability.

4. Prognosis. IVH occurs in 40% to 60% of neonates of less than 34 weeks gestation or very low birth weight ($\leq$1250 g). Hydrocephalus and death are more common in infants with the highest grades of hemorrhage.

5. Management of Anesthesia. Incomplete autoregulation of cerebral blood flow puts the premature neonate's normal blood pressure at the lower range of the auto regulatory limit. Blood pressures should be maintained within the normal range to decrease the risk of cerebral hyperperfusion. Hypotension, hypertensive spikes, and rapid volume expansion should be avoided.

D. Retinopathy of Prematurity (ROP), or retrolental fibroplasia, is a vasoproliferative retinopathy occurring almost exclusively in preterm infants. The risk is inversely related to birth weight and gestational age. Risk factors are not fully known but include hyperoxia, sepsis, congenital infections, congenital heart disease, mechanical ventilation, RDS, blood transfusions, IVH, hypoxia, hypercapnia and hypocapnia, asphyxia, and vitamin E deficiency.

1. Signs and Symptoms range from mild, transient changes to severe progressive extraretinal vasoproliferation (over the surface of the retina as well as into the vitreous humor), cicatrization, and subsequent retinal detachment (the primary cause of visual impairment and blindness in ROP).

2. Diagnosis. Ophthalmologic examination at 6 weeks of chronologic age or at 32 weeks' postconceptual age is recommended in infants weighing less than 1500 g at birth and those born before 28 weeks of gestation.

3. Treatment. Transscleral cryotherapy or laser photocoagulation destroys the peripheral avascular areas of the retina, resulting in slowing or reversing the abnormal growth of blood vessels and reducing risk of retinal detachment. Central vision is measured at the expense of some peripheral vision.

4. Prognosis. Approximately 80% to 90% of cases spontaneously regress with few effects or visual disability. Infants who develop ROP are at higher risk of developing ophthalmologic problems later in life (retinal tears, retinal detachment, myopia, strabismus, amblyopia, glaucoma).

5. Management of Anesthesia raises the dilemma of minimizing oxygen administration to a group of neonates susceptible to arterial hypoxemia. The use of supplemental oxygen at pulse oximetry saturations of 96% to 99% has not been shown to worsen preexisting ROP. Efforts should be made to maintain PaO_2 at 50 to 80 mm Hg, $PaCO_2$ at 35 to 45 mm Hg, and oxygen saturation at a pulse oximetry target of 89% to 94%. Infants undergoing peripheral retinal ablation have an increased incidence of apnea and bradycardia during the procedure and for up to 3 days afterward.

E. Apnea is defined as a cessation of breathing that is accompanied by cyanosis and bradycardia or that lasts longer than 20 seconds. Periodic breathing and apnea in preterm infants is usually caused by idiopathic apnea of prematurity but may also be a sign of other neonatal diseases. Idiopathic apnea of prematurity is a disorder of respiratory control and may be obstructive, central, or mixed.

1. Signs and Symptoms. In central apnea, there is complete cessation of airflow and respiratory efforts. In obstructive apnea, airflow is absent despite chest wall movements. The majority (50% to 75%) of apnea episodes in preterm neonates are of mixed etiology.

2. Diagnosis. Onset of idiopathic apnea typically occurs on the second to seventh days of life. Apnea must be differentiated from periodic breathing (regular breathing interrupted by short pauses lasting 5 to 10 seconds without cyanosis or changes in heart rate), which is a normal characteristic of neonatal respiration.

3. Treatment. Apnea monitors should be used on infants at risk of apnea.

a. Supplemental Oxygen improves CO_2 sensitivity, decreases hypoxic respiratory depression, decreases periodic breathing, and enhances diaphragmatic strength and activity. Obstructive or mixed apneas may be treated with high-flow nasal cannula therapy and nasal continuous positive airway pressure.

b. Theophylline (orally) or aminophylline (intravenously) is given as a loading dose of 5 mg/kg and maintenance regimen of 1 to 2 mg/kg every 6 to 8 hours. Caffeine can be given as a loading dose of 10 mg/kg and maintenance doses of 2.5 mg/kg per day orally.

c. Transfusions of packed red blood cells may be helpful in severely anemic infants.

4. Prognosis. Apnea of prematurity usually resolves by 36 weeks' postconceptual age. In the absence of significant life-threatening events, monitoring can often be discontinued at 44 to 45 weeks' postconceptual age.

5. Management of Anesthesia. Life-threatening apnea has occurred in former preterm infants following even minor surgeries. The risk is increased in infants with anemia (hematocrit <30) and after exposure to inhaled and injected anesthetics. Ex-premature infants should be admitted and monitored with pulse oximetry and apnea monitors for at least 12 hours after surgery. The risk of postoperative apnea appears to be significantly decreased after 50 to 52 weeks' gestational age. Elective surgery should be postponed if possible until that time.

F. Kernicterus. Jaundice is seen during the first week of life in up to 60% of term infants and 80% of premature infants. Kernicterus is a neurologic syndrome caused by the toxic effects of deposition of unconjugated bilirubin in the basal ganglia and brainstem nuclei.

1. Signs and Symptoms of kernicterus become apparent 2 to 5 days after birth in term infants and as late as day 7 in premature infants. Lethargy, poor feeding, and loss of the Moro reflex may progress to diminished tendon reflexes and respiratory distress, followed by hypotonia and hypertonia, opisthotonus, twitching of the face or limbs, and a shrill high-pitched cry. In advanced cases, convulsions and spasm occur. The classic sequelae of kernicterus is a tetrad of athetoid cerebral palsy, hearing loss, impairment of upward gaze, and enamel dysplasia of the primary teeth.

2. Diagnosis is made by a history of jaundice, characteristic neurologic symptoms, and confirmation of hyperbilirubinemia.

3. Treatment is phototherapy, exchange blood transfusions, and drugs that induce or enhance activity of the hepatic bilirubin conjugation system.

4. Prognosis. Neonates with overt neurologic signs have a grave prognosis (mortality >75%, choreoathetosis with involuntary muscle spasms in 80% of survivors). Mental retardation, deafness, and spastic quadriplegia are common sequelae.

5. Management of Anesthesia. Acidosis, hyperoxia, and hyperosmolarity should also be avoided or corrected. Normal saline diluents and flush solutions preserved with benzyl alcohol (a preservative implicated in causing kernicterus) should be avoided.

G. Hypoglycemia is the most common metabolic problem occurring in newborn infants. The risk is highest in small-for-gestational age infants. Causes include alterations in maternal metabolism, intrinsic neonatal problems, and endocrine or metabolic disorders (**Table 24-6**).

1. Signs and Symptoms are irritability, apnea, cyanotic spells, seizures, hypotonia, lethargy, and difficulty feeding. Many clinical manifestations are subtle or nonspecific, and a high index of suspicion is necessary.

2. Diagnosis. Signs of hypoglycemia occur when serum glucose concentrations are less than 20 mg/dL in premature infants, less than 30 mg/dL in term infants during the first 72 hours, and less than 40 mg/dL thereafter.

3. Treatment. Infants with symptoms other than seizures should receive an intravenous bolus of 2 mL/kg of 10% dextrose (4 mL/kg if seizures occur) followed by an infusion at 8 mg/kg per minute titrated to maintain the serum glucose at more than 40 mg/dL.

TABLE 24-6	Causes of Neonatal Hypoglycemia

Maternal Factors	Intrapartum administration of glucose
	Drug treatment
	  β-adrenergic blocking agents (terbutaline, ritodrine, propranolol)
	  Oral hypoglycemic agents
	  Salicylates
	Maternal diabetes/gestational diabetes

Neonatal Factors	Depleted glycogen stores
	  Asphyxia
	  Perinatal stress
	Increased glucose utilization (metabolic demands)
	  Sepsis
	  Polycythemia
	  Hypothermia
	  Respiratory distress syndrome
	  Congestive heart failure (cyanotic congenital heart disease)
	Limited glycogen stores
	  Intrauterine growth retardation
	  Prematurity
	Hyperinsulism/endocrine disorders
	  Infants of diabetic mothers
	  Erythroblastosis fetalis, fetal hydrops
	  Insulinomas
	  Beckwith-Wiedemann syndrome
	  Panhypopituitarism
	Decreased glycogenolysis, gluconeogenesis, or utilization of alternate fuels
	  Inborn errors of metabolism
	  Adrenal insufficiency

4. Prognosis is good in asymptomatic neonates with transient hypoglycemia. The prognosis is more guarded in symptomatic infants, particularly low-birth-weight infants, those with persistent hyperinsulinemic hypoglycemia, and infants of diabetic mothers.

5. Management of Anesthesia. Signs of hypoglycemia may be masked by anesthetic drugs, supporting the concept of intraoperative blood glucose monitoring and supplemental glucose administration (e.g., 5% dextrose and 0.2 normal saline at 4 mL/kg per hour). Serum glucose concentrations of 125 mg/dL can cause osmotic diuresis, subsequent dehydration, and further release of insulin with rebound hypoglycemia.

H. Hypocalcemia. Infants with intrauterine growth retardation, infants of insulin-dependent diabetics, and infants with birth asphyxia during prolonged, difficult deliveries are at risk. Late neonatal hypocalcemia occurring 5 to 10 days after birth is usually caused by ingestion of cow's milk, which contains high levels of phosphorus. Other notable causes of hypocalcemia in the newborn include maternal hypercalcemia and DiGeorge syndrome.

1. Signs and Symptoms are irritability, seizures, increased skeletal muscle tone, twitching, tremors, and hypotension. Additional nonspecific symptoms of neonatal hypocalcemia such as poor feeding, vomiting, and lethargy often prompt investigation for sepsis, intracranial hemorrhages, and meningitis.

2. Diagnosis. Hypocalcemia is serum calcium concentration less than 8 mg/dL in term neonates and less than 7 mg/dL in preterm neonates, or serum ionized calcium concentration less than 4.4 mg/dL (or 1.1 mmol/L). Hypoalbuminemia may falsely suggest hypocalcemia because the total serum calcium is low even though the ionized calcium concentration remains normal. The ionized calcium concentration, rather than the total calcium, is low in true hypocalcemia.

3. Treatment is administration of calcium. Calcium gluconate 10% is given as 100 to 200 mg/kg (1 to 2 mL/kg) repeated every 6 to 8 hours until the calcium level stabilizes. Cardiac monitoring is mandatory, and atropine should be available to treat possible bradycardia. Other potential complications of treatment include soft-tissue necrosis caused by extravasation of drug, precipitation in intravenous tubing and small veins when administered concomitantly with bicarbonate, and digitalis toxicity in patients on digoxin.

4. Prognosis. Early neonatal hypocalcemia usually resolves within a few days without treatment in asymptomatic newborns. Serum calcium levels typically normalize within 1 to 3 days with treatment in symptomatic early neonatal hypocalcemia.

5. Management of Anesthesia. Hypocalcemia should be corrected preoperatively. Events that precipitate hypocalcemia (alkalosis, sodium bicarbonate administration, or rapid infusion of albumin and citrated blood products) should be avoided.

I. Sepsis. Premature or low-birth-weight infants have a 3- to 10-fold higher incidence of sepsis than full-term, normal-birth-weight infants. Most nosocomial infections are bloodstream infections related to intravascular catheters.

1. Signs and Symptoms (Table 24-7)

2. Diagnosis. Fever and leukocytosis may be absent. Positive blood cultures help confirm the diagnosis. When clinical findings suggest an acute infection

TABLE 24-7	Signs and Symptoms of Infection in Neonates

Fever

Temperature instability

Hypoglycemia

Feeding intolerance

Apnea

Respiratory distress

Cyanosis

Tachycardia

Hypotension

Bradycardia

Poor perfusion with pallor and mottled skin

Metabolic acidosis

Lethargy

Seizures

in the absence of a clear etiology, additional studies including lumbar puncture, urine studies, and a chest radiograph are indicated.

3. Treatment.

a. Antibiotic Therapy should be instituted immediately. Initial empirical treatment of bacterial infections in neonates should consist of ampicillin and gentamicin (or another aminoglycoside).

b. Supportive Care includes ventilatory support, fluid resuscitation, and inotropic agents. Hyperbilirubinemia should be treated aggressively; the risk of kernicterus increases in the presence of sepsis.

4. Prognosis. Mortality approaches 50%. Complications include respiratory failure, pulmonary hypertension, endocarditis, cardiac failure, shock, renal failure, liver dysfunction, cerebral edema or thrombosis, adrenal hemorrhage and/or insufficiency, bone marrow dysfunction (neutropenia, thrombocytopenia, anemia), meningitis, and disseminated intravascular coagulation (DIC). Fatality rates are highest for patients with gram-negative and fungal infections.

5. Management of Anesthesia. Supportive therapy initiated prior to arrival in the operating room should be continued intraoperatively. Fluid, electrolyte, and glucose levels should be monitored and deficits corrected. Arterial cannulation and central vascular access may be necessary to obtain accurate blood pressure measurements and facilitate aggressive fluid resuscitation. Corticosteroids should be administered only for adrenal insufficiency that is proven or suggested by profound hypotension refractory to both volume expansion and inotropic therapy.

J. Neonatal Surgical Diseases

1. Congenital Diaphragmatic Hernia is usually associated with pulmonary hypoplasia caused by in utero compression of the developing lungs by the herniated viscera.

a. Signs and Symptoms are scaphoid abdomen, barrel-shaped chest, detection of bowel sounds in the chest, and profound arterial hypoxemia. Chest radiographs show loops of intestine in the thorax and mediastinal shift to the opposite side. Arterial hypoxemia is caused by right-to-left shunting through a PDA resulting from persistent fetal circulation. There is a high incidence of congenital heart disease and intestinal malrotation.

b. Diagnosis. The diagnosis is now commonly made prenatally because of routine ultrasonography. Prenatal findings that correlate with poor prognosis are polyhydramnios, displacement of the stomach above the diaphragm, and diagnosis made prior to 20 weeks of gestation.

c. Treatment. Immediate treatment includes decompression of the stomach with an orogastric or nasogastric tube and administration of supplemental oxygen. Positive-pressure mask ventilation should be avoided (gas inflation of the stomach further compromises pulmonary function). Positive airway pressures should not exceed 25 to 30 cm H_2O (excessive airway pressures can damage the neonate's normal lung). Sedation, skeletal muscle paralysis, mechanical ventilation of the lungs, or extracorporeal membrane oxygenation (ECMO) prior to surgery may decrease the mortality rate among unstable patients. Permissive hypercapnia (PCO_2 <60 mm Hg) with gentle ventilation to minimize airway inflation pressures and barotrauma is associated with improved survival. Inhaled nitric oxide does not improve survival with the pulmonary hypertension associated with congenital diaphragmatic hernia.

d. Prognosis. Survival ranges from 42% to 75% and is related to the degree of pulmonary hypoplasia and associated anomalies.

e. Management of Anesthesia begins with awake tracheal intubation after preoxygenation. Preductal arterial cannulation is useful or, if the neonate already has an umbilical arterial line, a pulse oximeter is applied to the right hand. Venous access should be avoided in the lower extremities (venous return may be limited because of compression of the inferior vena cava following reduction of the hernia). Nitrous oxide should be avoided (bowel distension compromises pulmonary function). Airway pressures should be maintained at less than 25 to 30 cm H_2O to minimize the risk of pneumothorax. A sudden decrease in lung compliance or deterioration in oxygenation or blood pressure suggests a pneumothorax. Hypothermia must be avoided (increased pulmonary vascular resistance with right-to-left shunting). After reduction of the hernia, inflation of the hypoplastic lung is not recommended. It is unlikely to expand, and contralateral lung damage may result.

f. Postoperative Course may include rapid improvement, followed by sudden deterioration with arterial hypoxemia, hypercapnia, and acidosis (because of reappearance of fetal circulatory patterns and right-to-left shunting through the foramen ovale and PDA) and, possibly, death. Sedation is necessary (stressful stimulus can further elevate pulmonary pressures, increasing shunt).

2. Esophageal Atresia (EA) and Tracheoesophageal Fistula (TEF). More than 90% of affected individuals with EA also have a TEF. The most common form of EA is a blind upper esophageal pouch plus a distal esophagus that forms a TEF (**Fig. 24-1**). Approximately 50% of infants with EA have other

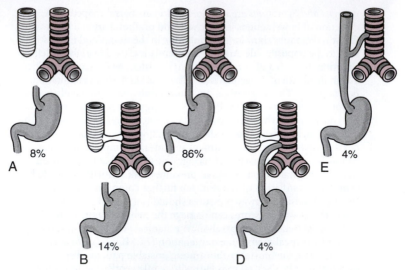

Figure 24-1 • Types of esophageal atresia (EA). *A*, Pure EA; *B*, proximal fistula; *C*, EA, distal fistula; *D*, proximal and distal fistula; *E*, pure tracheoesophageal fistula. (Adapted from Ravitch MM, et al. [eds]: Pediatric Surgery, Volume 1, 3rd ed. Chicago, Year Book Medical Publishers, 1979; and Smith BM, Matthes-Kofidis C, Golianu B, Hammer GB: Pediatric general surgery. In Jaffe RA, Samuels SI [eds]: Anesthesiologists Manual of Surgical Procedures, 3rd ed. Philadelphia, Lippincott Williams & Wilkins, 2004, p 1019.)

anomalies, most often VATER (*v*ertebral defects, imperforate *a*nus, *t*racheo*e*sophageal fistula, *r*enal dysplasia)/VACTERL (VATER plus cardiac and limb anomalies). Survival of neonates with EA and no associated defects approaches 100%.

a. Signs and Symptoms. The neonate with EA presents with respiratory distress (coughing, cyanosis, and frothing at the mouth and nose). Feeding exacerbates these symptoms and causes regurgitation.

b. Diagnosis. Prenatally, EA is suspected if maternal polyhydramnios is present. EA is usually diagnosed after birth when an oral catheter cannot be passed into the stomach or when the neonate exhibits cyanosis, coughing, and choking during oral feedings. Pure EA may present as an airless, scaphoid abdomen.

c. Treatment includes maintaining a patent airway, preventing aspiration, cessation of feedings, and placement in a head-up position to minimize regurgitation. Endotracheal intubation is avoided, if possible, because of the potential to worsen distension of the stomach. One-lung ventilation may be necessary if life-threatening gastric distension occurs. Surgical repair of a TEF is urgent. However, some neonates will require a staged surgical approach with an initial gastrostomy and later definitive repair.

d. Prognosis. Tracheal collapse after extubation and esophageal stricture are not uncommon. Chronic gastroesophageal reflux and dysphagia can predispose children to recurrent aspiration pneumonitis. Early deaths are caused by cardiac or chromosomal abnormalities, and later deaths are usually the result of respiratory complications.

e. Management of Anesthesia. Ideally, awake intubation with spontaneous ventilation allows the appropriate positioning of the endotracheal tube while minimizing the risk of ventilatory impairment from gastric distension caused by positive-pressure ventilation. But awake intubation may be difficult and traumatic in a vigorous infant. Inhalation induction allows spontaneous ventilation. If intravenous induction is chosen, PIP must be minimized during ventilation to avoid inflation of the stomach. Proper placement of the tracheal tube is critical (above the carina but below the TEF). A peripheral arterial catheter permits continuous monitoring of systemic blood pressure and measurement of arterial blood gases. Intraoperative insensible and third-space fluid losses should be replaced with crystalloid (6–8 mL/kg/hr). Blood loss may be replaced with 5% albumin and blood to maintain a hematocrit above 35%. Lung retraction may impair ventilation, surgical manipulation of the trachea may cause airway obstruction, and blood and secretions can obstruct the endotracheal tube, requiring frequent suctioning or even replacement of the tube. Extubation of term infants at the end of surgery is preferable, although continued intubation and ventilation are necessary if cardiac or pulmonary complications arise intraoperatively or if the adequacy of ventilation is in question. Excessive neck extension and reintubation can compromise the new anastomosis.

3. Abdominal Wall Defects: Omphalocele and Gastroschisis. Omphalocele is external herniation of abdominal viscera through the base of the umbilical cord. Gastroschisis is external herniation of abdominal viscera through a small (usually <5 cm) defect in the anterior abdominal wall (**Table 24-8**).

TABLE 24-8 Comparison of Omphalocele and Gastroschisis

	Omphalocele	Gastroschisis
Etiology	Failure of midgut migration from yolk sac into abdomen	Abnormal development of right omphalomesenteric artery or umbilical vein with ischemia to right paraumbilical area
Location	Within umbilical cord	Periumbilical (usually to right of cord)
Covering	Membranous sac	None (exposed viscera)
Associated conditions	Beckwith-Wiedemann syndrome Congenital heart disease Trisomies 13, 18, 21 Malrotation of gastrointestinal tract Pentalogy of Cantrell Exstrophy of bladder	Malrotation of gastrointestinal tract, prematurity Intestinal atresia

Adapted from Roberts JD Jr, Cronin JH, Todres ID: Neonatal emergencies. In Cote CJ, Todres ID, Goudsouzian NG, Ryan JF (eds): A Practice of Anesthesia for Infants and Children, 3rd ed. Philadelphia, Saunders, 2001, p 309.

a. Diagnosis. Omphalocele and gastroschisis can be diagnosed prenatally by fetal ultrasonography.

b. Treatment. Gastroschisis requires urgent repair. Placing the infant's lower body and exposed intestine immediately after delivery into a plastic drawstring bowel bag reduces evaporative fluid and heat loss from the large surface area of exposed bowel. While omphalocele also requires urgent corrective surgery, the association of cardiac anomalies warrants preoperative cardiology evaluation and echocardiography. If inspiratory pressures are greater than 25 to 30 cm H_2O or intravesical or intragastric pressures are greater than 20 cm H_2O, primary closure is not recommended. The viscera should be covered with a prosthetic silo and the abdominal viscera allowed to slowly reduce over a period of several days to 1 week.

c. Prognosis. The survival rate for gastroschisis is 90% or more. Survival rates for omphalocele range from 70% to 95%. Mortality is related to associated cardiac and chromosomal abnormalities.

d. Preoperative Management. The primary concerns are prevention of infections and minimization of fluid and heat loss from exposed abdominal viscera. The stomach should be decompressed with an orogastric tube to decrease the risk of aspiration. Fluid requirements are 2 to 4 times daily maintenance requirements ($\geq$8 to 16 mL/kg per hour). To maintain normal oncotic pressures, protein-containing solutions (5% albumin) should constitute 25% of the replacement fluids.

e. Management of Anesthesia. Important concerns are preservation of body temperature and fluid replacement. Primary closure may require the ability to ventilate the patient with high PIPs into the postoperative period. Repair of a large defect will require maximal relaxation intraoperatively and during the initial postoperative period. Nitrous oxide is avoided because of bowel distension. Tight surgical abdominal closure can result in compression of the inferior vena cava and decreased diaphragmatic excursion, resulting in impaired abdominal organ perfusion and decreased pulmonary compliance. Evidence of unacceptable intra-abdominal pressure requires removal of fascial sutures and closure of only the skin or addition of a prosthesis. Intensive intraoperative and postoperative monitoring is recommended. Direct monitoring of arterial blood gases and pH is helpful for guiding fluid therapy. Intraoperative fluid requirements of at least 25% of estimated blood volume are expected during surgical repair of large abdominal defects. Mechanical ventilation may be needed for 24 to 48 hours postoperatively.

4. Hirschsprung's Disease (congenital aganglionic megacolon) is the most common cause of lower intestinal obstruction in full-term neonates, characterized by the absence of parasympathetic ganglion cells in the large bowel.

a. Signs and Symptoms include constipation, dilation of the proximal bowel, and abdominal distension. Progressive bowel distension causes increasing intraluminal pressure, decreased blood flow, and deterioration of the mucosal barrier. Persistent intestinal stasis promotes bacterial proliferation, leading to enterocolitis (abdominal distension, fever, explosive diarrhea).

b. Diagnosis. Hirschsprung's is suspected in any full-term neonate with delayed passage of stool. A classic radiographic finding following a contrast enema is the presence of a transition zone between normal dilated proximal colon and a narrow, spastic distal colon segment caused by nonrelaxation of the aganglionic bowel. Rectal biopsy is the diagnostic gold standard, confirming the absence of ganglion cells and the presence of hypertrophied nerve bundles that stain positively for acetylcholinesterase.

c. Treatment is surgical, bringing ganglionated bowel down to the anus.

d. Prognosis. Most patients attain fecal continence. Patients with retained or acquired aganglionosis, severe strictures, dysfunctional bowel, and intestinal neuronal dysplasia may require reoperation.

e. Management of Anesthesia. Intraoperative blood loss is usually mild, but third-space fluid losses can be significant. Patients may require an initial bolus of 10 to 20 mL/kg IV of crystalloid to offset the volume deficit resulting from bowel preparation and fasting. Epidural anesthesia provides intraoperative and postoperative analgesia in patients undergoing open abdominal procedures. Extubation at the end of surgery is routine.

5. Anorectal Malformations include a spectrum of defects, most of which involve a fistula between the lower intestinal tract and genitourinary structures. Imperforate anus without fistula occurs in a small number of patients, especially in association with Down syndrome. Spinal and vertebral anomalies occur in up to 50% of patients with anorectal malformations. Cardiovascular anomalies (atrial septal defect, PDA, tetralogy of Fallot, ventricular septal defect [VSD]) are present in one third of patients with imperforate anus.

a. Signs and Symptoms. Inspection of the perineum reveals an anorectal malformation. The neonate may fail to pass meconium in the first 24 to 48 hours of life.

b. Diagnosis. Meconium seen on the neonate's perineum is evidence of a rectoperineal fistula. Meconium in the urine indicates a rectourinary fistula. Rectovaginal fistula in females and rectourethral fistula in males are the most common presentations.

c. Treatment. Preliminary treatment for high lesions is a diverting colostomy followed later by a definitive procedure. Low lesions (perineal fistulas) may be repaired during the neonatal period without a protective colostomy.

d. Prognosis. The greater the degree of sacral malformation, the greater the likelihood of fecal and urinary incontinence. Most patients with perineal fistula and rectal atresia are expected to be fully continent following repair.

e. Management of Anesthesia. Electrical muscle stimulation is used during the procedure to identify muscle structures and to define the anterior and posterior limits of the new anus. Blood loss and third-space fluid losses are usually moderate. Intravenous catheters should be placed in upper extremities because surgical positioning of the legs may impede venous flow or limit access to the intravenous site. Patients are usually extubated at the end of surgery.

6. Pyloric Stenosis is a common cause of gastric outlet obstruction in infants. Idiopathic hypertrophy of the circular muscle of the pylorus results in compression and narrowing of the pyloric channel.

a. Signs and Symptoms are nonbilious projectile vomiting at 2 to 5 weeks of age. Jaundice may occur in some infants, possibly because of hepatic glucuronyl transferase deficiency associated with starvation. The most common metabolic presentation is hypokalemic, hypochloremic primary metabolic alkalosis with secondary respiratory acidosis.

b. Diagnosis. An olive-like mass can usually be palpated in the epigastrium. After feeding, a gastric peristaltic wave may be seen progressing across the abdomen from left to right. Confirmation of the diagnosis is by abdominal ultrasonography.

c. Treatment is pyloromyotomy (either open or laparoscopic). Severely dehydrated infants require fluid resuscitation prior to surgery, which should be guided by measurement of serum electrolyte concentrations (essential for estimating the degree of dehydration, alkalosis, and metabolic derangements). Feedings can usually be initiated within 4 to 6 hours following surgery.

d. Management of Anesthesia. Pulmonary aspiration of gastric fluid is a definite risk in infants with gastric outlet obstruction. The stomach should be emptied with a large-bore orogastric catheter after premedication with atropine and before induction of anesthesia. Awake tracheal intubation is indicated if a difficult intubation is anticipated. Otherwise, rapid-sequence induction is recommended. Skeletal muscle relaxation is usually not needed. Infiltration of the incision sites with local anesthetics usually provides sufficient postoperative analgesia. Postoperative depression of ventilation of unknown cause often occurs and apnea monitoring for 12 hours after surgery is indicated. Hypoglycemia may occur 2 to 3 hours after surgical correction of pyloric stenosis, most likely because of inadequate liver glycogen stores and cessation of intravenous dextrose infusions.

7. Necrotizing Enterocolitis (NEC), characterized by various degrees of mucosal or transmural necrosis of the intestine, is the most common neonatal surgical emergency, and is associated with substantial perinatal morbidity and mortality. Although the greatest risk factor for NEC is prematurity, other risk factors include perinatal asphyxia, systemic infections, umbilical artery catheterization, exchange blood transfusions, hypotension, RDS, patent ductus arteriosus, cyanotic congenital heart disease, and aggressive hyperosmolar formula feeding.

a. Signs and Symptoms include recurrent apnea, lethargy, temperature instability, glucose instability, and shock. More specific signs of NEC are abdominal distension, high gastric residuals after feeding, and bloody or mucoid diarrhea. Metabolic acidosis, neutropenia, and thrombocytopenia are common.

b. Diagnosis is by clinical correlation with plain abdominal x-ray findings. Pneumatosis intestinalis, air in the intestinal wall, is diagnostic of NEC in newborns.

c. Treatment. Medical treatment (cessation of feeding, gastric decompression, intravenous fluids, antibiotics) is often successful. Mechanical ventilation, fluid resuscitation, transfusion, and inotropic support may be indicated. Surgery is reserved for neonates in whom medical management fails (50% of infants with NEC).

d. Prognosis is worse in the presence of pnuematosis intestinalis (20% fail medical management, 25% die). Short bowel syndrome, central venous catheter complications, and cholestatic jaundice may follow surgery.

e. Management of Anesthesia includes fluid resuscitation and transfusion if needed. Arterial pressure and blood gas monitoring is helpful. Rapid fluid administration in preterm infants may cause intracranial hemorrhage or reopening of the ductus arteriosus. Full stomach precautions are needed. High intra-abdominal pressures and decreased pulmonary compliance are likely during surgery. Inotropes may be required to maintain adequate cardiac output and bowel perfusion. Fluids and the operating room should be appropriately warmed to maintain normothermi. Postoperative mechanical ventilation is usually required because of abdominal distension and co-existing RDS.

8. Congenital Hyperinsulinism (persistent hyperinsulinemic hypoglycemia of infancy) is characterized by inappropriately elevated plasma insulin levels in relation to blood glucose levels.

a. Signs and Symptoms. Some hyperinsulinemic newborns may be macrosomic due to anabolic effects of insulin in utero and experience hypoglycemia within hours or days of birth. Infants with lesser degrees of hyperinsulinemia may not manifest symptoms until later, when the frequency of feedings is decreased to allow the infant to sleep through the night and hyperinsulinemia prevents glucose mobilization.

b. Diagnosis is based on evidence of excess insulin activity during a state of hypoglycemia. The diagnostic criteria include (1) serum insulin level above 10 μU/mL when blood glucose concentration is less than 50 mg/dL, (2) inappropriate suppression of lipolysis and ketogenesis, (3) requirement of a glucose infusion rate higher than 10 mg/kg per minute to maintain a blood glucose concentration of more than 35 mg/dL, and (4) a positive glycemic response to glucagon despite hypoglycemia.

c. Treatment. Prevention of hypoglycemia and its effects on central nervous system development is imperative in the neonatal period. Blood glucose levels less than 50 mg/dL should be vigorously treated. Pancreatectomy is performed in an attempt to prevent recurrent episodes of neuroglycopenia and long-term neurologic sequelae.

d. Prognosis. Results of pancreatectomy are unpredictable and hypoglycemia may persist postoperatively, especially following subtotal resection.

e. Management of Anesthesia. Supplemental glucose should be continued intraoperatively. Hyperglycemic response to surgery may reduce glucose requirements intraoperatively. An arterial catheter will facilitate frequent monitoring of blood gases and serum glucose. Blood glucose concentrations must be monitored closely postoperatively, as near-total pancreatectomy may result in hyperglycemia requiring insulin, whereas subtotal pancreatectomy may result in persistent hypoglycemia.

9. Congenital Lobar Emphysema is a rare cause of respiratory distress in neonates that results from localized bronchial obstruction, air trapping, and lobar overexpansion. Acquired lobar emphysema may result from barotrauma associated with the treatment of bronchopulmonary dysplasia. There is an increased incidence of congenital heart disease (VSD, PDA).

> *a. Signs and Symptoms* range from mild tachypnea and wheezing to severe dyspnea and cyanosis.
>
> *b. Diagnosis* is made by chest radiography, computed tomography (CT), and ventilation/perfusion scan.
>
> *c. Treatment* is resection of the diseased lobe. Some infants with only very mild symptoms and without evidence of progression may not require surgery.
>
> *d. Prognosis.* Long-term pulmonary growth and function are excellent following lobectomy.
>
> *e. Management of Anesthesia.* Infants are at greatest risk during induction of anesthesia, as positive-pressure ventilation of the lungs before the chest is opened may cause abrupt, exaggerated expansion of emphysematous lobes with sudden mediastinal shift and cardiac arrest. Tracheal intubation without muscle relaxants and maintenance of spontaneous breathing with minimal positive airway pressures is recommended. An arterial catheter allows serial blood gas monitoring and earlier detection of hemodynamic changes. Nitrous oxide should not be used, as its diffusion into the diseased lobes can cause further distension. Severely decompensated infants may require emergency needle aspiration or thoracotomy for decompression of the affected lobe or lobes.

K. Nervous System.

1. Cerebral Palsy (CP) is a symptom complex rather than a specific disease, comprising a group of nonprogressive motor impairment syndromes secondary to lesions or anomalies of the brain that arise during the early stages of development. CP is classified according to the extremity involved (monoplegia, hemiplegia, diplegia, quadriplegia) and the characteristics of the neurologic dysfunction (spastic, hypotonic, dystonic, athetotic). There is a high frequency of epilepsy and cognitive disorders associated with CP. The cause of most cases is unknown.

> *a. Signs and Symptoms.* The most common manifestation is skeletal muscle spasticity. Extrapyramidal CP is associated with choreoathetosis and atonic CP is characterized by dystonia and cerebellar ataxia. Varying degrees of mental retardation and speech defects may accompany CP.
>
> *b. Treatment.*
>
> > *1.) Surgical Treatment.* These children often undergo elective orthopedic corrective procedures (Achilles tendon lengthening, hip adductor and iliopsoas release, derotational osteotomy of the femur, correction of scoliosis); stereotactic surgery to decrease skeletal muscle rigidity, spasticity, and dyskinesia; and dental restorations requiring general anesthesia and antireflux operations due to increased incidence of reflux disease.
> >
> > *2.) Medications.* Medications to relieve muscle spasm include dantrolene, botulinum neurotoxin (Botox) injections, and baclofen. Baclofen should not be discontinued abruptly in the perioperative period because of potential withdrawal symptoms (seizures, hallucinations, delirium, pruritus), which may persist up to 72 hours. Valproic acid is associated with hepatotoxicity, bone marrow suppression, and platelet dysfunction.

c. Management of Anesthesia tracheal intubation is recommended (risk of aspiration due to reflux). Succinylcholine does not produce abnormal potassium release. Children on anticonvulsants may be resistant to nondepolarizing muscle relaxants because of hepatic enzyme induction. Emergence from anesthesia may be slow. Tracheal extubation should be delayed until these children are fully awake and body temperature is near normal.

2. Hydrocephalus is a congenital or acquired increase in CSF resulting in enlarged cerebral ventricles. Hydrocephalus can be caused by obstruction to the flow of CSF (e.g., tumor), as well as overproduction or decreased absorption of CSF. Patients with hydrocephalus usually present with an increase in intracranial pressure (ICP).

a. Signs and Symptoms depend on the age of the child and the presence of increased ICP. Congenital hydrocephalus presents at birth or soon thereafter with an enlarged head, separation of cranial sutures, inferiorly deviated eyes ("sunsetting eyes"), dilated scalp veins, and thin shiny skin. Normal pressure hydrocephalus is triad of abnormal gait, dementia, and urinary incontinence.

b. Diagnosis Serial head circumference measurements, skull radiographs, and CT confirm the diagnosis.

c. Treatment depends on the cause of the hydrocephalus. When surgical excision of obstructive lesions is not feasible or is unsuccessful, a shunting procedure (ventriculoperitoneal, ventriculoatrial, ventriculopleural) is necessary. The most common of these is the ventriculoperitoneal (VP) shunt. VP shunts often require revisions or replacement because of infections involving the shunt or shunt malfunction (80% at the proximal end of the shunt). Patients presenting with increased ICP secondary to shunt malfunction may have their ICP lowered acutely by tapping the proximal reservoir.

d. Management of Anesthesia

  1.) *Preoperative.* Delayed gastric emptying and vomiting are indications for a rapid-sequence induction technique.

  2.) *Intraoperative.* Arterial catheterization is reserved for the patient with uncontrolled ICP and hemodynamic instability. The child with increased ICP and/or delayed gastric emptying should have intravenous rapid sequence induction. Atropine premedication is recommended in infants because of the immaturity of the sympathetic autonomic system. Laryngoscopy may cause significant increases in ICP, and the benefit of lidocaine administration prior to laryngoscopy in preventing such increases has not been demonstrated in infants and small children. Sudden cardiac arrest in infants receiving 1.0 to 1.5 mg/kg IV lidocaine at time of induction has been reported. Mild hypocapnia (32 to 35 mm Hg) may prevent further elevation of the ICP. Normocapnia should be maintained in patients with normal ICP. Intraoperative spontaneous ventilation is not recommended because of the risk of air embolism and (in ventriculopleural shunts) the risk of pneumothorax. Nitrous oxide is not recommended because it increases cerebral blood flow and volume (raises ICP), and it is associated with nausea and emesis that may confuse evaluation of the patient postoperatively. Ventricular shunt procedures usually do not result in significant blood or third-space losses. Hypothermia can occur because of the large body surface areas exposed during surgical prep. Patients should be awake prior to extubation.

3.) *Postoperative.* Patients with severe neurologic deficits may be more prone to postoperative respiratory problems.

3. Intracranial Tumors. Neoplasms of the central nervous system are a major proportion of all solid tumors in children younger than 15 years of age. It is the second most common cancer in childhood after leukemia.

a. Supratentorial Tumors account for 50% of all pediatric brain neoplasms. Most of these tumors originate from midline structures and many impinge on the ventricular system, leading to obstructive hydrocephalus.

1.) *Signs and Symptoms* include evidence of increased ICP. The clinical presentation is usually either a subacute progression of a focal neurologic deficit, seizures, or a nonfocal disorder (headache, dementia, personality change, gait disorder). Patients with gliomas have an increased incidence of deep vein thrombosis and pulmonary embolism caused by release of procoagulant factors into the systemic circulation.

2.) *Diagnosis.* Computed tomography and magnetic resonance imaging confirm the presence of an intracranial mass effect. Positron emission tomography and single-photon emission tomography may distinguish tumor recurrence from tissue necrosis, especially after brain radiation. Lumbar puncture for CSF analysis is contraindicated in patients with brain tumors because of the risk of brain herniation in the presence of elevated ICP.

3.) *Treatment.* Glucocorticoids (dexamethasone 0.1 mg/kg up to 10 mg, 12 to 20 mg/day) improve neurologic function by reducing edema around the tumor. Anticonvulsants are used in patients presenting with seizures.

4.) *Management of Anesthesia*

a.) **Preoperative.** Patients with large mass lesions, significant tumor edema, or obstruction to CSF outflow require an anesthetic approach aimed at reducing ICP and improving cerebral perfusion. Preoperative evaluation should include notation of neurologic deficits, documentation of urine output (caused by possible syndrome of inappropriate antidiuretic hormone secretion [SIADH]) and examination of serum electrolyte values, serum osmolality, and urine osmolality.

b.) **Intraoperative.** Monitoring should include an arterial catheter for hemodynamic monitoring and blood chemistry sampling. A central venous catheter is indicated when there is a potential for significant blood loss or increased risk of air embolism. A urinary catheter is essential because of the duration of the surgical procedure, the use of diuretic therapy, and the possible development of diabetes insipidus. Stimulation during laryngoscopy should be minimized. Patients with increased ICP are generally hyperventilated ($PaCO_2$ should not be <30 mm Hg). If positive end-expiratory pressure (PEEP) is used, it should be implemented gradually to prevent impairment of venous return. Fluid management is via isotonic solutions to maintain normotonicity across the blood-brain barrier. If the child is to be extubated after surgery, it should be accomplished once they are awake.

c.) **Postoperative.** The most common contributor to postoperative increased ICP is uncontrolled hypertension (agitation, pain). Treatment is sedation, muscle relaxation (if postoperative ventilation is needed), appropriate treatment of pain, and control of hypertension with vasodilators and/or β-blocker (e.g., labetolol). Prophylactic administration of anticonvulsants is recommended.

b. Craniopharyngiomas (benign encapsulated tumors of the hypophysis cerebri) are the most common intracranial tumors of nonglial origin in pediatric patients. They may cause progressive neurologic deterioration and/or death because of their close relation to important structures such as the hypothalamus, optic nerves, and pituitary stalk.

1.) *Signs and Symptoms.* Headaches and endocrine dysfunction are pathognomonic of a sellar craniopharyngioma. Patients with prechiasmatic tumors have reduced visual acuity, field cuts, and optic atrophy. Obstructive hydrocephalus and increased ICP with papilledema are often observed with retrochiasmatic tumors.

2.) *Diagnosis.* CT is superior to magnetic resonance imaging in demonstrating intratumoral calcification.

3.) *Treatment.* The treatment of choice is total removal, which can be achieved in more than 65% of patients. Alternative therapy includes radiation therapy, sometimes in addition to surgery.

4.) *Management of Anesthesia*

a.) **Preoperative Evaluation** is focused on determining the presence of hydrocephalus and endocrine dysfunction (hypothyroidism, growth hormone deficiency, corticotropin deficiency, diabetes insipidus). Diabetes insipidus (DI) often occurs 4 to 6 hours postoperatively. Patients produce a copious quantity of dilute urine in association with an increasing serum osmolality and low urine osmolality (usually <200 mOsm · L^{-1}). Hypernatremia, hypovolemia and low urine specific gravity (<1.002) are characteristic.

b.) **Intraoperative.** In the presence of DI, fluid therapy must be started and hourly urine output must be measured. Maintenance fluids should be administered along with volume replacement equal to three fourths of the previous hour's urine output. The choice of solution is dictated by the serum electrolyte levels. Vasopressin (DDAVP) should be administered when the diagnosis is confirmed either IV (infusion of 0.5 mU/kg/hour) or intranasally. Postoperatively intranasal DDAVP 5 to 30 μg/day is given in two divided doses.

    c.) **Postoperative.** An endocrinologist should be consulted in the postoperative period for appropriate management of steroid, thyroid, and sex hormone replacement. Insulin-dependent diabetics may experience a reduction in insulin requirements after surgery. Anticonvulsant prophylaxis is indicated both intraoperatively and postoperatively.

c. Posterior Fossa Tumors. The four common types are medulloblastoma (30%), cerebellar astrocytoma (30%), brainstem glioma (30%), and ependymoma (7%).

    1.) Signs and Symptoms. Even small tumors can cause increased ICP, rapid obstruction of CSF flow, and hydrocephalus with negative effects on the brainstem respiratory and cardiovascular regulatory centers. The clinical history is one of worsening headaches, most often in the morning, accompanied by nausea and vomiting. Other signs include abnormal gait or unsteadiness of arm movements, rapid obtundation, stupor, and coma.

    2.) Diagnosis is by CT or magnetic resonance imaging scan with or without contrast enhancement. Astrocytomas are more likely to have calcifications (50%) and large cysts (>2 cm in diameter). Lumbar puncture is contraindicated.

    3.) Treatment is surgical resection.

    4.) Management of Anesthesia

        a.) **Preoperative.** The anesthesiologist must pay particular attention to neurologic symptoms, cerebellar dysfunction, evidence of upper airway obstruction (inspiratory stridor), cardiovascular instability, and increased ICP.

        b.) **Intraoperative.** The induction of anesthesia is aimed at preserving cerebral perfusion pressure and preventing sudden changes in ICP. Monitoring should include an arterial catheter and possibly a central venous line. The use of electrophysiologic somatosensory evoked potential monitoring helps detect intraoperative ischemia and/or compromised perfusion of the brainstem or cranial nerves. The surgery is usually performed in the prone posterior (kinking of tracheal tube).

        The goal of anesthesia is to provide a "slack brain." Intermittent positive pressure ventilation is initially adjusted to maintain $PaCO_2$ in the range of 28 to 30 mm Hg. Once the dura mater is opened, $PaCO_2$ should be increased to 32 mm Hg. Patients are typically awakened immediately at the end of the procedure to allow a neurologic evaluation.

4. Cerebrovascular Abnormalities

a. Arteriovenous Malformations (AVMs) are congenital vascular malformations characterized by direct arterial-to-venous communications without intervening capillary circulation. In the pediatric population AVMs often involve the posterior cerebral artery and the great vein of Galen.

    1.) Signs and Symptoms include those associated with intraparenchymal hemorrhage, thrombosis, and cerebral infarction, compression of adjacent neural structures, parenchymal ischemia as a result of circulatory "steal" from the low resistance vascular network, or congestive heart failure. Approximately 70% of pediatric patients presenting with spontaneous subarachnoid hemorrhage have AVMs as the cause. Seizure is the presenting symptom in 25% of patients. The neonatal presentation of cerebral AVM is often associated with congestive heart failure.

2.) *Diagnosis.* Approximately 50% of AVMs become symptomatic because of a small amount of bleeding. CT is the test of choice for the detection of ruptured AVMs. Four-vessel angiography is generally performed to localize and define the lesion. Lesions may be treatable using endovascular techniques at the time of the initial angiogram. The use of transcranial Doppler sonography is recommended to detect the onset of cerebral vasospasm and follow its course and response to therapy.

3.) *Treatment* is surgical excision, radiographic embolization of the arterial blood supply, or stereotactic radiosurgery as definitive or adjunctive therapy.

4.) *Anesthesia Considerations*

   a.) **Preoperative.** Patients without congestive heart failure can be premedicated to reduce agitation and systemic pressure changes during anesthetic induction.

   b.) **Intraoperative.** A primary goal is prevention of hypertension during laryngoscopy and tracheal intubation. Inhalation or intravenous induction may be performed in the child without evidence of increased ICP. Management for neonates and infants presenting with congestive heart failure is dictated by the severity of this problem and the need to maintain proper cardiac output and brain tissue perfusion. Hyperventilation might be required in patients with hydrocephalus to reduce ICP. Once the dura is opened, normocarbia must be maintained to avoid shunting blood flow to the low-resistance malformed vessels, increasing the risk of rupture and worsening congestive heart failure. In the absence of congestive heart failure, a hypotensive anesthesia technique may be indicated during ligation of the arteriovenous malformation and facilitate surgical manipulation. Preoperative attempts to decrease brain water can lead to rapid circulatory collapse in the event of brisk intraoperative bleeding and is therefore not recommended. It is essential to aggressively treat hyperthermia (shown to exacerbate cerebral ischemic injury). Two large-bore intravenous catheters, an indwelling arterial catheter and a central venous catheter, allow rapid control of blood pressure, infusion of vasoactive drugs, assessment of adequacy of fluid therapy, and monitoring of cerebral perfusion pressure. Urinary catheter placement is mandatory following induction of anesthesia.

   c.) **Postoperative.** Sudden changes in blood pressure must be avoided. Vasospasm is not a common postoperative complication in children but must be considered in the face of neurologic deterioration.

5. Myelomeningocele. Failure of the canal end of the neural tube to close during development can result in spina bifida, or saclike herniation of the meninges (meningocele), or herniation containing neural elements (myelomeningocele).

1.) *Signs and Symptoms.* Children with meningoceles are usually born without neurologic deficits; those with myelomeningoceles usually have varying degrees of motor and sensory deficits, including flaccid paraplegia, loss of sensation to pinprick, and loss of anal and bladder-sphincter tone. Associated congenital conditions include clubfoot, hydrocephalus, dislocation of the hips, extrophy of the bladder, prolapsed uterus, Klippel-Feil syndrome, and congenital cardiac defects. Patients are prone to recurrent urinary tract infections, gram-negative sepsis, and scoliosis.

2.) *Diagnosis.* These defects may be found at birth (Arnold-Chiari II malformation) or incidentally (spina bifida) when plain films are obtained for other reasons. Magnetic resonance imaging is the most useful radiographic test to confirm the presence of neural tube defects and/or spinal cord anomalies.

3.) *Treatment.* Early neurosurgical repair of a myelomeningocele will lead to restoration of a more normal configuration of the spine. The more severe anomalies will be detected at birth and will require a surgical intervention within the first 24 hours of life to reduce the risk of infection of exposed central nervous system tissue.

4.) *Management of Anesthesia*

    a.) **Preoperative.** Infants presenting for repair of a meningomyelocele defect rarely have increased ICP. Neonates with a myelomeningocele may have an abnormal ventilatory response to hypoxia and hypercarbia, gastroesophageal reflux, and abnormal vocal cord mobility. Intraoperative blood loss can be insidious, especially if the sac is large. Invasive monitoring is indicated for patients presenting with large defects, such as a multilevel myelomeningocele where significant cutaneous undermining will be needed. Hypothermia is common during these procedures considering the surface area of tissue exposed and the age of the patient.

    b.) **Intraoperative.** If general anesthesia is selected, awake tracheal intubation may be performed with these children in the lateral decubitus position (to avoid pressure on the meningocele sac) or in the supine position with the meningocele sac protected by elevating it on a doughnut-shaped support. Long-acting nondepolarizing muscle relaxants are avoided, as the surgeon may use a nerve stimulator to identify functional neural elements. Succinylcholine does not elicit a hyperkalemic response in these patients. Children with a myelomeningocele may have an increased incidence of sensitivity to latex because of chronic exposure to indwelling latex catheters. A preoperative history of itching, rashes, or wheezing after wearing latex gloves or inflating toy balloons suggests latex allergy.

    c.) **Postoperative.** Neonates should be maintained in the prone position, with a high index of suspicion maintained for the development of increased ICP.

6. Craniosynostosis refers to a condition where one or more cranial sutures fuse prematurely leading to focal or global growth delay of the skull, which can result in aesthetic abnormalities as well as functional problems (increased ICP, hydrocephalus, developmental delay, amblyopia).

    a. Diagnosis is suspected in the presence of abnormal head circumference and shape, fontanelle size, and palpable bony ridges along affected sutures. The diagnosis is confirmed with plain radiographs, ultrasonography, CT, and/or magnetic resonance imaging.

    b. Treatment is surgical intervention performed early in infancy to prevent further progression of the deformity and potential complications associated with increased ICP.

    c. Prognosis. More than half of the patients suffering from increased ICP show some signs of mental retardation. Intraoperative death is usually caused by massive blood loss.

    d. Anesthetic Management. Intracranial pressure may be elevated in syndromic children and airway management may be challenging (upper airway obstruction) because of other concomitant craniofacial anomalies. Alternative airway management techniques (e.g., laryngeal mask airway, fiberoptic bronchoscope) should be available. In the presence of increased ICP, specific anesthetic measures must be considered (avoiding hypercapnia, hypoxemia, arterial hypotension). Large-bore intravenous access is required and an arterial indwelling catheter is recommended to allow for real-time blood pressure measurements and repeated blood sampling. Techniques to reduce allogenic blood transfusions include cell saver, preoperative acute normovolemic hemodilution, and controlled arterial hypotension. Hypotensive anesthesia can be achieved by using volatile anesthetics, opioids, and/or adrenergic receptor-blocking drugs. Arterial hypotension should not be used in patients with increased ICP. A precordial Doppler ultrasound probe may be indicated to detect intraoperative venous air embolism. A long central venous catheter may be placed to evacuate air from the right side of the heart in case of significant air embolism. Because air embolism is common, nitrous oxide should be avoided. Facial swelling related to surgery can be quite pronounced (particularly when the surgery extends below the orbital ridge) and requires postoperative mechanical ventilation.

7. Down Syndrome (Trisomy 21) is the most common human chromosomal syndrome.

    a. Signs and Symptoms. Common features affect the head (brachycephaly, a flat occiput, dysplastic ears, epicanthal folds with typical up-slanting of the palpebral folds [mongoloid slanting] and strabismus, and Brushfield spots on the iris). The tongue is normal at birth but later becomes enlarged because of hypertrophy of the papillae. Midface hypoplasia, a high-arched palate, and micrognathia complicate this problem.

Skeletal anomalies may include short stature and a short, broad neck with occipitoatlantoaxial instability (approximately 20% of patients). The hands are usually short and broad with a simian crease, and the middle phalanx of the fifth finger is often hypoplastic. Muscle tone is reduced, and the joints are hypermobile. Respiratory problems can be caused by a floppy soft palate, enlarged tonsils, laryngotracheal or subglottic stenosis, obstructive sleep apnea, and recurrent pulmonary infections. Cardiac defects are common (atrial septal defect, ventricular septal defect [25%], endocardial cushion defect [50%], patent ductus arteriosus, or tetralogy of Fallot). Pulmonary hypertension should be suspected and may even lead to Eisenmenger complex. Visceral anomalies include gastroesophageal reflux, duodenal atresia, imperforate anus, and Hirschsprung's disease.

b. Diagnosis can be established antenatally by chorionic villous sampling or by amniocentesis. Postnatally, the diagnosis is based on the typical clinical features and confirmed by karyotyping.

c. Prognosis. There is a 10- to 20-fold increased risk of leukemia (acute myelocytic leukemia or acute lymphocytic leukemia). Hypothyroidism, precocious Alzheimer's disease, and conductive hearing loss are other common problems.

d. Management of Anesthesia Preoperative assessment includes evaluation of the current respiratory and cardiac status. Airway management can be difficult (macroglossia, micrognathia, narrow hypopharynx, muscular hypotonia). The risk of spinal cord compression resulting from occipitoatlantoaxial instability should be kept in mind during intubation or positioning for surgical procedures (neck radiographs do not reliably predict this). A history of gait anomalies, a preference for the sitting position, hyperreflexia, and signs of clonus could all be suggestive of spinal canal stenosis/cord compression. The anesthetic risk is increased in the presence of cardiac disease. Vascular access can be challenging secondary to xerodermia, atopic dermatitis, and obesity. Narrowing of the trachea (subglottic stenosis) is common and may require a smaller endotracheal tube than expected. These patients have reduced immune competence and require strict asepsis with all invasive procedures. Airway abnormalities increase the risk of obstructive sleep apnea and mandate close monitoring in the early postoperative period.

8. Craniofacial Abnormalities

a. Cleft Lip and Palate are among the most common congenital anomalies. Chromosomal abnormalities, drugs (steroids, antiepileptics [benzodiazepines]), chemotherapy, excessive maternal vitamin A intake), folic acid deficiency, maternal tobacco or alcohol abuse (fetal alcohol syndrome), maternal diabetes mellitus, and possibly maternal age (<20 years or >39 years old) and increased paternal age, have all been associated with orofacial clefting. The clefting may be an isolated anomaly or be part of a syndrome (e.g., Pierre Robin syndrome, Treacher Collins syndrome).

1.) *Signs and Symptoms* may include airway obstruction, feeding problems, aspiration, failure to thrive, and chronic otitis media.

2.) *Diagnosis* is most commonly made postnatally, sometimes requiring meticulous inspection and palpation of the hard and soft palate.

3.) ***Treatment*** is surgical correction, preferably before the development of speech.

4.) ***Prognosis*** is excellent, although several corrective surgeries may be required.

5.) ***Management of Anesthesia.*** In infants with nonsyndromic clefting, an inhalational induction is usually preferred, and after establishing venous access, a small dose of neuromuscular blocker and opioid (fentanyl or morphine) is administered followed by oral endotracheal intubation. In infants with syndromic clefting, spontaneous ventilation should be maintained until the airway has been secured. Local anesthetics should be used to minimize pain intraoperatively and postoperatively. The patient may be extubated once fully awake and after confirming that any throat pack inserted during surgery has been removed. Cool mist in the postoperative period may help keep these children comfortable and prevent airway complications.

b. *Mandibular Hypoplasia.* Upper airway obstruction and difficult tracheal intubation are likely.

1.) ***Pierre Robin Syndrome*** consists of micrognathia usually accompanied by glossoptosis (posterior displacement of the tongue) and cleft palate. Acute upper airway obstruction, feeding problems, failure to thrive, and cyanotic episodes are early complications. Associated congenital heart disease is common.

2.) ***Treacher Collins Syndrome*** is the most common of the mandibulofacial dysostoses and results in early airway problems similar to those experienced by infants with Pierre Robin syndrome. Congenital heart disease (VSD) often accompanies this syndrome. Other features include malar hypoplasia, colobomas (notching of the lower eyelids), and an antimongoloid slant of the palpebral fissures. Tracheal intubation, as in infants with Pierre Robin syndrome, is difficult and sometimes impossible.

3.) ***Goldenhar Syndrome*** is unilateral mandibular hypoplasia. Associated anomalies include eye, ear, and vertebral abnormalities on the affected side. Ease of tracheal intubation is highly variable.

4.) ***Nager Syndrome*** is a rare form of acrofacial dysostosis that includes characteristic craniofacial abnormalities (malar hypoplasia, severe micrognathia).

5.) ***Anesthesia Concerns***

a.) **Preoperative Evaluation** includes airway evaluation, plans for intubation, and assessment of the cardiovascular system and the hemoglobin concentration. Some patients with chronic airway obstruction experience chronic arterial hypoxemia and develop pulmonary hypertension. Premedication with anticholinergic drugs is recommended to decrease upper airway secretions. Opioids and other ventilatory depressants are usually avoided in the preoperative medication.

b.) **Intraoperative.** Equipment for emergency bronchoscopy, cricothyrotomy, or tracheostomy should be available. Preoxygenation should occur before initiation of direct laryngoscopy. Use of muscle relaxants is not recommended until the airway is secured. Awake tracheal intubation is a consideration, but more often, fiberoptic tracheal intubation is accomplished after inhalation induction of anesthesia with volatile anesthetics. Use of laryngeal mask airways is an alternative to tracheal intubation in selected patients or when tracheal intubation proves impossible. Tracheostomy under local anesthesia may be required when all other attempts to maintain the airway have failed. Tracheal extubation following surgery should occur when the patient is fully awake and alert. Equipment for urgent tracheal reintubation must be immediately available.

c. Hypertelorism (an increased distance between the eyes) is associated with many craniofacial anomalies, such as Crouzon (hypertelorism, craniosynostosis, shallow orbits with marked proptosis, and midface hypoplasia) and Apert syndromes (same features plus syndactyly). Other associated anomalies are cleft palate, synostosis of the cervical spine, hearing loss, and mental retardation.

1.) *Treatment* is complex surgical correction, preferably before ossification of the facial bones occurs.

2.) *Management of Anesthesia.* Tracheal intubation may be difficult. Blood loss generally occurs in a steady ooze averaging approximately 1 to 2 blood volumes. Measurement of serial hematocrits, central venous pressure, and urine output are helpful for estimating blood loss and guiding intravenous fluid replacement. Intravenous catheters must be of sufficient number and diameter to permit rapid transfusions of blood. Head up positioning may reduce blood loss. Controlled hypotension (nitroprusside) may be useful, although the mean arterial pressure, as measured at the level of the circle of Willis, should not be decreased to less than 50 mm Hg during controlled hypotension. Hypothermia during these lengthy operations can be minimized by placing children on warming blankets, warming intravenous fluids and blood, and using warmed, humidified inspired gases. Hyperventilation of the lungs to maintain the $PaCO_2$ between 30 to 35 mm Hg, maintenance of the head-up position, and administration of furosemide, mannitol, and corticosteroids minimize brain swelling. Drainage of lumbar CSF may also be used to minimize brain swelling. Corneal abrasions are likely; eye ointment should be used and the eyelids sutured closed. Placement of an arterial catheter (for continuous measurement of systemic blood pressure and monitoring of blood pH, blood gases, hematocrit, electrolytes, and plasma osmolarity) is mandatory. A central venous catheter and a Foley catheter are helpful for evaluating the adequacy of intravenous fluid replacement. Mechanical ventilation may be required for several days postoperatively.

9. Disorders of the Upper Airway

a. Acute Epiglottitis (supraglottitis) is a short-lived disease presenting most often in children 2 to 7 years of age. The most common pathogen is *Haemophilus influenzae* type B. Acute epiglottitis may be difficult to differentiate from laryngotracheobronchitis (croup) (**Table 24-9**).

1.) Signs and Symptoms of acute epiglottitis are acute difficulty swallowing, high fever, and inspiratory stridor, typically developing in less than 24 hours. Patients display a characteristic posture of sitting upright and leaning forward with the chin up and mouth open. Pulmonary edema, pericarditis, meningitis, and septic arthritis may accompany acute epiglottitis.

2.) Diagnosis. Acute epiglottitis is a medical emergency with diagnosis based on clinical signs. The history is quickly obtained and the child examined for signs of upper airway obstruction. No attempts to directly visualize the epiglottis should be made, because any instrumentation, even a tongue blade, may provoke laryngospasm.

3.) Treatment. Physicians skilled in airway management must accompany these children at all times. Definitive treatment of acute epiglottitis includes prompt establishment of a secure airway and administration of antibiotics effective against *H. influenzae,* once blood and throat cultures are obtained.

TABLE 24-9 Clinical Features of Acute Epiglottitis and Laryngotracheobronchitis

Parameter	Acute Epiglottitis	Laryngotracheobronchitis
Age group affected	2–7 yr	<2 yr
Incidence	Accounts for 5% of children with stridor	Accounts for about 80% of children with stridor
Etiologic agent	Bacterial (*Haemophilus influenzae*)	Viral
Onset	Rapid over 24 hr	Gradual over 24–72 hr
Signs and symptoms	Inspiratory stridor, pharyngitis, drooling, fever (often >39°C), lethargic to restless, insists upon sitting up and leaning forward, tachypnea, cyanosis	Inspiratory stridor, "barking" cough, rhinorrhea, fever (rarely >39°C)
Laboratory	Neutrophilia	Lymphocytosis
Lateral radiographs of the neck	Swollen epiglottis	Narrowing of the subglottic area
Treatment	Oxygen, urgent tracheal intubation or tracheostomy during general anesthesia, fluids, antibiotics, corticosteroids (?)	Oxygen, aerosolized racemic epinephrine, humidity, fluids, corticosteroids, tracheal intubation for severe airway obstruction

4.) *Prognosis.* Up to 6% of children with epiglottitis without an artificial airway (endotracheal tube or tracheostomy) die. Because the response to antibiotics is rapid, extubation may be achieved within 2 to 3 days in most cases.

5.) *Management of Anesthesia.* An otolaryngologist should be present at the time of induction and tracheal intubation, which are accomplished with the child in the sitting position, breathing the volatile anesthetic sevoflurane in oxygen. Before induction of anesthesia, the care team should be completely prepared to carry out emergency cricothyrotomy or tracheostomy. An intravenous line is placed after adequate depth of anesthesia is established. Direct laryngoscopy and intubation (with a styletted endotracheal tube that is one half size smaller than would ordinarily be selected) are performed. Tracheal extubation may be considered when the child's fever and other signs of infection have waned, and an air leak develops around the endotracheal tube. The airway is examined by direct laryngoscopy or flexible fiberoptic laryngoscopy during sedation or general anesthesia to confirm that inflammation of the epiglottis and other supraglottic tissues has resolved before the trachea is extubated.

b. *Laryngotracheobronchitis (Croup)* is a viral infection of the upper respiratory tract that typically afflicts children between 6 months and 6 years of age (see **Table 24-9**).

1.) *Signs and Symptoms.* Croup has a gradual onset over 24 to 72 hours, with signs of upper respiratory tract infection (rhinorrhea, pharyngitis, low-grade fever, "barking" cough, hoarse voice, inspiratory stridor). Leukocyte counts are normal or only slightly increased with lymphocytosis. Patients present with a characteristic "barking" cough, hoarse voice, and inspiratory stridor.

2.) *Diagnosis* is made clinically. Neck radiographs may show a characteristic subglottic narrowing or "steeple sign" on the anteroposterior view.

3.) *Treatment* of mild to moderate laryngotracheobronchitis is administration of supplemental oxygen and cool mist. In cases of severe respiratory distress with cyanosis and retractions, nebulized racemic epinephrine (0.05 mL/kg up to 0.5 mL of 2.25% epinephrine solution in 3 mL normal saline) in addition to oxygen may help relieve airway obstruction. Patients often require repeated treatments 1 to 4 hours apart and may experience a rebound obstruction following an initial state of improvement. Administration of corticosteroids, such as dexamethasone (0.5 to 1.0 mg/kg IV) or inhalation of budesonide, decreases edema in the laryngeal mucosa. Increasing $PaCO_2$ is an indication for tracheal intubation. The trachea should be intubated with a smaller than normal tube to minimize the edema associated with intubation.

4.) *Prognosis.* Most patients, especially older children, with croup experience only stridor and mild dyspnea before recovering.

5.) *Management of Anesthesia.* When intubation is necessary, the procedure should be performed in the operating room as for a child with epiglottitis. A surgeon should be present in case a tracheostomy becomes necessary.

c. Postintubation Laryngeal Edema is a potential complication of tracheal intubation in all children, but the incidence is highest in children 1 to 4 years old.

   1.) *Symptoms and Signs* are stridor, a "barking" or "brassy" cough, hoarseness, retractions, flaring of the ala nasi, hypoxemia, and mental status changes, and generally occur within 1 hour of extubation, with peak intensity within 4 hours and resolution of stridor within 24 hours.

   2.) *Diagnosis.* Inspiratory stridor suggests airway obstruction at or above the level of the vocal cords, whereas expiratory stridor suggests airway obstruction below the level of the vocal cords.

   3.) *Treatment* of postintubation laryngeal edema may include hourly administration of aerosolized racemic epinephrine (0.05 mL/kg [maximum 0.5 mL] in 3.0 mL of saline) until symptoms subside. In severe cases of postintubation laryngeal edema, helium and oxygen mixtures have proven to be useful. Steroids do not reliably prevent postintubation laryngeal edema, although the progression of airway edema may be prevented.

   4.) *Prognosis.* In most cases, postintubation laryngeal edema is self-limited. For those requiring racemic epinephrine, one or two treatments usually produce significant improvement.

   5.) *Management of Anesthesia.* The use of uncuffed endotracheal tubes has traditionally been recommended in children younger than 8 years old because of concerns that cuffed endotracheal tubes might contribute to the risk of subglottic edema. Extubation is considered when a leak around the endotracheal tube is demonstrated, indicating adequate improvement in the laryngeal edema.

d. Foreign Body Aspiration into the airways can produce a wide range of responses, from mild symptoms that are barely noticeable to death from asphyxiation.

   1.) *Signs and Symptoms* are cough, wheezing, and decreased air entry into the affected lung. The most common site of aspiration is the right mainstem bronchus. The type of foreign body aspirated influences the clinical course. For example, nuts and certain vegetable materials are highly irritating to the bronchial mucosa.

   2.) *Diagnosis.* Choking or coughing episodes accompanied by wheezing in a previously normal child are highly suggestive of an airway foreign body. Chest radiography provides direct evidence (radiopaque objects) or indirect evidence (hyperinflation of the affected lung [due to air trapping] and shifting of the mediastinum toward the opposite side on expiratory chest radiograph). Laryngeal foreign bodies present with complete obstruction and asphyxiation unless promptly relieved, or with partial obstruction and croup, hoarseness, cough, stridor, and dyspnea. Tracheal foreign bodies most commonly present with choking, stridor, and wheezing.

    3.) Treatment requires endoscopic removal using direct laryngoscopy and/or rigid bronchoscopy.

    4.) Prognosis. Fragmentation of the foreign body during the course of removal is extremely dangerous and can result in death if the pieces occlude both mainstem bronchi and prevent ventilation. Objects small enough to pass through the vocal cords rarely occlude the trachea.

    5.) Management of Anesthesia. When a laryngeal foreign body or airway obstruction is present, induction of anesthesia using only volatile anesthetics such as sevoflurane in oxygen is useful. Induction of anesthesia with intravenous drugs followed by inhalation of volatile anesthetics is acceptable if the airway is less tenuous. Spraying the larynx with a lidocaine solution is effective in preventing laryngospasm. Administration of atropine (10 to 20 μg/kg IV) or glycopyrrolate (3 to 5 μg/kg IV) decreases the likelihood of bradycardia from vagal stimulation during endoscopy. Positive airway pressures could contribute to distal migration of foreign bodies, complicating their extraction. Spontaneous ventilation is desirable until the nature and location of the foreign body have been identified by bronchoscopy. After completion of bronchoscopy, the patient is intubated with an endotracheal tube and extubated when appropriate criteria are met. Dexamethasone is often given prophylactically to decrease subglottic edema. Nebulized racemic epinephrine is useful for postintubation croup. Chest radiographs should be obtained after bronchoscopy to detect atelectasis or pneumothorax. Postural drainage and chest percussion enhance clearance of secretions and decrease the subsequent risk of infection.

e. Laryngeal Papillomatosis is the most common benign laryngeal neoplasm in children. The most likely cause is a tissue response to human papillomavirus.

    1.) Signs and Symptoms. A change in the character of the child's voice is the most common initial symptom. Children present with hoarseness, and infants may present with an altered cry and sometimes stridor.

    2.) Diagnosis is confirmed by microlaryngoscopy and biopsy of lesions.

    3.) Treatment includes surgical excision, cryosurgery, topical 5-fluorouracil, exogenous interferon, and laser ablation. Tracheostomy can be life saving and is usually reserved for cases with rapid recurrence and airway obstruction.

    4.) Prognosis. Distal involvement of the lower tracheobronchial tree represents an aggressive variant that may be fatal. Malignant degeneration of juvenile papillomas is rare but can occur in older children. Papillomas usually regress spontaneously at puberty.

    5.) Management of Anesthesia. Spontaneous ventilation is recommended until the extent and nature of airway obstruction is determined. Awake tracheal intubation is recommended for severe airway obstruction but is not always feasible. Intubating the trachea after inducing anesthesia with sevoflurane in oxygen is usually a safe approach. Skeletal muscle paralysis or deep anesthesia is required to immobilize the vocal cords during treatment. The usual safety precautions concerning laser use should be observed. The tracheal tube should be removed only when the child is fully awake and laryngeal bleeding has ceased. After tracheal extubation, inhalation of aerosolized racemic epinephrine and intravenous administration of dexamethasone may decrease subglottic edema.

f. Lung Abscess develops when localized infection in the lung parenchyma becomes necrotic and cavitates.

1.) *Signs and Symptoms* include fever, cough, pleuritic chest pain, productive sputum, anorexia, weight loss, hemoptysis, dyspnea, and tachypnea.

2.) *Diagnosis.* Chest radiograph, chest CT, and percutaneous needle aspiration of the abscess cavity under CT guidance may help isolate the causative organism.

3.) *Treatment* consists of parenteral antibiotic therapy that covers both aerobic and anaerobic organisms until a specific bacteriologic diagnosis is established. Surgical treatment is indicated in cases that do not respond to antibiotic therapy.

4.) *Prognosis.* Medical therapy is often unsuccessful in neonates and immunocompromised children. However, the prognosis for previously healthy patients is quite good, with most symptoms resolving within 7 to 10 days.

5.) *Management of Anesthesia.* Placement of a double-lumen endobronchial tube (or endobronchial intubation in infants and small children when a double-lumen tube is too large) is often used to isolate the affected lung and prevent cross-contamination.

g. Malignant Hyperthermia is a pharmacogenetic clinical syndrome. Susceptible patients have a genetic predisposition for the development of this disorder when they are exposed to triggering pharmacologic agents (all volatile inhalation anesthetic agents and succinylcholine) or stressful environmental factors. MH represents a spectrum of reactions from minor reactions to rapid temperature increase, muscle rigidity, acidosis, arrhythmias, and death. Some reactions may not occur until the postoperative period.

1.) *Signs and Symptoms (Table 24-10)*

2.) *Diagnosis.* Without hypercapnia and acidosis, the diagnosis of MH is questionable. If sufficiently sensitive measuring equipment is used, jaw stiffness after administration of succinylcholine can be detected in most patients but is often more pronounced in children (**Fig. 24-2**). Children in whom masseter muscle rigidity (MMR) develops have a 50% incidence of susceptibility to MH. Skeletal muscle biopsies are positive for MH susceptibility in all patients in whom plasma creatine kinase concentrations exceed 20,000 IU/L after succinylcholine-induced masseter spasm. Findings that support the diagnosis of MH include myoglobinuria, elevated serum creatine kinase, fever, hypoxemia, hypercarbia, respiratory and metabolic acidosis, hyperkalemia, and marked central venous

TABLE 24-10	Clinical Features of Malignant Hyperthermia		
Timing	Clinical Signs	Changes in Monitored Variables	Biochemical Changes
Early	Masseter spasm		
	Tachypnea	Increased minute ventilation	
	Rapid exhaustion of soda lime	Increasing end-tidal carbon dioxide concentration	Increased PaCO$_2$
	Warm soda lime canister		
	Tachycardia		Acidosis
	Irregular heart rate	Cardiac dysrhythmias, peaked T waves on ECG	Hyperkalemia
Intermediate	Patient warm to touch	Increasing core body temperature	
	Cyanosis	Decreasing oxygen saturation	
	Dark blood in surgical site		
	Irregular heart rate	Cardiac dysrhythmias, peaked T waves on ECG	Hyperkalemia
Late	Generalized skeletal muscle rigidity		Increased creatine kinase concentrations
	Prolonged bleeding		
	Dark urine		Myoglobinuria
	Irregular heart rate	Cardiac dysrhythmias, peaked T waves on ECG	Hyperkalemia

ECG, electrocardiogram.
Adapted from Hopkins PM: Malignant hyperthermia: Advances in clinical management and diagnosis. Br J Anaesth 2000:118–128.

oxygen desaturation. Late complications of untreated MH include disseminated intravascular coagulation, pulmonary edema, and acute renal failure. Central nervous system damage may manifest as blindness, seizures, coma, or paralysis.

3.) *Differential Diagnosis (Table 24-11)*

4.) *Treatment.* Intravenous dantrolene (2 to 3 mg/kg repeated every 5 to 10 minutes to a maximum dose of 10 mg/kg) is the only drug that is reliably effective treatment for MH (**Table 24-12**). The patient should respond to treatment within 45 minutes. Recrudescence may occur in 25% of patients, usually within

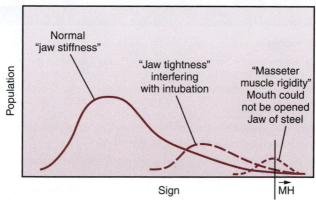

Figure 24-2 • The spectrum of masseter muscle responses to succinylcholine varies from a slight jaw stiffness that does not interfere with endotracheal intubation to the extreme "jaws of steel," which is masseter muscle tetany, not allowing the mouth to be opened. It is likely that the latter response is more highly associated with malignant hyperthermia. It should be noted that, even with the inability to open the mouth, the patient should still be able to be ventilated by bag and mask because all other muscles are relaxed. (Adapted from Kaplan RF. Malignant Hyperthermia. Annual Refresher Course Lectures. Washington, DC, American Society of Anesthesiologists, 1993.)

TABLE 24-11	Differential Diagnosis of Malignant Hyperthermia
Diagnosis	**Distinguishing Traits**
Hyperthyroidism	Symptoms and physical findings often present, blood gas abnormalities increase gradually
Sepsis	Usually normal blood gases
Pheochromocytoma	Similar to MH except marked blood pressure swings
Metastatic carcinoid	Same as pheochromocytoma
Cocaine intoxication	Fever, rigidity, rhabdomyolysis similar to malignant neuroleptic syndrome
Heat stroke	Similar to MH except that the patient is outside the operating room
Masseter spasm (MMR)	May progress to MH, total body spasm more likely than isolated MMR
Neuroleptic malignant syndrome	Similar to MH, usually associated with the use of dopamine antagonist antipsychotic drugs
Serotonin syndrome	Similar to MH and neuroleptic malignant syndrome, associated with the administration of serotoninergic drugs

Adapted from Bissonnette B, Ryan JF: Temperature regulation: Normal and abnormal [malignant hyperthermia]. In Cote CJ, Todres ID, Goudsouzian NG, Ryan JF, (eds): A Practice of Anesthesia for Infants and Children, 3rd ed. Philadelphia, Saunders, 2001, p 621.

463

TABLE 24-12	Treatment of Malignant Hyperthermia

Etiologic Treatment

Administer dantrolene (2–3 mg/kg IV) as an initial bolus, followed with repeat doses every 5–10 min until symptoms are controlled (rarely need total dose >10 mg/kg).

Prevent recrudescence (dantrolene 1 mg/kg IV every 6 hours for 72 hours).

Symptomatic Treatment

Immediately discontinue inhaled anesthetics and conclude surgery as soon as possible.

Hyperventilate the lungs with 100% oxygen.

Initiate active cooling (iced saline 15 mL/kg IV every 10 min; gastric and bladder lavage with iced saline; surface cooling).

Correct metabolic acidosis (sodium bicarbonate 1–2 mEq/kg IV based on arterial pH).

Maintain urine output (hydration, mannitol 0.25 g/kg IV, furosemide 1 mg/kg IV).

Treat cardiac dysrhythmias (procainamide 15 mg/kg IV).

Monitor in an intensive care unit (urine output, arterial blood gases, pH, electrolytes).

4 to 8 hours, but can occur as late as 36 hours. Dantrolene should probably be repeated even if the initial episode is under control at a dose of 1 to 2 mg/kg IV every 6 hours for a 24-hour period. Some recommend continuing oral dantrolene 1 mg/kg every 4 to 8 hours for 48 hours.

5.) *Prognosis.* After recovery from acute episodes of MH, patients should be closely monitored in an intensive care unit for up to 72 hours. Urine output, arterial blood gases, pH, and serum electrolyte concentrations should be determined frequently.

6.) *Identification of Susceptible Patients.* Detailed medical and family anesthetic histories should be obtained. MH appears to be linked with central core disease (most have mutation at the RYR1 locus). Other syndromes associated with multicore myopathy are Evan's myopathy and the King-Denborough syndrome/phenotype. An exceptionally rare phenomenon of stress-induced MH (triggered by trauma, anxiety, vigorous exercise, high ambient temperature) affects a small number of MH-susceptible patients. The mechanism of rhabdomyolysis in Duchenne muscular dystrophy now appears unrelated to MH. The creatine kinase level should be measured in patients being evaluated for susceptibility to MH, but this is not a definitive screening test. Skeletal muscle biopsies with in vitro contracture testing provide definitive confirmation of susceptibility to MH but are not appropriate in children younger than 6 years or those who weigh less than 20 kg, because of the amount of muscle needed for the test. It is preferable to take a biopsy sample from the patient with MMR before testing other family members. Follow-up of patients who have had MMR is summarized in **Table 24-13**.

TABLE 24-13	Follow-up of Patients with Masseter Muscle Rigidity

Medic-Alert bracelet or other conspicuous form of identification must be worn. The patient and first-degree relatives must be assumed to have malignant hyperthermia susceptibility (MHS) unless the patient is subsequently proved to have a negative caffeine halothane contracture test.

Refer the patient to malignant hyperthermia susceptible sites, Malignant Hyperthermia Association of the United States (MHAUS) (800-98MHAUS; www.mhaus.org). MHAUS can refer the patient to an MH diagnostic center.

Review the family history for adverse anesthetic events or suggestion of heritable myopathy.

Consider evaluation for temporomandibular joint disorder.

Consider neurologic consultation to evaluate for a potential myotonic disorder; if rhabdomyolysis is severe, consider evaluation for a muscular dystrophy (e.g., Duchenne or Becker muscular dystrophy) or a heritable metabolic disorder (e.g., carnitine palmitoyltransferase II deficiency or McArdle's disease).

7.) Management of Anesthesia

a.) **Dantrolene Prophylaxis** is unnecessary if one adheres to a nontriggering technique. If a severe MH reaction has previously occurred, dantrolene 2 to 4 mg/kg IV may be administered over 10 to 30 minutes just prior to induction of anesthesia, and one half the dose is repeated in 6 hours. Diuresis may accompany intravenous administration of dantrolene (caused by mannitol in the powder), and patients should have a urinary catheter placed. Dantrolene may cause nausea, diarrhea, blurred vision, and skeletal muscle weakness.

b.) **Drug Selections (Table 24-14).** Drugs that can trigger MH include volatile anesthetics and succinylcholine. Administration of calcium entry-blocking drugs in the presence of dantrolene has been associated with hyperkalemia and myocardial depression. Antagonism of nondepolarizing muscle relaxants has not been shown to trigger MH.

c.) **Anesthesia Machine.** A conventional anesthesia machine can be used with a disposable anesthesia breathing circuit and fresh gas outlet hoses, fresh carbon dioxide absorbent, no vaporizers (removed or taped), and a continuous flow of oxygen at 10 L/min for 10 to 60 minutes (see manufacturer's recommendations) before using the machine with patients susceptible to MH.

d.) **Regional Anesthesia** is acceptable in MH-susceptible patients. Both ester- and amide-based local anesthetics are now considered safe for regional or local anesthesia.

e.) **Postoperative Discharge Home.** It is acceptable to perform surgery in ambulatory centers on patients susceptible to MH as long as they are monitored for at least 1 hour after a nontriggering anesthetic.

TABLE 24-14	Nontriggering Drugs for Malignant Hyperthermia
Barbiturates	
Propofol	
Etomidate	
Benzodiazepines	
Opioids	
Droperidol	
Nitrous oxide	
Nondepolarizing muscle relaxants	
Anticholinesterases	
Anticholinergics	
Sympathomimetics	
Local anesthetics (esters and amides)	
α_2-Agonists	
Clonidine	
Dexmedetomidine	

h. Familial Dysautonomia (FD) or Riley-Day syndrome is an autosomal recessive inherited progressive neurodegenerative disorder that results in a loss of unmyelinated nerve fibers involved in central autonomic nervous system control and the perception of pain and temperature.

1.) *Signs and Symptoms.* Children affected with FD present in early infancy with feeding difficulties caused by pharyngeal dyscoordination. Other symptoms include generalized hypotonia, gastroesophageal reflux, recurrent vomiting and aspiration with pulmonary problems, absence of overflowing tears on emotion, a reduction or absence of lingual fungiform papillae, pallor, delayed developmental milestones, diminished response to nociceptive stimuli, seizures, body temperature instability, decreased or absent deep tendon reflexes, delayed walking, and ataxia. With increasing age, autonomic blood pressure dysregulation (profound orthostatic hypotension, supine hypertension), peripheral sensory dysfunction, and ataxia worsen. By age 3 to 6 years, many patients suffer from recurrent episodes of dysautonomic crises (nausea and cyclic vomiting, profuse sweating, mottled skin, agitation, and a rapidly changing pattern of arterial hypertension and hypotension with bradycardia and tachycardia) triggered by mild emotional or physical stress.

2.) *Diagnosis* is based on the five clinical features—(1) Ashkenazi Jewish origin and a reduction in or absence of (2) lacrimation, (3) deep tendon reflexes, (4) lingual fungiform papillae, and (5) axon flare after intradermal histamine injection—and is now confirmed by DNA analysis.

466

3.) *Treatment* is nutritional support and medical or surgical treatment of reflux.

4.) *Prognosis.* A newborn has a 50% chance of reaching the age of 40 years. Sudden death (with approximately two thirds occurring during sleep) and pulmonary and renal complications represent the main causes of death.

5.) *Management of Anesthesia.* Even moderate hypoxia results in central ventilatory depression with hypoventilation, arterial (systolic and diastolic) hypotension, bradycardia, and potentially respiratory arrest. Minor stress or events such as crying or laughing can trigger breath holding and decerebrate posturing. Preoperative testing should include an electrocardiogram (ECG) (association with long QT syndrome), serum electrolytes, creatinine, and blood urea nitrogen (sweating and vomiting lead to electrolyte disturbances). Prevention of stress episodes (pain, anxiety) is important. Patients are very sensitive to adrenergic and anticholinergic agents: The first-line treatment of hypotension is fluids. Because of the high incidence of gastroesophageal reflux, a rapid-sequence induction is recommended. Short-acting drugs allow titration to control pain and respiratory depression. Regional anesthesia alone or in combination with general anesthesia has been used safely. There should be a low threshold for invasive monitoring, given the frequency of hemodynamic instability (arterial catheter) and preoperative hypovolemia (central venous catheter). Eyes require lubrication and protection from alacrima. Postoperative management in the intensive care unit may be warranted. Diazepam is the drug of choice to control dysautonomic crises. Persistent arterial hypertension responds well to oral clonidine. More potent antihypertensive drugs (e.g., labetalol, hydralazine) may be required but should be used cautiously because hemodynamic instability can manifest as hypotension.

i. Solid Tumors. Cancer is second only to accidental trauma as a cause of death in children ages 1 to 14 years. Most intra-abdominal tumors in infants are benign and of renal origin. Retroperitoneal solid tumors are likely to be of renal origin (Wilms' tumor, neuroblastoma).

1.) *Neuroblastoma* is the most common extracranial solid tumor in infants and children, resulting from malignant proliferation of sympathetic ganglion cell precursors. Neuroblastoma may metastasize by direct invasion into surrounding structures, lymphatic infiltration, or hematogenous spread.

   a.) **Signs and Symptoms.** Children typically present with protuberant abdomens. Neuroblastomas are large, firm, nodular, sometimes painful flank masses that are usually fixed to surrounding structures. Paraspinal neuroblastomas may extend into the epidural space, producing paraplegia. Neuroblastomas may secrete vasoactive intestinal peptide causing persistent watery diarrhea with loss of fluid and electrolytes.

   b.) **Diagnosis.** Median age at diagnosis is 2 years, and 90% of cases are diagnosed by 5 years of age. Ultrasonography, CT, and magnetic resonance imaging are the primary diagnostic procedures. Urinary excretion of vanillylmandelic acid is increased in most children with neuroblastomas, reflecting the metabolism of catecholamines produced by these tumors (hypertension is rare).

c.) **Treatment** includes surgical removal, radiation therapy, and chemotherapy (cyclophosphamide, doxorubicin, cisplatin, vincristine).

d.) **Prognosis** depends on molecular markers and degree of tumor differentiation, patient age, and tumor stage. Infants younger than 1 year old at diagnosis have a significantly improved outcome across all tumor stages.

e.) **Management of Anesthesia** for resection of neuroblastoma is as described for children with nephroblastoma. Adequate intravenous access is essential because neuroblastomas are quite vascular and often adhere to or surround the great vessels, creating the potential for significant blood loss. Epidural analgesia is a beneficial adjunct as long as the tumor does not involve the spine.

2.) *Nephroblastoma (Wilms' Tumor)* is the most common malignant renal tumor and the second most common malignant abdominal tumor in children. Median age at onset is 3 years. Nephroblastoma is associated with WAGR syndrome (Wilms' tumor, aniridia, genitourinary malformations, and mental retardation), Beckwith-Wiedemann syndrome (hemihypertrophy, visceromegaly, macroglossia, and hyperinsulinemic hypoglycemia), and Denys-Drash syndrome (pseudohermaphroditism, progressive glomerulopathy, and Wilms' tumor).

a.) **Signs and Symptoms.** Nephroblastoma is usually found accidentally as an asymptomatic flank mass. Pain, fever, and hematuria are late manifestations. These children may exhibit malaise, weight loss, anemia, disturbed micturition, vomiting, or constipation. Systemic hypertension (mild to severe, caused by renin release directly or as an indirect effect of the tumor) may occur, particularly if the tumor involves both kidneys. Increases in systemic blood pressure are usually mild, but on rare occasions hypertension is so severe that encephalopathy and congestive heart failure develop. Secondary hyperaldosteronism and hypokalemia may be present.

b.) **Diagnosis** is via radiography, including intravenous pyelography (to examine the renal collecting system and assess the contralateral kidney), inferior vena cavagram (to examine tumor invasion), arteriogram, and chest radiographs or liver scans (to look for metastases).

c.) **Treatment** is nephrectomy, with or without subsequent radiation and chemotherapy. Preoperative chemotherapy is administered to patients with bilateral tumors who will undergo parenchyma-sparing procedures, patients with extensive intravascular (inferior vena caval) tumor extension, or those with inoperable tumors. Radiation therapy may be given initially to shrink the tumor, followed by surgery. Surgical treatment of bilateral disease may consist of bilateral partial nephrectomy or bilateral total nephrectomy followed by dialysis and eventually renal transplantation.

d.) **Prognosis.** Tumor size, stage, and histology are major prognostic factors. Survival rate approaches 90% in patients with favorable histology and stage and is more than 60% across all stages.

e.) **Management of Anesthesia.** Anemia and adverse effects of chemotherapy are considerations. Blood loss during surgery may be significant. Electrolyte and fluid abnormalities may exist secondary to diarrhea. Invasive monitoring with an arterial catheter and central venous catheter may be needed, and a Foley catheter should be placed to monitor urine output. Lower-extremity venous catheters should be avoided, as it may be necessary to ligate or partially resect the inferior vena cava. Measurement of central venous pressure is helpful for evaluating intravascular fluid volume and the adequacy of fluid replacement. Tumor extension into the suprahepatic vena cava and right atrium may require cardiopulmonary bypass. Epidural analgesia should be avoided in these patients because of potential complications associated with full heparinization.

Manipulation of the inferior vena cava containing a metastatic tumor can result in a tumor embolism to the heart or pulmonary artery.

k. *Oncologic Emergencies*

1.) *Mediastinal Tumors*

a.) **Signs and Symptoms.** Cardiovascular and respiratory symptoms depend on the size and location of the tumor. Tachypnea, orthopnea, and nocturnal dyspnea suggest airway compression. The patient's respiratory status may be normal in the sitting, decubitis, or prone position but poor in the supine position. Cardiovascular structures can be compressed or constricted by an enlarging mediastinal tumor. A Valsalva effect (which decreases venous return) may be associated with syncopal events. Superior vena cava (SVC) syndrome presents with facial and periorbital edema, shortness of breath, engorgement of jugular veins, and central nervous system symptoms (headache and visual disturbances) that worsen in the supine position.

b.) **Diagnosis.** Chest radiograph, computed axial tomography, and magnetic resonance imaging are static pictures of airway compression and may not accurately quantitate the degree of compression. Flow volume loops sitting and supine may give a dynamic assessment of the airway, as may flexible fiberoptic bronchoscopy under local anesthesia or sedation. Echocardiogram may help delineate cardiac compromise.

c.) **Treatment.** When SVC syndrome is present, radiation therapy is the treatment of choice. Procedures that may need general

469

anesthesia or sedation include computed axial tomography scan, biopsy of cervical nodes, and central venous catheter placement. Prior to surgical removal of tumor, preoperative chemotherapy, radiation therapy, and steroid therapy should be considered, to shrink tumor mass. Decreasing the size of the tumor prior to surgery is often beneficial.

d.) **Management of Anesthesia—Preoperative.** Limitations in respiratory and cardiovascular reserves must be evaluated and further deterioration anticipated.

e.) **Management of Anesthesia—Intraoperative.** Premedication should be avoided and intravenous access established prior to induction, preferably in a lower extremity if SVC obstruction is present. Inhalation or intravenous induction with maintenance of spontaneous ventilation at all times and avoidance of all muscle relaxants are recommended. If the child deteriorates during induction, turning him or her into the left lateral decubitus or prone position may improve cardiorespiratory function. Another option if collapse of the airway occurs is rigid bronchoscopy. Cardiopulmonary bypass (femorofemoral bypass) or venovenous bypass may be necessary if either complete airway obstruction or vessel occlusion is anticipated. A helium and oxygen mixture may be used to improve oxygenation in patients with airway compression caused by mediastinal tumors (lower density than oxygen, decreased airway resistance). Extubation is best when the patient is awake, ensuring adequate return of airway reflexes and prevention of laryngospasm.

f.) **Management of Anesthesia—Postoperative.** Recovery room personnel must be notified of the effect of position on the patient's cardiorespiratory status. Children with significant tracheomalacia may manifest tracheal obstruction and respiratory difficulties in recovery, necessitating reintubation. Unilateral pulmonary edema may be associated with lung re-expansion after mediastinal tumor removal.

l. Burn (Thermal) Injuries. Burns are classified according to the total body surface area involved, the depth of the burn (**Table 24-15**), and the presence or absence of inhalation injury. The total body surface area burned is calculated using the rule of nines, which accurately predicts the body surface area involved in adults (**Fig. 24-3**) but underestimates the extent of burn injury in children.

1.) *Signs and Symptoms.* Burn injuries produce predictable pathophysiologic responses (**Table 24-16**). Cytokines appear to be the primary mediators of systemic inflammation after burn injuries.

2.) *Treatment*

a.) **Intravascular Fluid Volume** deficits after burns are proportional to the extent and depth of the burn injury. On the first postburn

TABLE 24-15	Classification of Burn Injuries	
Classification	**Depth of Burn Injury**	**Outcome and Treatment**
First degree (superficial)	Epidermis	Heals spontaneously
Second degree (partial thickness) Superficial dermal burn	Epidermis and upper dermis	Heals spontaneously
Deep dermal burn	Epidermis and deep dermis	Requires excision and grafting for rapid return of function
Third degree (full thickness)	Destruction of epidermis and dermis	Wound excision and grafting required Some limitation of function and scar formation
Fourth degree	Skeletal muscles Fascia Bone	Complete excision Limited function

Adapted from MacLennan N, Heimbach DM, Cullen BF: Anesthesia for major thermal injury. Anesthesiology 1998;89:749–770.

day, extravasated plasma proteins exert an osmotic pressure that holds large volumes of fluid in the extravascular third space. Pulmonary capillary permeability does not increase unless smoke inhalation occurs. Colloids do not need to be withheld during the early phases of resuscitation. The loss of fluid from the vascular compartment on the first postburn day is roughly 4 mL/kg for each percent of body surface burned. On the second postburn day, capillary integrity is largely restored, and decreasing amounts of fluid are required to maintain intravascular fluid volume.

b.) **Airway Management.** Fiberoptic laryngoscopy is indicated if the diagnosis of upper airway edema is in doubt. The airway should be secured before respiratory decompensation occurs. Tracheostomy is reserved for patients with pulmonary complications requiring prolonged ventilatory support.

c.) **Smoke Inhalation.** Treatment of respiratory distress related to smoke inhalation is symptomatic. Administration of warm humidified oxygen and bronchodilators is indicated. Early institution of mechanical ventilation with positive end-expiratory pressure should be considered if the PaO_2 is less than 60 mm Hg while breathing room air. Prophylactic antibiotic administration is not beneficial, and the value of corticosteroids is controversial. The best treatment for carbon monoxide poisoning is ventilation with 100% oxygen.

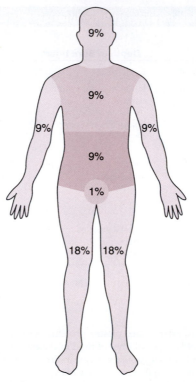

Figure 24-3 • Rule of nines for determining the percentage of body surface area burned in adults. (Adapted from MacLennan N, Heimbach DM, Cullen BF: Anesthesia for major thermal injury. Anesthesiology 1998;89:749–770.)

d.) **Metabolism and Thermoregulation.** The metabolic rate increases in proportion to the extent of burn injury. Total parenteral nutrition may be required to meet these increased metabolic requirements. Thermoregulatory functions of the skin, including vasoreactivity, sweating, piloerection, and insulation, are abolished or diminished by thermal injury.

e.) **Fluid, Electrolytes, and Blood Products.** Hourly urine output remains the best guide to the adequacy of fluid resuscitation. Urine output should be approximately 1.0 mL/kg per hour in adequately hydrated children. Increased serum potassium concentrations caused by tissue necrosis and hemolysis are common during the first 2 postburn days. Early transfusion is rarely necessary, but transfusions of erythrocytes are often needed by approximately the fifth postburn day. Serum concentrations of ionized calcium may be decreased during

TABLE 24-16	Pathophysiologic Responses Evoked by Burn Injuries

Cardiovascular Responses

Early: hypovolemia (burn shock), impaired myocardial contractility

Late: systemic hypertension, tachycardia, increased cardiac output

Pulmonary Responses

Early direct effects: upper airway obstruction, smoke inhalation (chemical pneumonitis, carbon monoxide poisoning), asphyxia

Early indirect effects: effects of inflammatory mediators, pulmonary edema

Late direct effects: chest wall constriction

Late indirect effects (complications of ventilation and airway management): oxygen toxicity, barotrauma, infection, laryngeal damage, tracheal stenosis

Metabolism and Thermoregulation

Increased metabolic rate

Increased carbon dioxide production

Increased oxygen utilization

Impaired thermoregulation

Renal and Electrolyte Responses

Early: decreased renal blood flow, myoglobinuria, hyperkalemia,

Late: increased renal blood flow, variable drug clearance, hypokalemia

Endocrine Responses

Increased serum norepinephrine concentrations

Hyperglycemia (susceptible to development of nonketotic hyperosmolar coma)

Gastrointestinal Responses

Stress ulcers

Impaired gastrointestinal barrier to bacteria

Endotoxemia

Coagulation

Early: activation of thrombotic and fibrinolytic systems, hemoconcentration, hemolysis

Late: anemia

Immune Responses

Impaired immune function (sepsis, pneumonia)

Endotoxemia

Multiple organ system failure

Adapted from MacLennan N, Heimbach DM, Cullen BF: Anesthesia for major thermal injury. Anesthesiology 1998;89:749–770.

postburn periods. Children with extensive burn injuries who are receiving large volumes of rapidly infused blood should receive 1 to 2 mg of calcium gluconate for every milliliter of infused blood.

f.) **Prognosis.** Survival in children with more than 80% total body surface area burn is now 80%. The most common cause of death remains severe multiorgan dysfunction resulting from overwhelming late sepsis.

g.) Management of Anesthesia (Table 24-17)

TABLE 24-17	Anesthetic Considerations for Excision and Grafting of Major Burn Injuries

Preoperative

- Provide adequate analgesia.
- Limit period of fluid fasting.

Vascular Access

- Sites may be limited by burns.
- Consider invasive monitoring.

Airway Management

- Upper airway edema may be present.
- Tracheostomy may be needed if prolonged intubation is anticipated.
- Consider alternative to direct laryngoscopy.
- Consider awake fiberoptic intubation (neck or facial contractures).

Ventilation and Oxygenation

- Minute ventilation requirements increased (increased metabolic rate, parenteral hyperalimentation).
- Mechanical ventilation may be necessary (smoke inhalation, acute respiratory failure).
- If carbon monoxide is present (smoke inhalation), 100% oxygen should be used.
- Consider PEEP if PaO_2 <60 mm Hg on room air.

Fluids and Blood

- Anticipate possibility of rapid and large blood loss.
- Maintenance fluid needs are dictated by timing of the burn (4 mL/kg for each percent of body surface burn, decreasing after the second postburn day).
- Evaluate coagulation status.
- Urine output should be 1.0 mL/kg/hr in adequately hydrated children.
- Beware of hypocalcemia with blood transfusion.

Temperature Regulation

- Increase ambient temperature of the operating room (25°C).
- Warm intravenous fluids.

TABLE 24-17	Anesthetic Considerations for Excision and Grafting of Major Burn Injuries—cont'd

Anesthetic Drugs

- Include opioids.
- Consider effects of increased circulating catecholamine concentrations.
- Muscle relaxants: Avoid succinylcholine (hyperkalemia). Anticipate resistance to neuromuscular blocking effects of nondepolarizing muscle relaxants.

Postoperative Period

- Anticipate increased analgesic (opioids) requirements.
- Await air leak around endotracheal tube before extubation.

Adapted from MacLennan N, Heimbach DM, Cullen BF: Anesthesia for major thermal injury. Anesthesiology 1998;89:749–770.

CHAPTER 25

Geriatric Disorders

The elderly population (>65 years of age) represented 12.4% of the U.S. population in 2004. The number of people 65 years and older will be 20% of the population by 2030. The aging of the U.S. population will result in significant growth in the demand for surgical services, which is predicted to increase 14% to 47%. Anesthesiologists will need to develop strategies to address this increased demand while maintaining quality of care for senior patients.

I. PHYSIOLOGY OF AGING (TABLE 25-1)

II. GERIATRIC SYNDROMES

A. Skeletal Changes

1. Osteoporosis is characterized by microarchitectural deterioration and decreased bone density, with increased bone fragility and susceptibility to fracture. Complications of hip fracture account for 37,000 deaths annually in the U.S. Prevention is key; weight-bearing exercises and adequate calcium and vitamin D intake are essential.

2. Osteoarthritis is the most common joint disease, characterized by degeneration of articular cartilage primarily of the weight-bearing joints. Diagnosis is based on clinical assessment and positive radiographic findings on the affected joints. Weight loss, physical therapy, occupational therapy, and reduction of joint stress, acetaminophen and nonsteroidal anti-inflammatory drugs, and selective use of muscle relaxants are primary therapy. Intra-articular glucocorticoid injections, narcotics, and arthroplasty are reserved for patients with the most severe pain.

a. Cervical Spinal Mobility and Stability carry special implications for the anesthesiologist when laryngoscopy and tracheal intubation is planned.

B. Emphysema.
In the United States, 4% to 6% of male adults and 1% to 3% of female adults have emphysema. Emphysema involves destruction of distal airways and small airway inflammation. Breathlessness ensues when FEV_1 has decreased to 30% of predicted. In advanced disease, cyanosis, elevated central

TABLE 25-1	Organ System Function and Aging
Nervous System	• Loss in neurons, reduced cerebral blood flow, diminished neurotransmitters
	• Cerebral atherosclerosis, Parkinson's disease, depression, dementia, Alzheimer's disease, delirium all more prevalent
	• Parasympathetic function declines, sympathetic outflow increases (increase in hypothermia, heat stroke, orthostatic hypotension, syncope)
	• Reduced anesthetic requirement
	• Increased postoperative cognitive dysfunction
Cardiovascular System	• Reduced exercise tolerance
	• Loss of vascular elasticity (HTN, LVH)
	• Decreased baroreceptor activity
	• Higher incidence of coronary and valvular heart disease
Respiratory System	• Decreased protective mechanisms (coughing, swallowing)
	• Loss of alveolar surface
	• Decreased responsiveness to hypercapnia and hypoxemia
	• Work of breathing increased (reduced chest wall elasticity, reduced FEV_1, FVC, increased RV)
	• Decreased mean arterial oxygen tension from 95 mm HG at age 20 to 70 mm Hg at age 80.
Hepatic, GI, Renal	• Decreased hepatic synthetic activity
	• Changes in drug clearance
	• Decreased renal blood flow
	• Reduced glomerular function (50% reduction by age 80)
Endocrine	• Diabetes, hypothyroidism, impotence, osteoporosis more common
	• Basal metabolic rate declines 1% per year after age 80
Hematology, Oncology, Immune Function	• Reduced production of bone marrow elements
	• Compromised cellular immunity
	• Increased rate of cancer
	• Increased prevalence of autoantibodies

FEV, forced expiratory volume; FVC, forced vital capacity; HTN, hypertension; LVH, left ventricular hypertrophy; RV, residual volume.

venous pressure, and anasarca can be observed. On chest radiographs, hyperinflation, flattening of diaphragms, increased retrosternal air space, and hyperlucency of the lungs are characteristic for this disease. Smoking cessation, bronchodilators, and supplemental oxygen therapy are the most commonly prescribed maintenance treatments for emphysema. Prognosis in patients with smoking-related emphysema shows a 40% 12-year survival rate in those with an initial FEV_1 of 1.25 L and approximately 5% for those with an initial FEV$_1$ of 0.75 L. Surgical treatment includes bullectomy and lung volume reduction.

C. Parkinson's Disease is a disorder of the extrapyramidal system. Age is the most consistent risk factor, with Parkinson's disease affecting approximately 3% of the population older than 66 years of age.

1. Characteristics of Parkinson's Disease are progressive depletion of dopaminergic neurons of the substantia nigra of the basal ganglia. Clinical presentation is the classic triad of rigidity, resting tremor, and bradykinesis.

2. Treatment is directed at allowing the patient to pursue normal daily activities using L-dopa or dopamine receptor agonists. Surgical treatment developed recently includes subthalamic deep brain stimulation and fetal mesencephalic tissue implantation.

3. Anesthestic Management includes aspiration prophylaxis and close monitoring of adequate perioperative respiratory function. The patient's usual drug regimen should be continued as close to the regular schedule as possible. Phenothiazines, butyrophenones, and metoclopramide should be avoided. Diphenhydramine may be effective if extrapyramidal signs develop.

D. Dementia. Intellectual decline is one of the early hallmarks of dementia. Mental status is often a barometer of health in the patient with dementia, and abrupt changes necessitate a search for additional superimposed problems that may be occurring (**Table 25-2**). Causes of reversible dementia include chronic

TABLE 25-2	Comparison of Different Central Nervous System Disorders		
Diagnosis	**Distinguishing Feature**	**Symptoms**	**Course**
Dementia	Memory impairment	Disorientation, agitation	Slow onset, progressive, chronic
Delirium	Decreased attention, fluctuating levels of consciousness	Disorientation, visual hallucination, agitation, withdrawal, memory and attention impairment	Acute; most cases remit with correction of underlying medical condition
Psychotic disorders	Deficit in reality testing	Social withdrawal, apathy	Slow onset with prodromal syndrome; chronic with exacerbations
Depression	Decreased pleasure in usual activities Sadness, loss of interest	Disturbances of sleep, appetite, concentration; suicidal ideation, decreased energy; feelings of hopelessness	Single episode, or recurrent episodes; may be chronic

TABLE 25-3	Components of Delirium

To establish a diagnosis of delirium, a patient must show each of the features listed:
- Disturbance of consciousness (i.e., reduced clarity of awareness about the environment) with reduced ability to focus, sustain, or shift attention
- Change in cognition (e.g., memory deficit, disorientation, language disturbance) or development of a perceptual disturbance that is not better accounted for by a preexisting, established, or evolving dementia
- Development over a short period (usually hours to days); tends to fluctuate during the course of the day
- Evidence from the history, physical examination, or laboratory findings indicating that the disturbance is caused by direct physiologic consequences of a general medical condition

drug intoxication, vitamin deficiencies, subdural hematoma, major depression, normal pressure hydrocephalus, and hypothyroidism.

1. Treatment is aimed at behavioral and sleep problems. Those treatments include vitamin E, nonsteroidal anti-inflammatory drugs, estrogen replacement, and centrally acting acetylcholinesterase inhibitors.

2. Informed Consent may be an issue.

3. Postoperative Cognitive dysfunction is strongly associated with increasing age; as many as one in every four elderly surgical patients may be affected. It usually resolves by 3 months after surgery, and presents as a failure to perform simple cognitive tasks or to complete mental tasks.

E. Delirium (Table 25-3). Risk factors include advanced age (>70), underlying dementia, various co-morbidities, drugs, and electrolyte abnormalities. Almost any acute illness, or an exacerbation of any chronic illness, may precipitate delirium (**Table 25-4**). Hospitalized patients with delirium demonstrate up to a 10-fold higher risk of developing other medical complications (including death), longer hospitalization, higher hospital costs, and increased need for long-term care after discharge. For acute control of delirium, 0.25 to 2 mg of oral haloperidol is the preferred treatment, but diazepam, droperidol, and chlorpromazine are also often used with good results.

TABLE 25-4	Factors That Can Precipitate Delirium

Drug use (especially when the dose is adjusted)

Electrolyte and physiologic abnormalities (hypoxemia, hyponatremia)

Lack of drugs (withdrawal)

Infection (especially urinary tract or respiratory infection)

Reduced sensory input (blindness, deafness, darkness, unfamiliar surroundings)

Intracranial problems (stroke, bleeding, meningitis, postictal state)

Urinary retention and fecal impaction

Myocardial problems (myocardial infarction, heart failure, arrhythmia)

III. GERIATRIC ANESTHESIA STRATEGIES (TABLE 25-5)

IV. ETHICAL CHALLENGES IN GERIATRIC ANESTHESIA AND PALLIATIVE CARE

A. Autonomy and Consent. The ultimate decision of what medical therapy is to be employed rests with the patient. Essential criteria for informed consent include sufficient information, patient competence, and voluntary decision-making. Patients with possible dementia may need referral for competency evaluations to assess mental functioning and decision-making capacity. Surrogate decision makers may be designated by living will or durable powers of attorney. Each state has a legal hierarchy to appoint a proxy decision maker if these documents are not available to guide the process.

B. DNR Orders in the Operating Room. Informed consent to or informed refusal of medical intervention is guided by the same moral principles during end-of-life care, regardless of location. Institutional protocols and policies regarding do-not-resuscitate status in the operating room and postanesthetic care unit should be consulted.

TABLE 25-5	Special Considerations in Anesthesia Management of Geriatric Patients
Increased co-morbidities	Take a thorough history and physical examination.
Sensory impairments	Be prepared for impaired vision and hearing.
Age-related alterations in drug clearance	Be aware of adverse drug effects and polypharmacy with increased risks.
Integumentary system	Avoid tape on thin, delicate skin and protect bony prominences.
Fluid status	Monitor for increased risk of dehydration due to diminished thirst sensation.
Decreased LV compliance	Monitor for increased risk of hypotension.
Increased risk of hypothermia	Use warming devices.
Prolonged clearance of anesthetic agents and decreased MAC with age	Patients are slower awakening; lower doses are needed. Short-acting agents may be advantageous.
Postoperative cognitive dysfunction	Regional anesthesia may be advantageous.
Postoperative respiratory complications are the most common	Postoperative supplemental oxygen, pulse oximetry monitoring, and capnography may be useful.
Thromboembolic events	Encourage early ambulation.

LV, left ventricle; MAC, minimum alveolar concentration.

C. Palliative Care is defined as the all-inclusive care of patients whose disease is not responsive to curative treatment (**Table 25-6**). It requires a multidisciplinary approach to treat symptoms, control pain, and address the psychological, social, and spiritual needs of the patient and his or her family. By training, anesthesiologists are invaluable experts at pharmacologic and procedural pain management.

TABLE 25-6	Definition of *Palliative Care* by the World Health Organization
Affirms life and regards dying as a normal process	
Neither hastens nor postpones death	
Provides relief from pain and other distressing symptoms	
Integrates the psychological and spiritual aspects of patient care	
Offers a support system to help the family cope during the patient's illness and their own bereavement	

Index